An Integrated Study of Drug Metabolism

An Integrated Study of Drug Metabolism

Edited by **Erica Helmer**

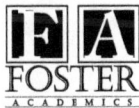

FOSTER
ACADEMICS

New Jersey

Published by Foster Academics,
61 Van Reypen Street,
Jersey City, NJ 07306, USA
www.fosteracademics.com

An Integrated Study of Drug Metabolism
Edited by Erica Helmer

International Standard Book Number: 978-1-63242-044-2 (Hardback)

Contents

Preface   VII

Chapter 1   **Pharmacogenetics and Metabolism:**
             Past, Present and Future   1
             Fabricio Rios-Santos and Luiz Alexandre V. Magno

Chapter 2   **Oral Absorption, Intestinal Metabolism**
             and Human Oral Bioavailability   27
             Ayman El-Kattan and Manthena Varma

Chapter 3   **Phase II Drug Metabolism**   61
             Petra Jančová and Michal Šiller

Chapter 4   **Altered Drug Metabolism and Transport**
             in Pathophysiological Conditions   87
             Adarsh Gandhi and Romi Ghose

Chapter 5   **Anticancer Drug Metabolism: Chemotherapy**
             Resistance and New Therapeutic Approaches   113
             Hanane Akhdar, Claire Legendre,
             Caroline Aninat and Fabrice Morel

Chapter 6   **Genetic and Epigenetic Factors**
             Affecting Cytochrome P450 Phenotype
             and Their Clinical Relevance   147
             Viola Tamási and András Falus

Chapter 7   **Transcription Factors Potentially Involved**
             in Regulation of Cytochrome P450 Gene Expression   171
             Piotr Czekaj and Rafał Skowronek

Chapter 8   **Determination of Cytochrome P450**
             Metabolic Activity Using Selective Markers   191
             Jan Jurica and Alexandra Sulcova

Chapter 9   **Microdosing Assessment to Evaluate
               Pharmacokinetics and Drug Metabolism
               Using Liquid Chromatography-Tandem
               Mass Spectrometry Technology**   **221**
               Jinsong Ni and Josh Rowe

Chapter 10   **Electrochemical Methods for
               the *In Vitro* Assessment of Drug Metabolism**   **239**
               Alejandro Álvarez-Lueje, Magdalena Pérez
               and Claudio Zapata

Chapter 11   **Label-Free Quantitative Analysis Using LC/MS**   **265**
               Atsumu Hirabayashi

Chapter 12   **Recent Advances in Pharmacogenomic
               Technology for Personalized Medicine**   **281**
               Toshihisa Ishikawa and Yoshihide Hayashizaki

               Permissions

               List of Contributors

Preface

Every book is a source of knowledge and this one is no exception. The idea that led to the conceptualization of this book was the fact that the world is advancing rapidly; which makes it crucial to document the progress in every field. I am aware that a lot of data is already available, yet, there is a lot more to learn. Hence, I accepted the responsibility of editing this book and contributing my knowledge to the community.

Late-stage drug failure can occur due to various factors like unwanted metabolic instability, drug-drug interactions, toxic metabolites, and polymorphic metabolism. To meet the purpose of preventing this failure; sincere effort has been employed by academia as well as the pharmaceutical industry for the development of more effective methods and screening analysis to recognize the metabolic enzymes and profiles involved in drug metabolism. The book elucidates detailed reviews of chosen topics in drug metabolism. The important topics that have been described in this book are: impact of genetic and epigenetic factors on drug metabolism; use of new microdosing methods and new LC/MS and genomic techniques to conclude the metabolic parameters and profiles of potential novel drug candidates; the interaction between metabolism and drug transport in oral biodiversity; and the effect of disease on metabolism and transport.

While editing this book, I had multiple visions for it. Then I finally narrowed down to make every chapter a sole standing text explaining a particular topic, so that they can be used independently. However, the umbrella subject sinews them into a common theme. This makes the book a unique platform of knowledge.

I would like to give the major credit of this book to the experts from every corner of the world, who took the time to share their expertise with us. Also, I owe the completion of this book to the never-ending support of my family, who supported me throughout the project.

Editor

Pharmacogenetics and Metabolism: Past, Present and Future

Fabricio Rios-Santos[1] and Luiz Alexandre V. Magno[2]
Federal University of Mato Grosso & Federal University of Minas Gerais,
Brazil

1. Introduction

Throughout history, humanity has referred to toxic reactions in response to food, plants, and more recently, medications or drugs. **Pythagoras** is thought to be one of the first to observe that some individuals, but not all, would get sick after eating fava beans. Introduction of the complex term *pharmakon* (a word used to designate substances that may produce beneficial or harmful effects to human health) by Hippocratic physicians brought with it a paradox: a compound may be served both as a drug and a poison at the same time. As it is currently known, administration of a substance may offer higher risk of toxic effects than when administered at a lower dose. But then, what about a drug dosage that induces toxicity in a patient, treats another well and had no effects on the other? This and other important observations such as the understanding of metabolic variability have started to unravel the mysteries behind these phenomena. For example, the ancient observation why different outcomes were regularly observed after Greek soldiers ate fresh fava beans (Nebert 1999).

The concept of **'variability in metabolism'** claims that biochemical processes within the organism are responsible for transformation of compounds from food or medicines, and that this process could be different among subjects leading to a range of organic responses. Alexander Ure (1841) seems to have been the first to report organism's ability to convert an exogenously administered compound into one or more different metabolites. In the study entitled *'On Gouty Concretions with a New Method of Treatment'*, Ure reported that benzoic acid was converted to hippuric acid by humans (Ure 1841). Then, it gradually began to be accepted that living systems have a "physiological chemistry" responsible for the modification of substances, and from the second part of 19th century, a significant number of metabolic pathways have been discovered.

At that time, however, the key answer to why there is individual variability in metabolism had not yet been answered, which only came to light after the rediscovery of Mendel's study about hereditary around the turn of the 20th century. A well-known example to illustrate this was the influence of the genetic findings of William Bateson on studies of Sir Archibald Garrod about alkaptonuria and phenylketonuria presented in the book entitled *"Inborn Errors of Metabolism"* (Garrod 1909). In fact, the results founded by Garrod were a milestone to explanation of metabolic variability from a genetic perspective. Thereafter, some forerunners separately described series of observations that preceded the conceptualization of the Pharmacogenetics (PGx). In 1932, Arthur Fox found a remarkable variation in the ability of some individuals to taste a foreign chemical phenylthiocarbamide (PTC) (the 'taste blindness') (Fox 1932). Interestingly, this finding was unexpectedly discovered when some of the PTC molecules escaped in to the air and Fox's co-worker C.R. Noller noticed a bitter taste, while Fox could not taste it. Intrigued by Fox's findings about bitter taste, L.H. Snyder published an important study (especially for the relevant quantity of participants) confirming the Fox's observation that some people perceive the bitter taste of PTC, while others do not. In addition, Snyder found that such non-tasting is a recessive genetic trait, and today it is one of the best-known Mendelian traits in human populations (Snyder 1932).

In a similar fashion, animal studies at that time also supported the genetic contribution in drug metabolism variability. Sawin and Glick (1943) in the study entitled *"Atropinesterase, a Genetically Determined Enzyme in the Rabbit"* demonstrated a genetically determined outcome in rabbits after ingestion of the belladonna leaves (Sawin & Glick 1943).

In the middle of 20th century, evidences necessary to support the transformation of the scattered "pharmacological heritability" in a new science finally appeared. First, Hettie Hughes described a relation between the level of isoniazid (an anti-tuberculosis drug) acetylation and occurrence of peripheral neuritis (Hughes et al. 1954), which absolutely was a landmark step for future demystification of the "one size fits all" system of drug prescribing. Another milestone in PGx was an independent investigation about death of patients caused by a generally safe, local anesthetic drug procaine (Kalow 1962). Further experiments enabled the authors to suggest that a genetically determined alteration in the enzyme structure may cause an abnormal and lethal low cholinesterase activity. The atypical enzyme does not hydrolyze the anesthetic with efficacy, resulting in a prolonged period of high levels of the drug in the blood and increased toxicity (Kalow 2005). Simultaneously, Alf Alving and co-workers observed that African-American soldiers presented an increased risk to develop acute haemolytic crises after primaquine (an antimalarial drug) administration, when compared with Caucasian ones (Clayman et al. 1952). As shown later, this sensitivity is caused by a genetically determined deficiency of glucose 6-phosphate dehydrogenase (G6PD), which alters erythrocyte metabolism (Alving et al. 1956). Thus, it took approximately 2,400 years to explain the Pythagoras observation about favism from a molecular perspective. It is now believed that defect in the *G6PD* gene is related with fava-induced hemolytic anemia in some individuals of Mediterranean descent.

Finally, opening a new era of pharmacological investigation, Arno Motulsky in 1957 published a masterpiece paper entitled *"Drug reactions, enzymes and biochemical genetics"*, highlighting the genetic basis of "how hereditary gene-controlled enzymatic factors determine why, with identical exposure, certain individuals become 'sick', whereas others are not affected" (Motulsky 1957). The works of Kalow and Motulsky were (and still are) an unequivocal scientific catalyzer for understanding of the genetic influence in drug metabolism. Friedrich Vogel, a German Pharmacologist in 1959 was the first to coin the term 'Pharmacogenetics' (PGx) for the emergent new area of scientific discoveries, that unifies different conceptions on pharmacotherapy and xenobiotic-induced disease risk (Vogel 1959).

Despite the terms *Pharmacogenetics* and *Pharmacogenomics* are used interchangeably, most authors prefer to use PGx when inherited differences in drug response are being evaluated. On the other hand, Pharmacogenomics is usually used to study general aspects of drug response involving genomic technologies to determine a drug profile or even a new drug. Although is common association between PGx and drug metabolism variation, many others inherited differences in drug response are investigated by PGx, such as polymorphisms in genes that encode molecules transporters (Vaalburg et al. 2005) and drug targets (Johnson & Liggett 2011; Maggo et al. 2011). For practical purposes, preference will be given to the use of the term Pharmacogenetics throughout this chapter.

2. Metabolizers subpopulations, a brief review

Since physiological responses associated with a particular drug have been linked to biochemical attributes in the body of the recipient, several studies have attempted to elucidate which factors modify the clinical response to a greater or lesser extent. There is now a general understanding that variability in the function of **drug-metabolizing enzymes (DME)** is responsible for many differences in the disposition and clinical consequences of drugs. Although it is a central issue to PGx, in clinical practice most decisions about a medicine prescription are mainly based on the classic factors responsible for drug variability, including co-existing disease (especially those that affect drug distribution, absorption or elimination), body mass, diet, alcohol intake, interaction with others drugs and mechanisms to improve patient compliance. In fact, all of these have been demonstrated to directly affect the indicated dose of the drug. However, they only partly explain why most major drugs are effective in only 25 to 60 percent of patients. Furthermore, taking into account patients with same physical and demographic characteristics, why does a standard dose is toxic to some patient but not to others? Why not all patients demonstrate the expected efficacy in drug treatment trials? Undoubtedly, these and many others questions opened the door for a new era of the personalized medicine and treatment perspectives (Nair 2010).

It is well-know that drug levels can be raised by increasing the dose or by more frequent administration in a non-responder patient. Conversely, if a higher plasmatic drug level with a standard dose administration is expected (in a patient with cirrhosis or malnutrition, for example), increasing the time of administration or suspending the dose may be a reasonable attitude. Although advances in medical technology and potential predictive models have improved the choice of dose, they are not yet sufficient to prevent high level of morbidity and mortality caused by **adverse drug reactions (ADR)**, as shown in the clinical practice (Wu et al. 2010). Thus, it is believed that the study of how genetic variation interface with drug metabolism, especially in genes codifying DMEs, may also lead to improve drug safety.

A variety of factors affecting the expression and activity of DMEs are classified into three major groups: **genetic factors, non-genetic host factors** (such as diseases, age, stress, obesity, physical exercise, etc.) and **environmental factors** (environmental pollutants, occupational chemicals, drugs, etc.). Recent studies clearly indicate that interindividual variation in drug metabolism is one of the most important causes of drug response differences. In general, common pharmacokinetic profile is a lighthouse for most prescribers in clinical practice. Figure 1A exemplify a simplified model of a drug biotransformation route. Most pharmaceuticals compounds or molecules (M1 in figure 1) when administrated orally are lipid-soluble enough to be reabsorbed (in the kidneys) and eliminated slowly in small amounts in an unchanged form in urine. Therefore, drug biotransformation by enzymes (represented by E1) has a key role in the control of plasmatic drug concentration. It should be remembered that the metabolites (M2) might also exert pharmacological effect (which will be discussed later). In addition, low activity of the

	MOST EXPECTED CLINICAL RESULT	**TIME FOR BIOTRANSFORMATION**

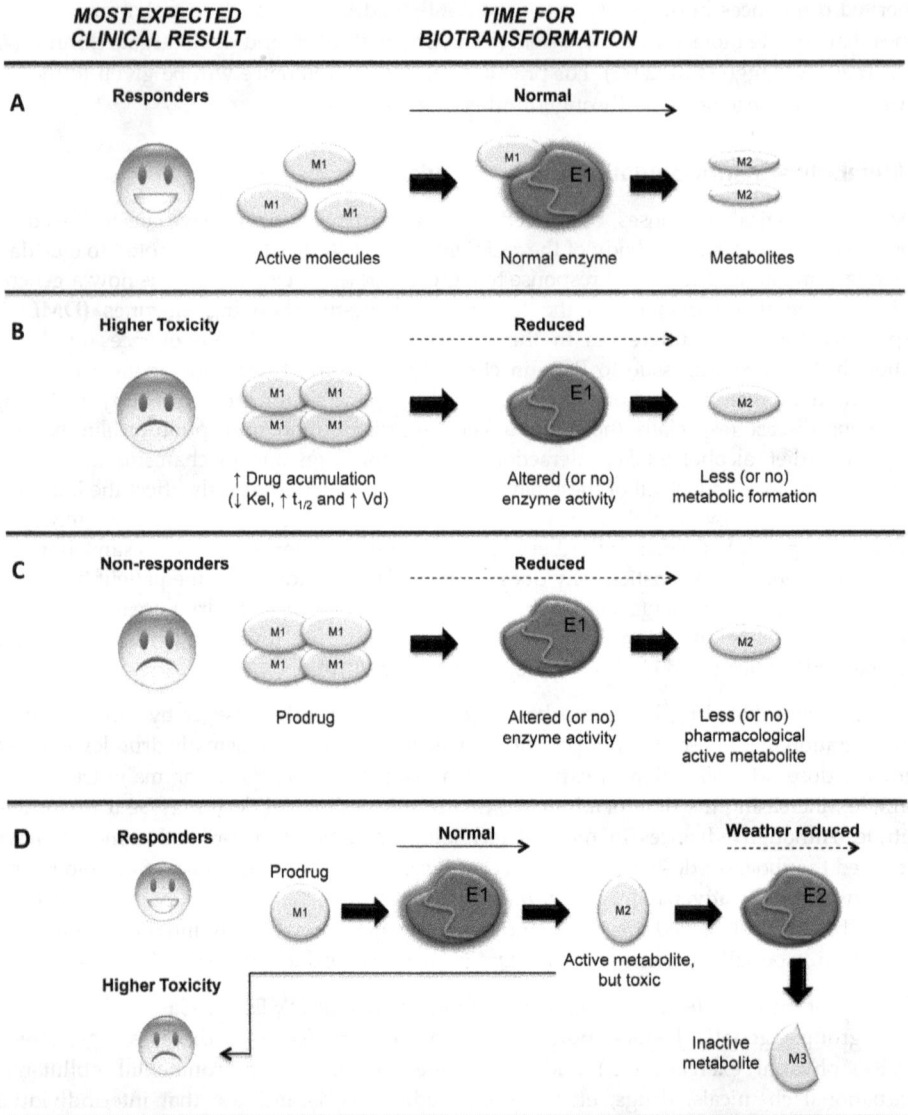

Fig. 1. Overview of the expected clinical result and its relation with activity of drug metabolizing enzymes. M1: pharmaceuticals compounds; E1: phase I biotransformation; M2 and M3: metabolites; E2: phase II biotransformation

metabolic step might cause accumulation of the drug and/or its metabolites in the body if the medicine continues to be taken (Figure 1B). As discussed earlier, genetic mutations in coding and noncoding regions may be involved in such inborn altered enzymatic activity (Ingelman-Sundberg 2001). Some relevant examples come from polymorphisms in CYPs (cytochrome P450) genes, which may result in absence of protein synthesis (2A6*4, 2D6*5), no enzyme activity (2A6*2, 2C19*2, 2C19*3, 2D6*4), altered substrate specificity (2C9*3), reduced affinity for substrate (2D6*17, 3A4*2), decreased stability (2D6*10) or even increased enzyme activity (2D6*2xn) (Tang et al. 2005). It is important to note that such genetically determined enzyme variation may directly interfere in the drug concentration at the target tissue, and though the pharmacological effect may be observed, the risk of toxicity will also be higher in "poor metabolizers" since it might accumulate to possibly harmful levels. Reduction in drug biotransformation, as observed in drug-drug interactions, will also result in altered expected values for the constant of elimination (Ke), half-life of the drug (t½), volume of distribution (Vd), area under the curve (AUC) and others common useful pharmacokinetic parameters used in therapeutic drug monitoring and adjustment. Based on these reasons, PGx approaches may contribute to the enhancement of clinical outcomes by providing a more effective match between patient and drug dose or type, and consequently reducing the probability of an adverse drug reaction.

Since the effect of inherited variation (genotype) on enzymatic activity isresult of changes in DNA sequence (will be discussed in more details later), it is plausible that there are distinct subgroups of subjects who have different metabolic capabilities (**phenotype**). IIndeed, epidemiologic studies have revealed at least two sub-populations of individuals based on drug metabolizing profile, classified as either "rapid", or "slow" metabolizers. Importantly to note that each metabolic group (rapid or slow) has advantages and disadvantages, and potential outcomes have been related to the type of drug studied. For example, administration of a prodrug may have higher therapeutic efficacy in a rapid than in slow metabolizer phenotype, as the metabolization of such drug is necessary to make it active. In addition, drug biotransformation is fundamental to generate an active-molecule (M2) from a less (or not) active form (M1) (Figure 1C). Despite controversies that exist in the literature about the real impact of pharmacogenetics on clinical practice (Padol et al. 2006), studies have reported different therapeutic response in patients treated with proton pump inhibitors (Tanigawara et al. 1999; Furuta et al. 2001; Klotz 2006). These examples illustrate how important PGx is, on a case-by-case basis.

Furthermore, it is evident that PGx approaches cited here are simplified assumptions of metabolism. Actually, many drugs are sequentially metabolized (Figure 1D) by parallel pathways or a broad range of enzymes to other intermediary metabolites. For practical purposes, two main classes of reactions are considered in the biotransformation of drugs. Exclusively for readability, some basic generalities of each phase reactions will be introduced below from a PGx perspective.

3. Lessons from phase I and II reactions

As discussed elsewhere in this book, the "**phase I**" metabolizing enzymes (or "nonsynthetic reactions") can convert drugs in reactive electrophilic metabolites by oxidation, hydrolysis, cyclization, reduction, and decyclization. The major and the most common phase I enzyme involved in drug metabolism are the microsomal cytochrome P450 (CYP) superfamily. CYPs mediate monooxygenase reactions that generate polar metabolites that may be readily excreted in the urine. Major CYP isoforms responsible for biotransformation of drugs include CYP3A4, CYP2D6, CYP2C9, CYP2C19, CYP1A2 and CYP2E1. However, CYP2D6, a member of this family, has been a true landmark in phase I reactions and also a common target of study in PGx.

Following the scientific vision of Evans and Sjöqvist concerning the inheritability of metabolism profile, Alexanderson continued the refining of the pharmacogenetic studies using twin models. Metabolism of some drugs such as nortriptiline (tricyclic antidepressant) were demonstrated to be under genetic control (Alexanderson et al. 1969). Later, Robert Smith (Mahgoub et al. 1977) and Michel Eichelbaum (Eichelbaum et al. 1979) and their co-workers independently attributed variability in debrisoquine/sparteine oxidation to feasible genetic polymorphisms in debrisoquine hydroxylase or sparteine oxidase (now known as CIP2D6, the same metabolizing enzyme of nortriptiline). In these studies, they suggested that at least two phenotypic subpopulations could be distinguished as "poor" and "extensive" metabolizers. This association between genotype and phenotype was explored only almost ten years after, when the gene encoding CYP2D6 was identified (Gonzalez et al. 1988). Nowadays, it is well recognized that *CYP2D6* polymorphisms may result in four phenotypes according to enzyme activity: **poor metabolizers** (PMs); **intermediate metabolizers** (IMs); **extensive metabolizers** (EMs); and **ultrarapid metabolizers** (UMs). The EM phenotype, considered as "reference", is the most frequent in worldwide populations. PMs inherit two deficient *CYP2D6* alleles, which result in a significant slower CYP2D6 metabolism rate (characterized by increase of the plasma drug levels) (Figure 2). Individuals carrying only one defective *CYP2D6* allele are considered IMs, the "functional" phenotype. Since IMs still have some CYP2D6 metabolic activity, pharmacological responses in those patients are considered marginally better than those observed in PM phenotype.

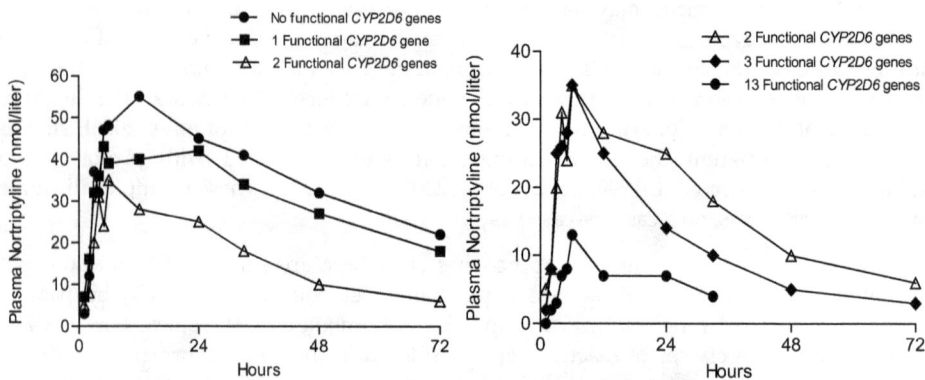

Fig. 2. Effect of functional *CYP2D6* genes in mean plasma concentrations of nortriptyline after a 25-mg oral dose administration. (Dalen et al. 1998).

The UM phenotype results from a gene duplication or even multiduplications. Individuals UMs tend to metabolize drugs at an ultrarapid rate (Ingelman-Sundberg et al. 2007). The relevance of such genetic variation in the biotransformation of drugs is very impressive. First, at least one fifth of all drugs used in clinical practice (or their active metabolites) share a pathway in CYP2D6 route. Among them, include those used to treat heart disease, depression and schizophrenia, for example (Ingelman-Sundberg & Sim 2010; Lohoff & Ferraro 2010). Second, phenotype status directly affects clinical response. Analgesic effects of some prodrugs, such as tramadol, codeine and oxycodone are CYP2D6-dependent, and PMs present low analgesic efficacy (Poulsen et al. 1996; Stamer et al. 2003; Stamer & Stuber 2007; Zwisler et al. 2009). On the other hand, loss of therapeutic efficacy at standard doses can also be observed in UMs since the drug metabolization occurs at a fast rate (Davis & Homsi 2001). Finally, UM may also present either improved therapeutic efficacy or more frequently severe adverse effects, due to a higher rate of toxic metabolites formation (Kirchheiner et al. 2008; Elkalioubie et al. 2011).

An interesting point is that many chemicals become more toxic (even carcinogenic) only when they are converted to a reactive form by phase 1 enzyme (represented by M2 in Figure 1D). Thus, subsequent biotransformation pathway has a critical role in protecting cells from damage by promoting elimination of such potentially dangerous compounds. In this context, many phase I products are not rapidly eliminated and they may undergo a subsequent reaction, known as **phase II** (represented by E2 in Figure 1D). Phase II reactions are characterized by incorporation of an endogenous substrate (for this reason are called "conjugation reactions") such as glutathione (GSH), sulfate, glycine, or glucuronic acid within specific sites in the target containing mainly carboxyl (-COOH), hydroxyl (-OH), amino (-NH$_2$), and sulfhydryl (-SH) groups to form a highly polar conjugate (represented by M3 in the figure 1D). As phase I, most phase II reactions generally produces more water-soluble metabolites, increasing the rate of their excretion from the body. However, it is important to notice that the conjugation of reactive compounds by phase 2 metabolizing enzymes will not necessarily convert them into inactive compounds before elimination. Actually, "phase I" and "phase II" terminologies have been more related to a historical classification rather than a biologically based one, since phase II reactions can occur alone, or even precede phase I reactions. In general, more complex routes are involved in drug metabolism though some pathways are preferentially used.

It is worthwhile to mention some clinical considerations with regard to recent advances seen in PGx. First, although genotyping may be useful in predicting a drug response or toxicological risk, classical factors related with variability in drug response (age, organic status, patient compliance and others) must also be considered at every stage of the therapeutic individualization (Vetti et al. 2010). Second, it is widely accepted that genetic variability in DMEs are also directly correlated with susceptibility to unexpected outcomes, such as suicide (Penas-Lledo et al. 2011), cancer (Di Pietro et al. 2010) and other complex diseases (Ma et al. 2011). In others words, PGx approaches are not limited to drug response.

Knowledge of the relevance of phase II enzymes for PGx precedes the CYP2D6 findings. The final touch of this association was done by Price Evans in an elegant and well-designed research on the Finish in 1950`s (Evans et al. 1960). Although his studies about variation of isoniazid metabolism had more impact on public health, Evans advanced the ideas of Hughes and McCusick about the influence of Mendelian inheritance on drug metabolism. In this regard, his findings allowed introduction of the 'fast' and 'slow' metabolizers nomenclature, and which finally provided evidences that genetic variation in drug metabolism could be shown using random families. Subsequent studies demonstrated that the common trimodal profile in plasma isoniazid levels as a result of genetically determined forms of hepatic **N-acetyltransferase (NAT)**. Particularly NAT2 (EC 2.3.1.5), catalyzes not only N-acetylation, but following N-hydroxylation also catalyzes subsequent O-acetylation and N,O-acetylation. NAT2 is a crucial enzyme to convert some environmental carcinogens such as polycyclic aromatic hydrocarbons (PAHs), aromatic amines (AAs), heterocyclic amines (HAs) and nitrosamines (NAs) in more water-soluble metabolite, avoiding accumulation of potentially dangerous metabolites (Hein et al. 2000).

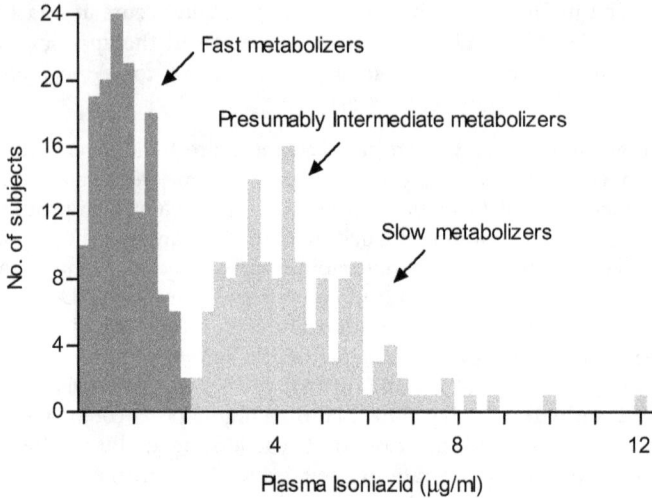

Fig. 3. Polymodal distribution of plasmatic concentrations after an oral dose of isoniazid in 267 subjects (Price-Evans 1962).

Other important phase II enzymes are **Glutathione S-transferases** (**GSTs**; EC 2.5.1.18), which constitute a superfamily of ubiquitous and multifunctional enzymes. As NAT2, GSTs play a key role in cellular detoxification, protecting macromolecules from attack by reactive electrophiles, including environmental carcinogens, reactive oxygen species and chemotherapeutic agents (Ginsberg et al. 2009). One common feature of all GSTs is their ability to catalyze the nucleophilic addition of the tripeptide glutathione (GSH; γ-Glu-Cys-Gly) to a wide variety of exogenous and endogenous chemicals with electrophilic functional groups, thereby neutralizing such sites, and similar with NAT2, rendering the products more water-soluble, facilitating their elimination from the cell. Besides NATs and GSTs, other enzymes are also important in phase II metabolism, such as UDP-glucuronosyl transferases (UGTs), sulfotransferases (SULTs), methyltransferases (as TPMT) and acyltransferases (as GNPAT).

Assumptions between functional variability in DMEs and heritable genetic polymorphisms have allowed recent studies to evaluate, for example, why exposition to a particular toxic substance does not result in the same degree of risk for all individuals. This approach called **toxicogenetics** is considered another arm of PGx. Additionally, toxicological perspectives provide opportunities to evaluate the interindividual variability in susceptibility to a number of disorders such as cancer (Orphanides & Kimber 2003; Di Pietro et al. 2010). As discussed later, it is inevitable that this knowledge would bring out endless debates about ethical questions.

4. Genetic variability in drug response

At this point, it is clear that variability in drug response depends on the complex interplay between multiple factors (including age, organ function, concomitant therapy, drug interactions, and the nature of the disease) and genetic background. Now, we will focus on the basic principles of genetics to get a better understanding of key issues addressed in PGx, and how genotype data may be used to infer phenotypic designations.

DNA sequence variations that are common in the population (present at frequencies of 1% or higher) are known as polymorphisms (not just "mutations") and they influence the function of their encoded protein, consequently altering human phenotypes. Among such genetic variations, there are at least two common polymorphisms having a substantial influence on the interindividual variation in human metabolism: Single Nucleotide Polymorphisms (**SNPs**) and insertions/deletions (**indels**). SNPs are polymorphisms that occur when a single nucleotide (A, T, C, or G) is altered in the genome sequence. They are largely distributed and account for most variations found in the genome. However, those that occur in genes and surrounding regions of the genome controlling gene expression are notoriously related to susceptibility to diseases or have a direct effect on drug metabolism. SNPs are classified as **nonsynonymous** (or missense) if the base pair change results in an amino acid substitution, or **synonymous** (or sense) if the base pair substitution within a codon does not alter the encoded amino acid. In comparison to base pair substitutions, indels are much less frequent in the genome, especially in coding regions. Most indels within exons (representative nucleotide sequences that code for mature RNA), may cause a frame shift in the translated protein and thereby changing protein structure or function, or result in an early stop codon, which makes an unstable or nonfunctional protein. Important to state that the functional effects of structural genomic variants are not limited by SNPs and indels, but also related to others process such as inversion and multiple copies of genes (as observed in *CYP2D6*), and even the occurrence of a new gene-fusion products.

As presented earlier, population studies have shown the frequency of an appropriate measure of *in vivo* enzyme activity frequently bimodal (with two phenotypes generally termed rapid and slow metabolizers). However, as observed in *CYP2D6* gene, additional phenotypes such as the ultrarapid (those with markedly enhanced activity) or intermediate metabolizers can be detected, resulting in subsets of individuals who differ from the majority (polymodal). As this phenotypic distribution is determined by genetic polymorphisms, the knowledge of alleles variants in selected genes may provide a basis for understanding and predicting individual differences in drug response. Here, we selected the *NAT2* gene, a clinically relevant gene example, to illustrate how PGx data may provide molecular diagnostic methods to improve drug therapy.

4.1 NAT2: Genetic determinants to a range of phenotypes

The gene coding for *NAT2* is located within 170 kb mapped to the short arm of human chromosome 8p22. *NAT2* codifies a 290 amino acid product from the intronless 870 base pair open reading frame (Blum et al. 1990). Numerous allelic variants have been described for *NAT2*. Although the SNPs in the coding exon causing amino acid changes remain most investigated, recent studies have described some *NAT2* SNPs that do not change amino acid codon but may have functional consequences in transcript stability and splicing. *NAT2* SNPs are described in detail on the website http://louisville.edu/medschool /pharmacology/consensus-human-arylamine-n-acetyltransferase-gene-nomenclature).

A number of studies have attempted to relate *NAT2* SNPs to interindividual differences in response to drugs or in disease susceptibility, however some inconsistencies were observed.

A reasonable explanation for this contradictions is that genotyping of individuals SNPs alone may not always provide enough information to reach these goals at genes containing multiple SNPs in high linkage disequilibrium such as *NAT2* (Sabbagh & Darlu 2005). Therefore, it seems more desirable that various combinations of *NAT2* SNPs, known as **haplotypes**, rather than individual SNPs can be required to infer phenotypes of NAT2 acetylation in a trimodal distribution of rapid, intermediate and slow (Vatsis et al. 1995). Thus, genetic alterations in *NAT2* described so far stem primarily from various haplotypes of 20 nonsynonymous (*C29T, G152T, G191A, T341C, G364A, C403G, A411T, A434C, A472C, G499A, A518G, C578T, G590A, G609T, T622C, C638T, A803G, G838A, A845C,* and *G857A*) and seven synonymous SNPs (*T111C, C228T, C282T, C345T, C481T, A600G* and *C759T*) in the *NAT2* coding exon.

Metabolic phenotyping assays are generally more time-consuming, more expensive, and not suitable in many situations. In this regard, many studies have successfully shown that phenotype prediction of NAT2 activity from genotype data is useful and accurate. However, this requires that all relevant SNPs and/or alleles be analyzed in the population studied since inference of NAT2 phenotypes is assigned based on co-dominant expression of rapid and slow acetylator *NAT2* SNPs, as previously shown (Xu et al. 2002). For example, individuals that have one or more slow acetylator *NAT2* SNPs such as *A191G, T341C, G590A* or *G857A* are deduced as slow acetylators since these substitutions are diagnostic for defective NAT2 function. However, if at least one rapid *NAT2* SNP is also present, an intermediate acetylator is observed. Failure to detect this hypothetical rapid SNP may explain, in part, an unreliable enzymatic prediction or even unexpected clinical outcomes. On the other hand, there is still no consensus about the number of *NAT2* SNPs considered necessary to infer accurately the human acetylator status. Many studies have performed genotyping using 4 SNPs (*A191G, C341T, A590G* and *A857G*), but some authors demonstrated that analysis at least of seven SNPs (adding *C282T, C481T* and *A803G*) seems more accurate to infer the NAT2 acetylator phenotypes (Deitz et al. 2004). It is important to note that this accuracy may vary depending on the ancestral background of the population under study because the SNP prevalence differs among ethnic groups. For example, our research group found that *G590A*, common to the *NAT2*6* slow haplotype, is present in almost all Afro-Brazilians and Caucasians, but present only in half of Amerindians (Talbot et al. 2010). In fact, even the reference haplotype considered "wild-type" is not common in all ethnic groups. The most common and clinically relevant *NAT2* haplotypes that have been the subject of most studies in recent years are illustrated in Table 1.

4.2 Why computational approach is valuable to infer haplotypes?

Haplotype approaches combining the information of adjacent SNPs into composite multilocus are more informative, robust and valuable in the study of human traits than single-locus analyses. However, problems may occur when *NAT2* SNPs are assigned to a particular combination of two multilocus haplotypes because most *NAT2* SNPs are found in high **linkage disequilibrium** and haplotype assembly from available genotype data which may a challenging task. In other words, the gametic phase of haplotypes is inherently ambiguous when individuals are heterozygous at more than one locus (Figure 4).

Haplotype	SNP and rs identifiers	Amino-acid change	Acetylator phenotype
NAT2*4	Reference	Reference	High
NAT2*5A	T341C (rs1801280) C481T (rs1799929)	I114T L161L	Slow
NAT2*5B	T341C (rs1801280) C481T (rs1799929) A803G (rs1208)	I114T L161L K268R	Slow
NAT2*5C	T341C (rs1801280) A803G (rs1208)	I114T K268R	Slow
NAT2*6A	C282T (rs1041983) G590A (rs1799930)	Y94Y R197Q	Slow
NAT2*6B	G590A (rs1799930)	R197Q	Slow
NAT2*7A	G857A (rs1799931)	G286E	Slow*
NAT2*7B	G857A (rs1799931) C282T (rs1041983)	G286E Y94Y	Slow
NAT2*12A	A803G (rs1208)	K268R	Rapid
NAT2*12B	A803G (rs1208) C282T (rs1041983)	K268R Y94Y	Rapid
NAT2*12C	A803G (rs1208) C481T (rs1799929)	K268R L161L	Rapid
NAT2*13A	C282T (rs1041983)	Y94Y	Rapid
NAT2*14A	G191A (rs1801279)	R64Q	Slow
NAT2*14B	G191A (rs1801279) C282T (rs1041983)	R64Q Y94Y	Slow

Common non-synonymous nucleotide and amino-acid change are bolded.
*Substrate dependent.

Table 1. Common studied NAT2 haplotypes and associated acetylator phenotype.

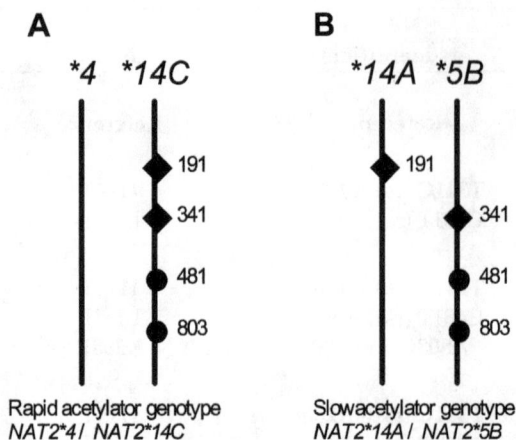

Fig. 4. Haplotype classification is depend on gametic phase and may induce equivocally phenotype. Subject can be either rapid (A) or slow (B) acetylator depending on whether these mutations are located in the same or different chromosome.

As current routine genotyping and sequencing methods typically provide unordered allele pairs for each marker, *NAT2* haplotypes must be determined by inferring the phase of the alleles in order to assign an acetylator phenotype to a particular individual. **Haplotype Phase Inference** is based on transfer of ordered genotypes to all members in the pedigree at all loci, consistent with all observed genotype data and Mendelian segregation (readers may refer to an article by Slatkin 2008 for more details). In this regard, statistical and computational methods for haplotype construction from genotype data of random individuals received considerable attention due to several approaches have been developed to infer the true haplotype phase (Stephens & Donnelly 2003; Scheet & Stephens 2006). For example, there is a web server that implements a supervised pattern recognition approach to infer NAT2 acetylator phenotype (slow, intermediate or rapid) directly from the observed combinations of 6 *NAT2* SNPs (Kuznetsov et al. 2009). Although haplotype data may also be obtained in family studies and experimentally from general population, these methods are considered laborious and expensive.

4.3 From genetic alterations to protein function: Moving from pharmacogenetics to pharmacogenomics

Given that genetic alteration may influence a protein function, several studies were conducted to assess how polymorphisms in genes of the corresponding DME can modify drug efficacy/toxicity and disease risk. In general, results have been obtained in epidemiologic or clinical studies and for better understanding of the population's PGx. Consequently, in order to investigate these associations, both *in vitro* and *in vivo* studies using a variety of substrates have been performed to assign phenotypes to many identified genotypes.

Functional studies and intracellular tracking of polymorphic variants are contributing to appreciation of how individual mutations modify protein function. In general, these studies support the idea that different combinations of polymorphisms in the gene coding region result in proteins with altered stability, degradation, and/or kinetic characteristics. For example, slow acetylator *NAT2* alleles showed reduced levels of NAT2 protein when compared with reference *NAT2*4* allele, and possible mechanisms SNP-induced protein alteration are discussed elsewhere (Zang et al. 2007). Moreover, reductions in catalytic activity for the N-acetylation of sulfamethazine and 2-aminofluorene, a sulfonamide drug and an aromatic amine carcinogen respectively, were observed in *NAT2* alleles possessing *G191A, T341C, A434C, G590A, A845C* or *G857A* (Fretland et al. 2001). As many chemicals cannot be tested *in vivo*, including certain human carcinogens, physiological effects of genetic alterations as SNPs and haplotypes, have been investigated *in vitro* in recombinant expression systems to determine the corresponding phenotypes.

The effects of genetic alteration on proteins are the basis for bimodal or polymodal phenotypes. With these relations between genotype and phenotype recognized, studies have shown promising pathways supposed to be susceptibility molecular targets for a number of drug side effects and certain malignancies predisposed by DME genes polymorphisms.

Furthermore, the molecular homology modeling techniques, including SNP locations and computational docking of substrates, have increased the understanding of the protein structure-function relationship. In this context, PGx has been a universal discipline providing many of the driving forces behind of the scientific development of the human genetics, pharmacology, clinical medicine and epidemiology. Additional evidences from laboratory-based experiments, haplotype mapping and clinical tests, lead us to believe that PGx will be a major contributor in the preventive and curative modern medicine.

5. Clinical pharmacogenetics and potential applications

Individual variability in plasma drug levels has been considered by many studies as a primary cause of therapeutic inefficacy and pharmacologic toxicity. Thus, matching patients to the drugs and dose that are most likely to be effective (maximizing drug efficacy) and least likely to cause harm (enhancing drug safety) is the main purpose of the novel contributions PGx.

Clinically relevant examples of inherited variation that may influence the individual's drug-metabolizing capacity and consequently pharmacokinetic properties of a drug are available in the literature. One of the earliest pharmacogenetic tests resulting in clinically important side effects was on the enzyme **thiopurine methyltransferase (TPMT)** (Krynetski et al. 1996). TPMT metabolizes two thiopurine drugs: azathioprine (AZA) and its metabolite 6-mercaptopurine (6-MP), used in the treatment of autoimmune diseases and acute lymphoblastic leukemia. Polymorphism in *TPMT* gene causes some individuals to be particularly deficient in TPMT activity, and then thiopurine metabolism must proceed by other pathways, one of which leads to cytotoxic 6-thioguanine nucleotide analogues. This metabolite can lead to bone marrow toxicity and myelosuppression. Such genetic variation in TPMT affects a small proportion of people (approximately 0.3% of the population), though seriously. As empiric dose-adjustments of AZA and 6-MP is risky, *TPMT* genotyping before institution pharmacotherapy by identifying individuals with low or absent TPMT enzyme activity may provide useful tools for optimizing therapeutic response and prevent toxicity (myelosuppression) (Krynetski & Evans 2003). In addition, *TPMT* genotype and drug adjustment may reduce the risk of secondary malignancies, including brain tumors and acute myelogenous leukemia (McLeod et al. 2000; Stanulla et al. 2005).

NAT2 pharmacogenetics has attracted significant attention as N-acetylation polymorphism seems to predispose to an increased risk of drug-induced hepatotoxicity in patients administered **isoniazid** for the treatment of tuberculosis. Although exact mechanism of isoniazid-induced hepatotoxicity is unknown, recent studies have provided exciting results. Until recently, findings have proposed that metabolite responsible for isoniazid-induced hepatotoxicity was acetylhydrazine (AcHZ) which can undergo further metabolism by CYPs to toxic reactive acetyl free radicals in patients with slow NAT2 acetylation capacities (figure 5). These toxic metabolites can form covalent bonds with liver cell macromolecules, interfering with their function and hepatocellular necrosis. In addition to this reason, some studies have also suggested that patients carrying both slow acetylator NAT2 and fast CYP2E1 isoforms may have a severe exacerbation outcome. Furthermore, it is believed that hydrazine (Hz) is also responsible for the isoniazid-induced hepatotoxicity based on results that metabolic activation of Hz causes hepatic disorder. Also in this second proposition, slow acetylators may be injured since Hz is metabolized by NAT2 to the less toxic derivative diacetylhydrazine (DiAcHZ), which is then excreted in the urine. On the other hand, fast acetylation of AcHZ and Hz in NAT2 rapid acetylators should theoretically form DiAcHZ efficiently and therefore reducing the oxidative metabolites accumulation from AcHZ. In fact, several studies found an increased risk in slow versus fast acetylators through genetically determined phenotype (Higuchi et al. 2007). However, there are conflicting data on whether *CYP2E1* genotypes do or do not increase the risk of isoniazid-induced (Cho et al. 2007).

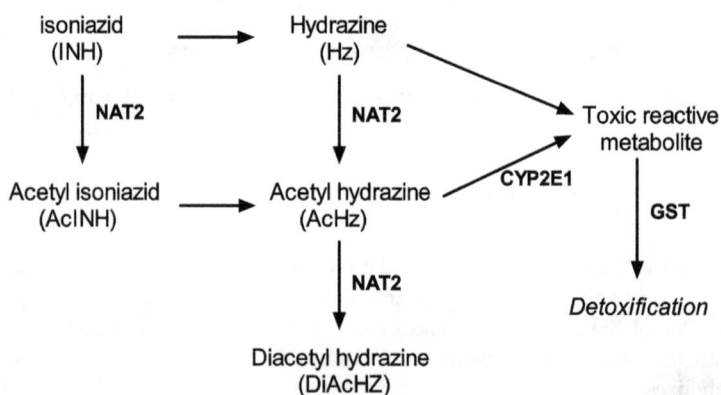

Fig. 5. Major enzymes involved in isoniazid biotransformation and relevant metabolites.

Isoniazid metabolic pathways clearly exemplify that elimination of most drugs involves the participation of several families of drug metabolizing enzymes. Therefore, it is incoherent thought that one or few isolated host factors that only response to drugs. However, there are few studies focusing on the relationship between the genotypes of related enzymes and susceptibility to drug adverse reactions. As shown in Figure 5, is theoretically possible that GST isoforms, which are genetically determined to a great extent, may also influence INH metabolism. In this way, a study found that well known *GSTM1* null genotype influenced the serum concentration of Hz in the NAT2 slow acetylators independently of their CYP2E1 phenotype (Fukino et al. 2008). Thus, more efforts are necessary to uncover the important question: interactions between *NAT2* and *CYP2E1* phenotypes, in addition to the GSTs, may have potential risks for isoniazid-induced hepatotoxicity? Thus, as a general rule, a better understanding of genetic factors in a more studies manner will be useful to demonstrate that prediction of toxicity is possible and consistently reliable.

In addition to significant number of publications available in the scientific literature, others comprehensive, public online resources are also available for beginners and experts in PGx. Undoubtedly, one of the most important is **Pharmacogenomics Knowledge Base** (**PharmGKB**, http://www.pharmgkb.org). The reader will find up-to-date information about the most important genes involved in drug response, highlighted summaries, pathway diagrams, and accurate literature (Sangkuhl et al. 2008). In general, the ultimate goal of such services is to guide appropriate PGx knowledge. Common data collected (with few modifications) from PharmGKB in regard to PGx polymorphisms of phase I DMEs and clinical associations are summarized in Table 2. Since we discussed earlier about PGx of *CYP2D6*, we purposely excluded it this table.

Gene	Common Alleles/Effect	Common substrates	Clinical evidences	References
CYP2A6	*2 (L160H) *5 (G479V) *7 (I471T) *11 (S224P) *12 (10 aa substitutions) *17 (V365M) *18 (Y392F) *20 (196 frameshift)	Coumarin, SM-12502, Tegafur#, Nicotine and 5-Fluorouracil	Influence on nicotine adverse effects and variability in quit smoking	(Malaiyandi et al. 2006; Ozaki et al. 2006; Ho et al. 2008)
			Altered therapeutic responses to antineoplastic Tegafur	(Daigo et al. 2002; Kong et al. 2009)
CYP2B6	*2 (R22C) *4 (K262R) *5 (R487C) *6 (Q172H; K262R)	Tamoxifen, Clopidogrel#, Carbamazepine#, Cyclophosphamide, Nicotine and Diazepan	Efavirenz effect and central nervous system side effects	(Haas et al. 2004; Ribaudo et al. 2010)
			Sub-therapeutic plasma concentrations of efavirenz	(Rodriguez-Novoa et al. 2005; ter Heine et al. 2008)
			Benefits of efavirenz dose adjustment	(Gatanaga et al. 2007; ter Heine et al. 2008)

Gene	Common Alleles/Effect	Common substrates	Clinical evidences	References
CYP2C9	*2 (R144C) *3 (I359L) *5 (D360E) *6 (273 frameshift) *13 (L90P)	Warfarin, Phenytoin, Tolbutamide, Glibenclamide, Gliclazide, Fluvastatin, Losartan, Ritonavir and Tipranavir.	Variability in warfarin therapy and elevated risk of severe bleeding	(Aithal et al. 1999; Takahashi et al. 2006; Gan et al. 2011)
			Elevated risk of hypoglycemia attacks during oral antidiabetic treatment.	(Kidd et al. 1999; Tan et al. 2010; Gokalp et al. 2011)
			More frequent symptoms of overdose in phenytoin therapy	(Ninomiya et al. 2000; van der Weide et al. 2001; Kesavan et al. 2010)
CYP2C19	*2A (splic; I331V) *2B (splic; E92D) *2C (splic; A161P; I331V) *3A (W212X; I331V) *3B (W212X; D360N; I331V) *9 (R144H; I331V) *17 (I331V)	Mephenytoin, Lansoprazole, Omeprazole, Selegiline, Imipramine, Fluoxetine Diazepan, Phenobarbital and Proguanil	Inadequate response to clopidogrel* and higher rate of major adverse cardiovascular events (thrombosis)	(Mega et al. 2009; Mega et al. 2010; Kelly et al. 2011)
			Increased risk of proguanil treatment failures	(Kaneko et al. 1997)
			Differences in clinical efficacy of proton pump inhibitors.	(Zhao et al. 2008; Furuta et al. 2009; Sheng et al. 2010; Yang & Lin 2010)
			Nelfinavir pharmacokinetics and virologic response in HIV-1-infection.	(Saitoh et al. 2010)

#prodrugs; aa: amino acid; splic: splicing defect. More information about allele, protein, nucleotide changes, trivial name and effect of the gene of polymorphism on enzyme activity may be found in http://www.cypalleles.ki.se/index.htm and http://www.snpedia.com/index.php/SNPedia.

Table 2. Common alleles, substrates and clinical evidences of some CYPs.

6. Ethnic characterization is not sufficient to reach pharmacogenetic goals: Focus on personal genomics

Inherited determinants generally remain stable throughout a person's lifetime (unlike other factors influencing drug response), making the pharmacogenetics approach attractive. However, both interethnic and intraethnic variability for a specific allele in human populations are extremely large and may have relevant clinical implications. *NAT2* is a good example of such gene. Several *NAT2* SNPs causing defective enzymes are heterogeneity distributed in the world making 50% of Caucasians but only 10% of Japanese slow acetylators, for example. Moreover, our research group demonstrated that some discrepancies in allelic frequencies in an important DME, even within the same population. (Magno et al. 2009).

Undoubtedly, PGx variability explains in part why there are important differences in response to conventional drug-based therapies among different ethnic groups. But, from a biological standpoint, what are the probability to predict efficiently and accurately an individual response to drug from a multi-ethnic study? Low, at least. Several evidences have provided enough data to concern about it. Attempts to predict genotypes and phenotypes from ethnic perspectives have been become less meaningful, mainly in parts of the world in which people from different regions have mixed extensively. Thus, recent studies have pointed out that ethnicity not always serves as a start point to define drug regimes because it typically not emphasizes biological components. To group individuals in only a same category based in non-biological criteria, is to assume that people from these groups have same biological backgrounds. For example, clinical and pharmacological trials have traditionally considered the different geographical regions of Brazil as being very heterogeneous. However, a recent study found that the genomic ancestry of subjects from these different regions of Brazil is more homogeneous than anticipated (Pena et al. 2011). In the same way, individual categorization depends not on physical appearance of the subjects (Parra et al. 2003).

Therefore, it is evident that results from population studies could be useful in some situations, but the fact that subjects have their own variations reinforce the necessity to study an individual's genetic profile and not ethnic populations.

7. Are PGx approaches cost-effective?

Unquestionably, some success has been achieved in recent years in establishing the clinical utility of the pharmacogenetic testing. However, it remains questionable whether it is cost-effective or not. To justify routine testing, PGx technology must be more practical than the available approaches and involve a clinical benefit higher than those reported and sufficiently to cover expenditures in genetic testing. Unfortunately, data on cost-effectiveness of PGx are currently limited and have been the subject of controversy in the literature. A possible explanation is that therapeutic outcomes depend on many poorly defined factors other than pharmacogenetic variation, such as the cost of therapeutic failure and circumstances surrounding patient therapy. Furthermore, to address the issue of "effectiveness" is difficult, considering that PGx purposes not only attempt save time and money, but also avoids any unnecessary physical suffering and emotional traumas.

In general, studies have shown that PGx is potentially cost-effective under certain circumstances (Carlson et al. 2009; Vegter et al. 2009; Meckley et al. 2010). Some authors consider that findings showing non-robust benefit of PGx testing are due to limited knowledge of its therapeutic application since access to technology and genotyping expenses are no longer limiting factors. Influence of *CYP2D6* alleles on therapeutic efficacy of psychiatry drugs clearly illustrates this. Besides the influence of *CYP2D6* alleles on metabolism of most antipsychotics drugs, studies investigating the association between *CYP2D6* genotypes and antipsychotic response have reported no predicted clinical improvement (Zhang & Malhotra 2011). Probably, this enzyme only has a significant clinical impact on a smaller non-investigated subgroup of drugs. In fact, a genetic variation that merely affects the drug elimination, modestly increase the frequency of an adverse effect or a common side effect that is well tolerated may still not be of sufficient importance to justify pharmacogenetic testing.

Presumably, cost-effectiveness of PGx also can vary from high to low depending on the illness and gene involved. According to this proposition, important support of the cost-effectiveness of PGx comes from clinical situations where PGx variations have major impact on therapeutic outcomes and clinical cost. Genotyping of *TPMT* before starting azathioprine treatment (Hagaman et al. 2010), *HTR2A* (serotonin 2A receptor) in selective serotonin reuptake inhibitors therapy (Perlis et al. 2009) and *CYP2C9* plus *VKORC1* (vitamin K epoxide reductase complex subunit 1) before warfarin treatment (Leey et al. 2009; You 2011) are well-known examples.

Important to date that economic evaluations of PGx have all highlighted the need to improve the quality of the evidence-based economics (Payne & Shabaruddin 2010), since a number of studies have been inconclusive (Verhoef et al. 2010). Finally, it is possible that the rapidly decreasing cost of genetic analysis and knowledge of the therapeutic application of PGx will be able systematically to make PGx approaches more and more cost-effective technology.

8. Ethics in PGx and final considerations

Past lessons had enabled us to see the rising of personalized prescriptions in improving prevention of serious adverse drug reactions, therapeutic effect and patient compliance. However, they have not resolved the ethical issues that are emerging in PGx research. Although the barriers between technological advances and the view of human well-being are not so clear-cut, both perspectives will be discussed below.

The first issue comes from the source of PGx data: human samples. Samples and data collected as a part of the research are stored and offer robust information about genome, cells, biological functions, life-style, previous diseases, and many others. Although it seems like a conspirator theory or just an ideological issue, because historical facts unfortunately have failed to clearly show this fact. A businessman from Seattle called John Moore developed hairy cell leukemia and was treated by a highly qualified team from a notorious research center of an American University. Then, Moore returned to the center in order monitor his condition seven years later, fearing a recurrence of the leukaemia. However, he was shocked to learn that besides his physician's preoccupation about his health, there indeed was another interest at stake. And that was a million dollar contract that was already negotiated and signed, to develop a cell line from Moore blood sample (now known as "Mo-cell line") without Moore's consent. It became a court case. Surprisingly, California Supreme Court decided the case in favour of the physician. This landline decision gave a clear impetus to commercialization of samples from human and led to patents developed from human samples. After that, new patents based on human samples gave a new gold rush treasure. It is obvious that the chapter's purpose is not to go deeper in this kind of philosophical issues, but the reader must think about the real impact of what the informed consent really represent and what should guide its free applications. Moreover, many studies involving thousands of individuals with application of "reconsents" and "tiered consent" aiming to obtain specimens to future research will also new clinical directives in PGx research.

A second bioethical hallmark allow the subject or patient confidentiality. How, for whom and why will the information be accessed? As a part of clinical diagnosis, it seems more reasonable that the patients themselves have special interest and the confidentiality is not different as in the case of other diseases. However, could patients' relatives know about inherited disorders or increased disease risk? Could employers and health insurances companies have access to this genetic information? For instance, we may suppose a company looking for employees based on the "tolerance levels" to exposure of occupational toxicants. In this regard, studies have shown a wide range of carcinogenic toxicants such as arsenic (Hernandez et al. 2008; Paiva et al. 2010), benzene (Sapienza et al. 2007) and polycyclic aromatic hydrocarbons (Rihs et al. 2005) in which detoxification is genetically influenced. Thus, should this information be used for admission or even resignation? Defenders of the breaking of genomic confidentiality usually have highlighted the cost-benefit of "protecting his/her own health", but some health insurance companies may use these data to introduce different fares depending on individual susceptibility such as "high costs" for subjects defined as "higher disease risk", for example. Actually there is no novelty on that since many worldwide apply different rates for automobiles or health insurance based on age, gender, life-style, previous disease and some others. In fact, companies, regulatory and public funding agencies are discussing how to integrate PGx practice into public health care (Robertson et al. 2002; Evans 2010).

Examples above illustrated lead to a third reflection: Equity. As discussed by Peterson-Iyer, "market forces do not guarantee justice in the distribution of health care". In a different way of the "one-size-fits-all" (a blind approach for drug prescription with regard to their pharmacokinetic profile), PGx approaches improving drug safety and efficacy are already beginning to be performed only in some private and medical centers. It is unquestionable that in short time clinical practice of PGx will favor highly sophisticated higher one's economic status. If currently there are a significant numbers of subjects uninsured for basic health care, would PGx rectify or exacerbate the profoundly disturbing those with higher economic status inequalities in the health care system? (Peterson-Iyer 2008). Indeed many other bioethical questions might be relevant, which we may not be able to treat here. We encourage the readers to read further on this subject from various excellent articles on these issues (Williams-Jones & Corrigan 2003; Weijer & Miller 2004; Patowary 2005; Sillon et al. 2008; Howard et al. 2011).

In conclusion, unequivocally DMEs still remain helping to elucidate the well-known mechanisms of variability in drug response and have been the major contributor in the successful advances in PGx (Freund et al. 2004; Jaquenoud Sirot et al. 2006; Swierkot &

Slezak 2011). Past lessons have taught us to consider each individual as a unique person from metabolic perspective. Currently, PGx is leading us to uncover several and potential applications of PGx in the clinical practice, which involves an interconnected puzzle pieces with patients, health professionals, industry and governmental regulatory agencies. Finally, PGx starts to tell us that all its benefits should also be applied in a close future for all members of the society and though differences in our DNA, pharmacogeneticians always worked together in the same perspective to improve the health of people without distinction.

9. Acknowledgment

Authors acknowledge the contributions of all investigators and students from Laboratory of Pharmacogenome and Molecular Epidemiology from Santa Cruz State University (UESC). Authors also acknowledge the relevant grants of Bahia State Research Foundation (*Fundação de Amparo a Pesquisa do Estado da Bahia - FAPESB*). LAVM is CAPES Ph.D. fellow (Proc. 2230/11-9).

10. References

Aithal, G. P., C. P. Day, et al. (1999). "Association of polymorphisms in the cytochrome P450 CYP2C9 with warfarin dose requirement and risk of bleeding complications." *Lancet* 353(9154): 717-719.

Alexanderson, B., D. A. Evans, et al. (1969). "Steady-state plasma levels of nortriptyline in twins: influence of genetic factors and drug therapy." *Br Med J* 4(5686): 764-768.

Alving, A. S., P. E. Carson, et al. (1956). "Enzymatic deficiency in primaquine-sensitive erythrocytes." *Science* 124(3220): 484-485.

Blum, M., D. M. Grant, et al. (1990). "Human arylamine N-acetyltransferase genes: isolation, chromosomal localization, and functional expression." *DNA Cell Biol* 9(3): 193-203.

Caldwell, J. (2006). "Drug metabolism and pharmacogenetics: the British contribution to fields of international significance." *Br J Pharmacol* 147 Suppl 1: S89-99.

Carlson, J.J., Garrison, L.P., et al. (2009). "The potential clinical and economic outcomes of pharmacogenomic approaches to EGFR-tyrosine kinase inhibitor therapy innon-small-cell lung cancer." *Value Health* 12(1): 20-7.

Cho, H. J., W. J. Koh, et al. (2007). "Genetic polymorphisms of NAT2 and CYP2E1 associated with antituberculosis drug-induced hepatotoxicity in Korean patients with pulmonary tuberculosis." *Tuberculosis (Edinb)* 87(6): 551-556.

Clayman, C. B., J. Arnold, et al. (1952). "Toxicity of primaquine in Caucasians." *J Am Med Assoc* 149(17): 1563-1568.

Daigo, S., Y. Takahashi, et al. (2002). "A novel mutant allele of the CYP2A6 gene (CYP2A6*11) found in a cancer patient who showed poor metabolic phenotype towards tegafur." *Pharmacogenetics* 12(4): 299-306.

Dalen, P., M. L. Dahl, et al. (1998). "10-Hydroxylation of nortriptyline in white persons with 0, 1, 2, 3, and 13 functional CYP2D6 genes." *Clin Pharmacol Ther* 63(4): 444-452.

Davis, M. P. & J. Homsi (2001). "The importance of cytochrome P450 monooxygenase CYP2D6 in palliative medicine." *Support Care Cancer* 9(6): 442-451.

Deitz, A. C., N. Rothman, et al. (2004). "Impact of misclassification in genotype-exposure interaction studies: example of N-acetyltransferase 2 (NAT2), smoking, and bladder cancer." *Cancer Epidemiol Biomarkers Prev* 13(9): 1543-1546.

Di Pietro, G., L. A. Magno, et al. (2010). "Glutathione S-transferases: an overview in cancer research." *Expert Opin Drug Metab Toxicol* 6(2): 153-170.

Eichelbaum, M., N. Spannbrucker, et al. (1979). "Influence of the defective metabolism of sparteine on its pharmacokinetics." *Eur J Clin Pharmacol* 16(3): 189-194.

Eichelbaum, M., N. Spannbrucker, et al. (1979). "Defective N-oxidation of sparteine in man: a new pharmacogenetic defect." *Eur J Clin Pharmacol* 16(3): 183-187.

Elkalioubie, A., D. Allorge, et al. (2011). "Near-fatal tramadol cardiotoxicity in a CYP2D6 ultrarapid metabolizer." *Eur J Clin Pharmacol.*

Evans, B. J. (2010). "Establishing clinical utility of pharmacogenetic tests in the post-FDAAA era." *Clin Pharmacol Ther* 88(6): 749-751.

Evans, D. A., K. A. Manley, et al. (1960). "Genetic control of isoniazid metabolism in man." *Br Med J* 2(5197): 485-491.

Fox, A. L. (1932). "The Relationship between Chemical Constitution and Taste." *Proc Natl Acad Sci U S A* 18(1): 115-120.

Fretland, A. J., M. A. Leff, et al. (2001). "Functional characterization of human N-acetyltransferase 2 (NAT2) single nucleotide polymorphisms." *Pharmacogenetics* 11(3): 207-215.

Freund, C. L., D. F. Gregory, et al. (2004). "Evaluating pharmacogenetic tests: a case example." *Arch Pediatr Adolesc Med* 158(3): 276-279.

Fukino, K., Y. Sasaki, et al. (2008). "Effects of N-acetyltransferase 2 (NAT2), CYP2E1 and Glutathione-S-transferase (GST) genotypes on the serum concentrations of isoniazid and metabolites in tuberculosis patients." *J Toxicol Sci* 33(2): 187-195.

Furuta, T., N. Shirai, et al. (2001). "Effect of genotypic differences in CYP2C19 on cure rates for Helicobacter pylori infection by triple therapy with a proton pump inhibitor, amoxicillin, and clarithromycin." *Clin Pharmacol Ther* 69(3): 158-168.

Furuta, T., M. Sugimoto, et al. (2009). "CYP2C19 genotype is associated with symptomatic recurrence of GERD during maintenance therapy with low-dose lansoprazole." *Eur J Clin Pharmacol* 65(7): 693-698.

Gan, G. G., M. E. Phipps, et al. (2011). "Contribution of VKORC1 and CYP2C9 polymorphisms in the interethnic variability of warfarin dose in Malaysian populations." *Ann Hematol* 90(6): 635-641.

Garrod, A. E. (1909). "The inborn errors of metabolism." (Oxford Univ. Press, London, UK).

Gatanaga, H., T. Hayashida, et al. (2007). "Successful efavirenz dose reduction in HIV type 1-infected individuals with cytochrome P450 2B6 *6 and *26." *Clin Infect Dis* 45(9): 1230-1237.

Ginsberg, G., S. Smolenski, et al. (2009). "Genetic Polymorphism in Glutathione Transferases (GST): Population distribution of GSTM1, T1, and P1 conjugating activity." *J Toxicol Environ Health B Crit Rev* 12(5-6): 389-439.

Gokalp, O., A. Gunes, et al. (2011). "Mild hypoglycaemic attacks induced by sulphonylureas related to CYP2C9, CYP2C19 and CYP2C8 polymorphisms in routine clinical setting." *Eur J Clin Pharmacol.*

Gong, L., R. P. Owen, et al. (2008). "PharmGKB: an integrated resource of pharmacogenomic data and knowledge." *Curr Protoc Bioinformatics* Chapter 14: Unit14 17.

Gonzalez, F.J., Skoda, R.C., et al. (1988). "Characterization of the common genetic defect in humans deficient in debrisoquine metabolism." *Nature* 4;331(6155): 442-446.

Haas, D. W., H. J. Ribaudo, et al. (2004). "Pharmacogenetics of efavirenz and central nervous system side effects: an Adult AIDS Clinical Trials Group study." *AIDS* 18(18): 2391-2400.

Hagaman, J.T., Kinder, B.W., et al. (2010). "Thiopurine S- methyltransferase [corrected] testing in idiopathic pulmonary fibrosis: a pharmacogenetic cost-effectiveness analysis." *Lung* 188(2): 125-32.

Hein, D. W., M. A. Doll, et al. (2000). "Molecular genetics and epidemiology of the NAT1 and NAT2 acetylation polymorphisms." *Cancer Epidemiol Biomarkers Prev* 9(1): 29-42.

Hernandez, A., N. Xamena, et al. (2008). "High arsenic metabolic efficiency in AS3MT287Thr allele carriers." *Pharmacogenet Genomics* 18(4): 349-355.

Higuchi, N., N. Tahara, et al. (2007). "NAT2 6A, a haplotype of the N-acetyltransferase 2 gene, is an important biomarker for risk of anti-tuberculosis drug-induced hepatotoxicity in Japanese patients with tuberculosis." *World J Gastroenterol* 13(45): 6003-6008.

Ho, M. K., J. C. Mwenifumbo, et al. (2008). "A novel CYP2A6 allele, CYP2A6*23, impairs enzyme function in vitro and in vivo and decreases smoking in a population of Black-African descent." *Pharmacogenet Genomics* 18(1): 67-75.

Howard, H. C., Y. Joly, et al. (2011). "Informed consent in the context of pharmacogenomic research: ethical considerations." *Pharmacogenomics J* 11(3): 155-161.

Hughes, H. B., J. P. Biehl, et al. (1954). "Metabolism of isoniazid in man as related to the occurrence of peripheral neuritis." *Am Rev Tuberc* 70(2): 266-273.

Ingelman-Sundberg, M. (2001). "Genetic susceptibility to adverse effects of drugs and environmental toxicants. The role of the CYP family of enzymes." *Mutat Res* 482(1-2): 11-19.

Ingelman-Sundberg, M. & S. C. Sim (2010). "Pharmacogenetic biomarkers as tools for improved drug therapy; emphasis on the cytochrome P450 system." *Biochem Biophys Res Commun* 396(1): 90-94.

Ingelman-Sundberg, M., S. C. Sim, et al. (2007). "Influence of cytochrome P450 polymorphisms on drug therapies: pharmacogenetic, pharmacoepigenetic and clinical aspects." *Pharmacol Ther* 116(3): 496-526.

Jaquenoud Sirot, E., J. W. van der Velden, et al. (2006). "Therapeutic drug monitoring and pharmacogenetic tests as tools in pharmacovigilance." *Drug Saf* 29(9): 735-768.

Johnson, J. A. & S. B. Liggett (2011). "Cardiovascular pharmacogenomics of adrenergic receptor signaling: clinical implications and future directions." *Clin Pharmacol Ther* 89(3): 366-378.

Kalow, W. (1962). "Pharmacogenetics. Heredity and the Response to Drugs." W. B. Saunders Co. Philadelphia, London

Kalow, W. (2005). "Pharmacogenomics: historical perspective and current status." *Methods Mol Biol* 311: 3-15.

Kaneko, A., O. Kaneko, et al. (1997). "High frequencies of CYP2C19 mutations and poor metabolism of proguanil in Vanuatu." *Lancet* 349(9056): 921-922.

Kelly, R. P., S. L. Close, et al. (2011). "Pharmacokinetics and Pharmacodynamics Following Maintenance Doses of Prasugrel and Clopidogrel in Chinese Carriers of CYP2C19 Variants." *Br J Clin Pharmacol.*

Kesavan, R., S. K. Narayan, et al. (2010). "Influence of CYP2C9 and CYP2C19 genetic polymorphisms on phenytoin-induced neurological toxicity in Indian epileptic patients." *Eur J Clin Pharmacol* 66(7): 689-696.

Kidd, R. S., A. B. Straughn, et al. (1999). "Pharmacokinetics of chlorpheniramine, phenytoin, glipizide and nifedipine in an individual homozygous for the CYP2C9*3 allele." *Pharmacogenetics* 9(1): 71-80.

Kirchheiner, J., J. T. Keulen, et al. (2008). "Effects of the CYP2D6 gene duplication on the pharmacokinetics and pharmacodynamics of tramadol." *J Clin Psychopharmacol* 28(1): 78-83.

Klotz, U. (2006). "Clinical impact of CYP2C19 polymorphism on the action of proton pump inhibitors: a review of a special problem." *Int J Clin Pharmacol Ther* 44(7): 297-302.

Kong, S. Y., H. S. Lim, et al. (2009). "Association of CYP2A6 polymorphisms with S-1 plus docetaxel therapy outcomes in metastatic gastric cancer." *Pharmacogenomics* 10(7): 1147-1155.

Krynetski, E. & W. E. Evans (2003). "Drug methylation in cancer therapy: lessons from the TPMT polymorphism." *Oncogene* 22(47): 7403-7413.

Krynetski, E. Y., H. L. Tai, et al. (1996). "Genetic polymorphism of thiopurine S-methyltransferase: clinical importance and molecular mechanisms." *Pharmacogenetics* 6(4): 279-290.

Kuznetsov, I. B., M. McDuffie, et al. (2009). "A web server for inferring the human N-acetyltransferase-2 (NAT2) enzymatic phenotype from NAT2 genotype." *Bioinformatics* 25(9): 1185-1186.

Leey, J.A., McCabe, S., et al. (2009). "Cost-effectiveness of genotype-guided warfarin therapy for anticoagulation in elderly patients with atrial fibrillation." *Am J Geriatr Pharmacother* 7(4): 197-203.

Lohoff, F. W. & T. N. Ferraro (2010). "Pharmacogenetic considerations in the treatment of psychiatric disorders." *Expert Opin Pharmacother* 11(3): 423-439.

Ma, Y., W. Ni, et al. (2011). "Association of genetic polymorphisms of CYP 2C19 with hypertension in a Chinese Han population." *Blood Press* 20(3): 166-170.

Maggo, S. D., M. A. Kennedy, et al. (2011). "Clinical implications of pharmacogenetic variation on the effects of statins." *Drug Saf* 34(1): 1-19.

Magno, L. A., J. Talbot, et al. (2009). "Glutathione s-transferase variants in a brazilian population." *Pharmacology* 83(4): 231-236.

Mahgoub, A., J. R. Idle, et al. (1977). "Polymorphic hydroxylation of Debrisoquine in man." *Lancet* 2(8038): 584-586.

Malaiyandi, V., C. Lerman, et al. (2006). "Impact of CYP2A6 genotype on pretreatment smoking behaviour and nicotine levels from and usage of nicotine replacement therapy." *Mol Psychiatry* 11(4): 400-409.

McLeod, H. L., E. Y. Krynetski, et al. (2000). "Genetic polymorphism of thiopurine methyltransferase and its clinical relevance for childhood acute lymphoblastic leukemia." *Leukemia* 14(4): 567-572.

Mega, J. L., S. L. Close, et al. (2009). "Cytochrome p-450 polymorphisms and response to clopidogrel." *N Engl J Med* 360(4): 354-362.

Mega, J. L., T. Simon, et al. (2010). "Reduced-function CYP2C19 genotype and risk of adverse clinical outcomes among patients treated with clopidogrel predominantly for PCI: a meta-analysis." *JAMA* 304(16): 1821-1830.

Meckley, L.M., Gudgeon, J.M., et al. (2010). "A policy model to evaluate the benefits, risks and costs of warfarin pharmacogenomic testing." *Pharmacoeconomics* 28(1): 61-74.

Motulsky, A. G. (1957). "Drug reactions enzymes, and biochemical genetics." *J Am Med Assoc* 165(7): 835-837.

Nair, S. R. (2010). "Personalized medicine: Striding from genes to medicines." *Perspect Clin Res* 1(4): 146-150.

Nebert, D.W. (1999). "Pharmacogenetics and pharmacogenomics: why is this relevant to the clinical geneticist?" *Clin Genet* 56: 247-258.

Ninomiya, H., K. Mamiya, et al. (2000). "Genetic polymorphism of the CYP2C subfamily and excessive serum phenytoin concentration with central nervous system intoxication." *Ther Drug Monit* 22(2): 230-232.

Orphanides, G. & I. Kimber (2003). "Toxicogenetics: applications and opportunities." *Toxicol Sci* 75(1): 1-6.

Ozaki, S., T. Oyama, et al. (2006). "Smoking cessation program and CYP2A6 polymorphism." *Front Biosci* 11: 2590-2597.

Padol, S., Y. Yuan, et al. (2006). "The effect of CYP2C19 polymorphisms on H. pylori eradication rate in dual and triple first-line PPI therapies: a meta-analysis." *Am J Gastroenterol* 101(7): 1467-1475.

Paiva, L., A. Hernandez, et al. (2010). "Association between GSTO2 polymorphism and the urinary arsenic profile in copper industry workers." *Environ Res* 110(5): 463-468.

Payne, K., Shabaruddin, F.H. (2010). "Cost-effectiveness analysis in pharmacogenomics." *Pharmacogenomics* 11(5): 643-6.

Parra, F. C., R. C. Amado, et al. (2003). "Color and genomic ancestry in Brazilians." *Proc Natl Acad Sci U S A* 100(1): 177-182.

Patowary, S. (2005). "Pharmacogenomics - therapeutic and ethical issues." *Kathmandu Univ Med J (KUMJ)* 3(4): 428-430.

Pena, S. D., G. Di Pietro, et al. (2011). "The genomic ancestry of individuals from different geographical regions of Brazil is more uniform than expected." *PLoS One* 6(2): e17063.

Penas-Lledo, E. M., P. Dorado, et al. (2011). "High risk of lifetime history of suicide attempts among CYP2D6 ultrarapid metabolizers with eating disorders." *Mol Psychiatry* 16(7): 691-692.

Perlis, R.H., Patrick, A. (2009). "When is pharmacogenetic testing for antidepressant response ready for the clinic? A cost-effectiveness analysis based on data from the STAR*D study." *Neuropsychopharmacology* 34(10): 2227-36.

Peterson-Iyer, K. (2008). "Pharmacogenomics, ethics, and public policy." *Kennedy Inst Ethics J* 18(1): 35-56.

Poulsen, L., L. Arendt-Nielsen, et al. (1996). "The hypoalgesic effect of tramadol in relation to CYP2D6." *Clin Pharmacol Ther* 60(6): 636-644.

Price-Evans, D. A. (1962). "Pharmacogenetics." *Acta Genet Med Gemellol (Roma)* 11: 338-350.

Ribaudo, H. J., H. Liu, et al. (2010). "Effect of CYP2B6, ABCB1, and CYP3A5 polymorphisms on efavirenz pharmacokinetics and treatment response: an AIDS Clinical Trials Group study." *J Infect Dis* 202(5): 717-722.

Rihs, H. P., B. Pesch, et al. (2005). "Occupational exposure to polycyclic aromatic hydrocarbons in German industries: association between exogenous exposure and urinary metabolites and its modulation by enzyme polymorphisms." *Toxicol Lett* 157(3): 241-255.

Robertson, J. A., B. Brody, et al. (2002). "Pharmacogenetic challenges for the health care system." *Health Aff (Millwood)* 21(4): 155-167.

Rodriguez-Novoa, S., P. Barreiro, et al. (2005). "Influence of 516G>T polymorphisms at the gene encoding the CYP450-2B6 isoenzyme on efavirenz plasma concentrations in HIV-infected subjects." *Clin Infect Dis* 40(9): 1358-1361.

Sabbagh, A. & P. Darlu (2005). "Inferring haplotypes at the NAT2 locus: the computational approach." *BMC Genet* 6: 30.

Saitoh, A., E. Capparelli, et al. (2010). "CYP2C19 genetic variants affect nelfinavir pharmacokinetics and virologic response in HIV-1-infected children receiving highly active antiretroviral therapy." *J Acquir Immune Defic Syndr* 54(3): 285-289.

Sangkuhl, K., D. S. Berlin, et al. (2008). "PharmGKB: understanding the effects of individual genetic variants." *Drug Metab Rev* 40(4): 539-551.

Sapienza, D., A. Asmundo, et al. (2007). "[Genetic polymorphisms (GSTT1 e GSTM1) and urinary excretion of t,t-muconic acid among refinery workers]." *G Ital Med Lav Ergon* 29(3 Suppl): 541-542.

Sawin, P. B. & D. Glick (1943). "Atropinesterase, a Genetically Determined Enzyme in the Rabbit." *Proc Natl Acad Sci U S A* 29(2): 55-59.

Scheet, P. & M. Stephens (2006). "A fast and flexible statistical model for large-scale population genotype data: applications to inferring missing genotypes and haplotypic phase." *Am J Hum Genet* 78(4): 629-644.

Sheng, Y. C., K. Wang, et al. (2010). "Effect of CYP2C19 genotypes on the pharmacokinetic/pharmacodynamic relationship of rabeprazole after a single oral dose in healthy Chinese volunteers." *Eur J Clin Pharmacol* 66(11): 1165-1169.

Snyder, L.H. (1932). "Studies in human inheritance IX. The inheritance of taste deficiency in man." Ohio J Sci 32: 436-468.

Slatkin, M. (2008). "Linkage disequilibrium--understanding the evolutionary past and mapping the medical future." *Nat Rev Genet* 9(6): 477-85.

Sillon, G., Y. Joly, et al. (2008). "An ethical and legal overview of pharmacogenomics: perspectives and issues." *Med Law* 27(4): 843-857.

Stamer, U. M., K. Lehnen, et al. (2003). "Impact of CYP2D6 genotype on postoperative tramadol analgesia." *Pain* 105(1-2): 231-238.

Stamer, U. M. & F. Stuber (2007). "Codeine and tramadol analgesic efficacy and respiratory effects are influenced by CYP2D6 genotype." *Anaesthesia* 62(12): 1294-1295; author reply 1295-1296.

Stanulla, M., E. Schaeffeler, et al. (2005). "Thiopurine methyltransferase (TPMT) genotype and early treatment response to mercaptopurine in childhood acute lymphoblastic leukemia." *JAMA* 293(12): 1485-1489.

Stephens, M. & P. Donnelly (2003). "A comparison of bayesian methods for haplotype reconstruction from population genotype data." *Am J Hum Genet* 73(5): 1162-1169.

Sultana, R. & D. A. Butterfield (2004). "Oxidatively modified GST and MRP1 in Alzheimer's disease brain: implications for accumulation of reactive lipid peroxidation products." *Neurochem Res* 29(12): 2215-2220.

Swierkot, J. & R. Slezak (2011). "[The importance of pharmacogenetic tests in evaluation of the effectiveness of methotrexate treatment in rheumatoid arthritis (part 1)]." *Postepy Hig Med Dosw (Online)* 65: 195-206.

Takahashi, H., G. R. Wilkinson, et al. (2006). "Different contributions of polymorphisms in VKORC1 and CYP2C9 to intra- and inter-population differences in maintenance dose of warfarin in Japanese, Caucasians and African-Americans." *Pharmacogenet Genomics* 16(2): 101-110.

Talbot, J., L. A. Magno, et al. (2010). "Interethnic diversity of NAT2 polymorphisms in Brazilian admixed populations." *BMC Genet* 11: 87.

Tan, B., Y. F. Zhang, et al. (2010). "The effects of CYP2C9 and CYP2C19 genetic polymorphisms on the pharmacokinetics and pharmacodynamics of glipizide in Chinese subjects." *Eur J Clin Pharmacol* 66(2): 145-151.

Tang, C., J. H. Lin, et al. (2005). "Metabolism-based drug-drug interactions: what determines individual variability in cytochrome P450 induction?" *Drug Metab Dispos* 33(5): 603-613.

Tanigawara, Y., N. Aoyama, et al. (1999). "CYP2C19 genotype-related efficacy of omeprazole for the treatment of infection caused by Helicobacter pylori." *Clin Pharmacol Ther* 66(5): 528-534.

ter Heine, R., H. J. Scherpbier, et al. (2008). "A pharmacokinetic and pharmacogenetic study of efavirenz in children: dosing guidelines can result in subtherapeutic concentrations." *Antivir Ther* 13(6): 779-787.

Ure, A. (1841). "On gouty concretions, with a new method of treatment." *Med Chir Trans* 24: 30-35.

Vaalburg, W., N. H. Hendrikse, et al. (2005). "P-glycoprotein activity and biological response." *Toxicol Appl Pharmacol* 207(2 Suppl): 257-260.

van der Weide, J., L. S. Steijns, et al. (2001). "The effect of genetic polymorphism of cytochrome P450 CYP2C9 on phenytoin dose requirement." *Pharmacogenetics* 11(4): 287-291.

Vatsis, K. P., W. W. Weber, et al. (1995). "Nomenclature for N-acetyltransferases." *Pharmacogenetics* 5(1): 1-17.

Vegter, S., Perna, A., et al. (2009). "Cost-effectiveness of ACE inhibitor therapy to prevent dialysis in nondiabetic nephropathy: influence of the ACE insertion/deletion polymorphism." *Pharmacogenet Genomics* 19(9): 695-703.

Verhoef, T.I., Redekop, W.K., et al. (2010). "A systematic review of cost-effectiveness analyses of pharmacogenetic-guided dosing in treatment with coumarin derivatives." *Pharmacogenomics* 11(7): 989-1002.

Vetti, H. H., A. Molven, et al. (2010). "Is pharmacogenetic CYP2D6 testing useful?" *Tidsskr Nor Laegeforen* 130(22): 2224-2228.

Vogel, F. (1959). "Moderne problem der humangenetik." Ergeb Inn Med U Kinderheilk 12: 52-125.

Weijer, C. & P. B. Miller (2004). "Protecting communities in pharmacogenetic and pharmacogenomic research." *Pharmacogenomics J* 4(1): 9-16.

Williams-Jones, B. & O. P. Corrigan (2003). "Rhetoric and hype: where's the 'ethics' in pharmacogenomics?" *Am J Pharmacogenomics* 3(6): 375-383.

Wu, T. Y., M. H. Jen, et al. (2010). "Ten-year trends in hospital admissions for adverse drug reactions in England 1999-2009." *J R Soc Med* 103(6): 239-250.

Xu, C. F., K. Lewis, et al. (2002). "Effectiveness of computational methods in haplotype prediction." *Hum Genet* 110(2): 148-156.

Yang, J. C. & C. J. Lin (2010). "CYP2C19 genotypes in the pharmacokinetics/ pharmacodynamics of proton pump inhibitor-based therapy of Helicobacter pylori infection." *Expert Opin Drug Metab Toxicol* 6(1): 29-41.

You, J.H. (2011). "Pharmacoeconomic evaluation of warfarin pharmacogenomics." *Expert Opin Pharmacother* 12(3): 435-41.

Zang, Y., M. A. Doll, et al. (2007). "Functional characterization of single-nucleotide polymorphisms and haplotypes of human N-acetyltransferase 2." *Carcinogenesis* 28(8): 1665-1671.

Zhang, J.P., Malhotra, A.K. (2011). "Pharmacogenetics and antipsychotics: therapeutic efficacy and side effects prediction." *Expert Opin Drug Metab Toxicol.* 7(1): 9-37.

Zhao, F., J. Wang, et al. (2008). "Effect of CYP2C19 genetic polymorphisms on the efficacy of proton pump inhibitor-based triple therapy for Helicobacter pylori eradication: a meta-analysis." *Helicobacter* 13(6): 532-541.

Zwisler, S. T., T. P. Enggaard, et al. (2009). "The hypoalgesic effect of oxycodone in human experimental pain models in relation to the CYP2D6 oxidation polymorphism." *Basic Clin Pharmacol Toxicol* 104(4): 335-344.

2

Oral Absorption, Intestinal Metabolism and Human Oral Bioavailability

Ayman El-Kattan and Manthena Varma
*Pharmacokinetics, Dynamics and Metabolism Department, Pfizer Inc.,
USA*

1. Introduction

Most of the drugs that are available in the marketplace are administered via the oral route, which is a convenient and cost effective route of administration (Lipinski 1995; Lipinski 2000; Lipinski et al. 2001; Lipinski 2004; Abrahamsson and Lennernas 2005). Thus, oral bioavailability is one of the key considerations for discovery and development of a new chemical entity (NCE). It is well recognized that poor oral bioavailability is one of the major causes of therapeutic variability, associated with the variable drug exposure (Beierle et al. 1999; Bardelmeijer et al. 2000; Katsura and Inui 2003). This is particularly important for drugs with narrow therapeutic window or potential for resistance development such as antibiotics and cytotoxic drugs (Bardelmeijer et al. 2000). Hellriegel *et al.* reported a significant inverse relationship between the oral bioavailability of drugs from several therapeutic classes and the coefficient of inter-individual variability in their oral bioavailability (Hellriegel et al. 1996).

Oral bioavailability is a product of fraction absorbed, fraction escaping gut-wall elimination, and fraction escaping hepatic elimination; and the factors that influence bioavailability can be divided into physiological, physicochemical, and biopharmaceutical factors. It has been well established that physicochemical properties determine oral absorption and drug metabolism. The "rule-of-five" devised by Lipinski and co-workers provided an important advance, with analysis of a large data set showing that compounds within certain physicochemical space tended to be more successful in clinical development than others. Using a dataset of 309 drugs, Varma *et al.* studied the interrelation of physicochemical properties and the individual parameters of oral absorption to define the physicochemical space for optimum human oral bioavailability (Varma et al. 2010). This analysis, which may provide a rational judgment on the physicochemical space to optimize oral bioavailability, will be discussed. Furthermore, the solubility and permeability as the fundamental properties of oral absorption will be discussed in-line with biopharmaceutics classification system. Uptake and efflux transporters are implicated as facilitating or limiting intestinal absorption. This book chapter will touch up on the latest findings on several chemistry approaches that has be directed to target the uptake transporters and circumvent the efflux transporters. Overall, this chapter will provides a better understanding of the interplay between gastrointestinal tract physiology/anatomy and drug physicochemical /biopharmaceutical factors in the absorption and metabolism mechanisms that affect oral bioavailability humans; and enable a rational approach to design NCE with better absorption in humans.

2. Concepts and theoretical calculations of oral bioavailability

Bioavailability (F) is the extent to which an active moiety is absorbed from a pharmaceutical dosage form and becomes available in the systemic circulation (Thomas et al. 2006). Bioavailability is usually determined by calculating the respective plasma drug exposure assessed as the total area under the drug plasma concentration versus time curve (AUC) after oral and intravenous administration as:

$$\text{Absolute Bioavailability } = \frac{AUC_{oral}}{AUC_{IV}} \times \frac{Dose_{IV}}{Dose_{oral}} \tag{1}$$

In general, determinants of oral drug bioavailability include fraction of dose absorbed in the gastrointestinal tract (GIT) and fraction of dose that escapes elimination by the intestinal tract, liver, and lung. Thus, oral bioavailability can be defined mathematically by the following equation:

$$F = F_{abs} \cdot F_g \cdot F_h \tag{2}$$

Where F_{abs} is the fraction of the dose that is absorbed from the intestinal lumen to the intestinal enterocytes; F_g is the fraction of the dose that escapes pre-systemic intestinal first pass elimination; and F_h is the fraction of the dose that passes through the liver and escapes pre-systemic liver first-pass elimination. The fraction of the dose that escapes first-pass elimination across the intestine (F_g) and liver (F_h) can be estimated experimentally via the comparison of systemic exposures (AUC ratios) where the dosing routes are selected to isolate the contribution by a particular organ.

F_g can be estimated (Eq. 3) for a compound when doses are given orally and via a cannulated hepatic portal vein (h.p.v.) with the fraction absorbed (F_{abs}) either assumed to be complete or is known.

$$F_{abs} \cdot F_g = \frac{AUC_{oral}}{AUC_{h.p.v.}} \times \frac{Dose_{h.p.v}}{Dose_{oral}} \tag{3}$$

Similarly, F_h can be estimated for a compound when doses are given via a cannulated hepatic portal vein and intravenously (Eq. 4).

$$F_h = \frac{AUC_{h.p.v.}}{AUC_{i.v.}} \times \frac{Dose_{i.v}}{Dose_{h.p.v.}} \tag{4}$$

The details on scientific background and factors that influence F_h are outside the scope of this book chapter; interested readers are encouraged to refer to our recent reviews in these areas (Thomas et al. 2006; Hurst et al. 2007; Varma et al. 2010) and other chapters in this book that focus on metabolism and related topics such as induction and inhibition of drug metabolism, pharmacogenetics and metabolism: past, present and future, and effect of pharmaceutical excipients on drug metabolism.

3. Mechanism of oral absorption

Following oral dosing, drug molecules can cross the luminal membrane through various mechanisms that involve passive diffusion or active transport. Passive diffusion is comprised of two pathways: the paracellular pathway, in which drug diffuses through the aqueous pores at the tight junctions between the intestinal enterocytes; and the transcellular (lipophilic) pathway, which requires drug diffusion across the lipid cell membrane of the enterocyte. The active transport pathway is mediated by transporters and is divided into active drug influx and efflux. It is important to note that the relevance of each route is determined by the compound's physicochemical properties and its potential affinity for various transport proteins (Thomas et al. 2006; Hurst et al. 2007; Varma et al. 2010; Varma et al. 2010).

3.1 Passive diffusion

In paracellular diffusion, drug molecules are absorbed by diffusion and convective volume flow through the water-filled intercellular space (Lennernas 1995). In general, drugs that are absorbed through this pathway are small molecules (e.g., molecular weight [MW] < 250 g/mol) and hydrophilic in nature (Log P < 0). Because the junctional complex has a net negative charge, positively charged molecules pass through more readily, whereas negatively charged molecules are repelled (Karlsson et al. 1999). Furthermore, the paracellular pathway offers a limited window for absorption since it accounts for < 0.01% of the total surface area of intestinal membrane. In addition, the tight junctions between cells become tighter traveling from the jejunum towards the colon.

The transcellular pathway is the major route of absorption for most of drug molecules. In general, the rate of passive transcellular permeability is mainly determined by the rate of transport across the apical cell membrane, which is controlled by the physicochemical properties of the absorbed compound. Unlike the paracellular pathway, compounds that are absorbed through the transcellular pathway are unionised, with lipophilicity of Log P > 0 and MW > 300 g/mole. In addition, the hydrogen-bonding capacity determined by the number of hydrogen bond donors and hydrogen bond acceptors is < 10 and 5, respectively (Lipinski 1995; Lipinski 2000; Avdeef 2001).

3.2 Active transport

Enterocytes express several transporters, belonging to the adenosine triphosphate (ATP) binding cassette (ABC) superfamily and the solute carrier (SLC) superfamilies, on the apical and basolateral membranes for the influx or efflux of endogenous substances and xenobiotics (Table 1). Although a variety of transporters are expressed in the enterocytes, only a few are known to play a key role in the intestinal absorption of drugs. ABC transporters utilize ATP to drive the transport and are called primary active transporter. However, SLC transporters majorly use the ion gradients (H+, Na+ and Ca++ gradients) created across the membrane by primary active carriers (Na+/K+-ATPase, Na+/H+-ATPase) (Tsuji and Tamai 1996). ABC transporters expressed in the intestine include P-glycoprotein (P-gp; *ABCB1*), breast cancer resistance protein (BCRP; *ABCG2*), multidrug resistance proteins (MRP1-6; *ABCC1-6*). P-gp, BCRP, MRP2 and MRP4 are localized on brush-border (apical) membrane while certain MRPs are expressed on the basolateral membrane of the enterocytes. These efflux transporters functionally limit the enterocytic levels of their substrates by reducing uptake and facilitating efflux. SLC transporters suggested as relevant at the intestinal apical surface of epithelial cells include, peptide transporter (PepT1; *SLC15A1*), organic anion polypeptide transporters (OATP1A2, *SLCO1A2*; OATP2B1,*SLCO2B1*), monocarboxylate transporters (MCT1; *SLC16A1*), sodium-multivitamin transport (SMVT; *SLC5A6*) and organic cation/zwitterion transporters (OCTN1, *SLC22A4*; OCTN2, *SLC22A5*). Several other SLC transporters including organic anion or cation transporters (OATs or OCTs; *SLC22*) have also been identified in the intestine, but seem to be of less importance in oral drug absorption (Englund et al. 2006; Seithel et al. 2006).

Transporter protein	Gene	Orientation	Drug Substrates
P-gp/MDR1	ABCB1	Apical efflux	Actinomycin D, cerivastatin, colchicine, cyclosporine A, daunorubicin, digoxin, docetaxel, doxorubicin, erythromycin, etoposide, fexofenadine, imatinib, indinavir, irinotecan, ivermectin, lapatinib, loperamide, losartan, nelfinavir, oseltamivir, paclitaxel, quinidine, ritonavir, saquinavir, sparfloxacin, tamoxifen, terfenadine, topotecan, verapamil, vinblastine, vincristine.
BCRP	ABCG2	Apical efflux	Abacavir, ciprofloxacin, dantrolene, dipyridamole, enrofloxacin, erlotinib, etoposide, furosemide, gefitinib, genistein, glyburide, grepafloxacin, hydrochlorothiazide, imatinib, irinotecan, lamivudine, lapatinib, methotrexate, mitoxantrone, prazosin, rosuvastatin, tamoxifen, triamterene, zidovudine.
MRP1	ABCC1	Basolateral efflux	Daunorubicin, doxorubicin, epirubicin, grepafloxacin, methotrexate, vincristine.
MRP2	ABCC2	Apical efflux	Indinavir, methotrexate, ritonavir, saquinavir, vinblastine.
MRP3	ABCC3	Basolateral efflux	Etoposide, methotrexate.
MRP4	ABCC4	Apical efflux	Ceftizoxime, topotecan.
PepT1	SLC15A1	Apical uptake	Ampicillin, bestatin, captoril, cephalexin, enalapril, fosinopril, oseltamivir, valciclovir.
OATP 1A2	SLCO1A2	Apical uptake	Fexofenadine, levofloxacin, methotrexate, ouabain, rosuvastatin, saquinavir.

Transporter protein	Gene	Orientation	Drug Substrates
OATP 2B1	SLCO2B1	Apical uptake	Atorvastatin, bosentan, fluvastatin, glyburide, pitavastatin, pravastatin, montelukast, rosuvastatin.
MCT1	SLC16A1	Apical uptake	Arbaclofen placarbil, carindacillin, gabapentin enacarbil, ketoprofen, naproxen, phenethicillin, propicillin.
SMVT	SLC5A6	Apical uptake	Gabapentin enacarbil
OCTN1	SLC22A4	Apical uptake	Quinidine, verapamil.
OCTN2	SLC22A5	Apical uptake	Cephaloridine, imatinib, ipratropium, tiotropium, quinidine, verapamil.
CNT1	SLC28A1	Apical uptake	Cytarabine, gemcitabine, zidovudine.
CNT2	SLC28A2	Apical uptake	Clofarabine, fluorouridine, ribavirin.
ENT1	SLC29A1	Basolateral efflux	Cladribine, clofarabine, cytarabine, gemcitabine, ribavirin.
ENT2	SLC29A2	Basolateral efflux	Clofarabine, gemcitabine, zidovudine.

Table 1. Major human intestinal efflux and uptake transorters involved in drug transport. Gene, transport orientation and the clinical drug substrates of each transporter is included (Polli et al. 2001; Mahar Doan et al. 2002; Murakami and Takano 2008; Giacomini et al. 2010; Klaassen and Aleksunes 2010).

4. Absorption kinetics

When an active uptake process is involved, the overall transport of a drug across the intestinal enterocytes can be defined by model incorporating saturable and nonsaturable components (Eq. 5).

$$J = \frac{J_{max,inf} \cdot C}{K_{m,inf} + C} + K_D C \qquad (5)$$

As outlined in the equation above, the total flux (J) of a compound across intestinal membrane is determined by four variables: J_{max}, which is the maximal uptake rate, K_m, which is the transporter substrate binding affinity, K_D, which is the kinetic constant for nonsaturable transport, and C, which is the luminal drug concentration. The impact of intestinal transporters on the overall absorption of drug across the intestine is determined by the percentage component of the active process ($J_{max}C/(K_m+C)$) to the total flux, J, of the drug molecule. In general hydrophilic drug have low K_D values and therefore there transport rates are mainly driven by the transporter activity, while for lipophilic drugs the passive component is usually high and the role of transporters is expected to be minimal.

5. Physiological, physicochemical and biopharmaceutical factors that impact oral drug absorption

The factors that alter the rate and extent of oral drug absorption can be divided into three main categories: physiological, physicochemical and biopharmaceutical factors (Sabnis 1999; Horter and Dressman 2001; Kramer and Wunderli-Allenspach 2001; Zhou 2003; Pouton 2006).

5.1 Physiological factors that impact oral drug absorption

5.1.1 Gastro-intestine anatomy and physiology

In humans, the GIT consists mainly of the stomach, small intestine (the duodenum, jejunum, and ileum) and large intestine (cecum, colon and rectum). The total length of the human GIT is 8.35 m and the relative size of the human small intestine, which is considered the primary site of drug absorption, to the total length of the GI tract is 81%. As for the large intestine, its relative size in humans is 19%. It may also be pointed out that the cecum, which is the major site of microbial digestion, forms only 5% of the length of the human large intestine (DeSesso and Jacobson 2001).

The surface area is attributed to the fact that the human small intestine has three anatomical modifications that significantly increase the surface area of the human small intestine (Shargel and Yu 1999). The human small intestine has grossly observable folds of mucosa (plicae circularis or folds of kerckring) that increase the surface area threefold. From the plicae circularis, microscopic finger-like pieces of tissue called villi project, which increase the surface area by 10-fold for humans. Each villus is covered in microvilli, which increase the surface area by 20-fold. Unlike the small intestine, the large intestine surface area does not have villi and is divided into geographical areas by transverse furrows. In addition, the large intestine enterocytes differ slightly from that of the small intestine and its microvilli are less packed (Kararli 1995). Overall, this significantly contributes to the smaller surface area of the large intestine in humans and is consistent with the fact that small intestine is the major site of drug absorption in humans.

5.1.2 Unstirred water layer

Adjacent to the intestinal membrane is an unstirred water layer, which is a potential barrier for the absorption of various drug molecules across the intestinal membrane (Winne 1976; Hayton 1980). The thickness of this layer in humans is only 25 µm (Strocchi et al. 1996). Chiou et al. quantitatively studied the impact of the unstirred water layer adjacent to the intestinal membrane on the rate and extent of absorption of passively absorbed drugs with different membrane absorption half-lives (10 – 300 min) in humans (Chiou 1994). Results of this analysis suggested that the presence of the unstirred water layer is generally expected to have a relatively mild or insignificant effect on the rate of absorption and an insignificant effect on the extent of absorption (Kimura and Higaki 2002).

5.1.3 Gastrointestinal transit times

The absorption rate of a drug molecule is generally a function of drug absorption through the GIT, which is determined by the residence time and absorption in each GIT segment

(Kimura and Higaki 2002). In general, gastric transit time impacts the systemic exposure of rapidly dissolved and well absorbed drugs. However, intestinal transit time influences the absorption of drugs with limited mucosal permeability, carrier mediated uptake, drugs subject to intestinal degradation, or products whose dissolution is the rate limiting step for systemic absorption (Martinez and Amidon 2002). In contrast to gastric transit time, intestinal transit time is independent of the feeding conditions and the physical composition of the intestinal contents (Garanero et al. 2005) . The human intestinal transit time is ~3 – 4 h (DeSesso and Jacobson 2001; Kimura and Higaki 2002). Several studies suggested that in human small intestine, there is a gradient of velocity where the small intestinal transit in the proximal intestine was faster compared with the distal intestine. The transit time in human large intestine can vary in the range of 8 – 72 h (DeSesso and Jacobson 2001).

5.1.4 The GIT pH

The extent of ionization plays a pivotal role in determining the drug dissolution rate and passive permeability across the GIT. Therefore, it becomes clear that the pH at the absorption site is a critical factor in facilitating or inhibiting the dissolution and absorption of various ionizable drug molecules (DeSesso and Jacobson 2001). It should be stressed that the pH of the luminal content (chyme) is altered by the luminal secretions. The pH of chyme is acidic and can be as low as 2.3. When the chyme arrives in the duodenum, it is quickly neutralized by the secretion of the pancreatic bicarbonate and bile. The pH values of chyme become progressively more alkaline in the distal portion of the small intestine in humans. However, the pH of chyme in the large intestine is generally more acidic than the pH observed in the small intestine in humans, possibly due to the fermentation mediated by the microbial flora (Kararli 1995).

5.1.5 Bile fluid

Bile is produced by hepatocytes and drained through the many bile ducts that penetrate the liver (DeSesso and Jacobson 2001). During this process, the epithelial cells add a watery solution that is rich in bicarbonates which increases the alkalinity of the solution. In humans, the bile is stored and concentrated up to five times its original potency in the gall bladder. It is to be noted that the human gall bladder secrets bile at a rate of 2 – 22 ml/kg/day. In humans, bile acts as a detergent to emulsify fats by increasing the surface area to help enzyme action, and thus aid in their absorption in the small intestine. In addition to bicarbonate solution, bile is composed of bile salts, such as the salts of taurocholic acid and deoxycholic acid, which are combined with phospholipids to break down fat globules in the process of emulsification by associating their hydrophobic side with lipids and the hydrophilic side with water. Emulsified droplets are then organized into many micelles which increases their absorption. Because bile increases the absorption of fats, it also plays a pivotal role in the absorption of the fat-soluble vitamins and steroids (Hanano 1993; Kirilenko and Gregoriadis 1993).

5.1.6 Bacterial microflora

In humans, bacterial microflora exists in most of the GIT and become an important component of the luminal content. However, there is no bacterial microflora in the stomach and upper small intestine. This is mainly attributed to the low pH of the human gastric content. However, a large number of bacterial microflora populates the human's distal small and large intestines (Cummings and Macfarlane 1997). These bacterial microflora play a role in the metabolism of various chemicals and xenobiotics through hydrolysis, dehydroxylation, deamidation, decarboxylation and reduction of azide groups (Lichtenstein 1990; Cummings and Macfarlane 1997; Blaut et al. 2003). Among these reactions, hydrolysis of the glucuronide conjugates is the most important metabolic reaction that is mediated by the glucronidase enzyme and produced by the bacterial microflora found in the GIT of humans.

5.1.7 Lymphatic absorption

The intestinal lymphatic route plays a key role in the absorption of drugs that are highly lipophilic. It has many advantages, such as increase in the oral bioavailability of highly lipophilic drugs by avoiding hepatic first pass effect, direct targeting of lymphoid tissue, indirect targeting of specific sites associated with low-density lipoprotein receptors, and alteration in the rate of oral drug input to the systemic circulation thereby providing opportunity for controlled release drug formulation (Cheema et al. 1987; Trevaskis et al. 2005; Trevaskis et al. 2006; Trevaskis et al. 2006).

5.1.8 Intestinal drug transporters

P-glycoprotein (P-gp)

P-gp (MDR1; *ABCB1*), an ATP-dependent transmembrane efflux pump belonging to ABC superfamily, shows affinity to a wide variety of structurally unrelated compounds (Juliano and Ling 1976). It is expressed as a 1280 amino acid long (MW ~170 kDa) single chain glycoprotein with two homologous portions of equal length, each containing six transmembrane (TM) domains and two ATP binding regions separated by a flexible linker polypeptide region (Schinkel et al. 1993; Ambudkar et al. 1999).

Immunohistochemical analysis using monoclonal antibody provided evidence for localization of P-gp in a wide range of tissues, particularly in columnar epithelial cells of the lower GIT, capillary endothelial cells of brain and testis, canalicular surface of hepatocytes and apical surface of proximal tubule in kidney (Thiebut et al. 1987). Due to selective distribution at the port of drug entry and exit, P-gp has been speculated to play a major physiological role in the absorption, distribution and excretion of xenobiotics and endogenous substrates. Overall, P-gp functions as a biochemical barrier for entry of drugs across intestine and brain, as well as a vacuum cleaner to expel drugs from the intestine, liver, kidney, etc. A number of clinically important drugs are P-gp substrates (Table 1), which are as diverse as anthracyclines (doxorubicin, daunorubicin), alkaloids (reserpine, vincristine, vinblastine), specific peptides (valinomycin, cyclosporine), steroid hormones (aldosterone, hydrocortisone) and local anesthetics (dibucaine) (Polli et al. 2001; Mahar Doan et al. 2002; Varma et al. 2003; Takano et al. 2006). P-gp substrates, digoxin and talinolol, show pharmacokinetic changes in human upon coadministration with P-gp inhibitors (Gramatte et al. 1996; Fenner et al. 2009). Greiner *et al.*, studied the effect of rifampicin pretreatment on the oral pharmacokinetics of digoxin and suggested that rifampicn induced duodenal P-gp expression and thus significantly reduced AUC of digoxin (Greiner et al. 1999). Similarly, rifampicn decreased talinolol oral exposure, which is consistent with ~4 fold increase in duodenal P-gp expression (Westphal et al. 2000).

P-gp affinity screening using various *in vitro* culture models is now an integral part of drug discovery due to wide substrate specificity and clinical relevance in drug disposition and associated drug-drug interactions (DDIs) (Varma et al. 2004a). Tailoring of molecules to reduce substrate specificity to P-gp may help in improving the oral bioavailability of drugs. Seelig and coworkers suggested that the partitioning into the lipid membrane is the rate-limiting step for the interaction of a substrate with P-gp and that dissociation of the P-gp-substrate complex is determined by the number and strength of the hydrogen bonds formed between the substrate and the transporter (Seelig and Landwojtowicz 2000). Several studies have related the binding affinity (K_m) of P-gp for substrates and modulators to their lipid-water partition coefficient (Log P). Evidence suggests that a drug with high Log P will accumulate to a high concentration within the cytoplasmic membrane and favors binding to P-gp with low K_m value, while a drug with low partitioning will have a lower membrane concentration and a high K_m value. Three-dimensional structures of a large number of drugs revealed that the minimal common binding element consisting of two or three hydrogen bond acceptor (HBA) groups in a specific spatial distance. Since the TM sequences of P-gp are rich in hydrogen bond donor (HBD) groups, it is hypothesized that P-gp recognizes the HBA groups of the substrates through hydrogen bond formation in the lipid membrane environment (Seelig 1998; Seelig 1998). Didziapetris *et al.* studied 220 substrates and 1000 non-substrates and proposed the 'rule of four', which states that compounds with the HBA ≥ 8, a molecular weight (MW) > 400 g/mol and most acidic pK_a < 4 are likely to be P-gp substrates, while compounds with HBA ≤ 4, MW < 400 g/mol and most basic pK_a > 8 are not substrates to P-gp (Didziapetris et al. 2003). Although many such models describe the physicochemical attributes of P-gp interaction and are shown to have high predictability, existence of multiple binding sites and other complicating factors has prevented the development of a definitive SAR (Stouch and Gudmundsson 2002).

Breast Cancer Resistance Protein (BCRP)

BCRP (ABCP/MXR; *ABCG2*), a member of the ABC family of transporters, is considered a half-transporter with six TM domains and one ATP-binding domain at the amino terminus and is believed to homodimerize in order to function (Staud and Pavek 2005). It is composed of 655 amino acids with a MW of 72 kDa (Graf et al. 2003). An atomic model of BCRP was predicted by homology modeling based on the crystal structure of the bacterial multidrug exporter Sav1866, which suggested that BCRP had multiple drug binding sites (Hazai and Bikadi 2008; Muenster et al. 2008). BCRP expression can be traced to placenta, kidney, liver, testis, brain, mammary tissue, and intestine (Doyle and Ross 2003). Unlike P-gp, the expression of BCRP along the length of the small intestine does not vary significantly (Bruyere et al. 2010). Additionally, the mRNA level of BCRP is notably higher than other efflux transporters such as P-gp and MRP2 in the human intestine (Taipalensuu et al. 2001). Since BCRP is highly expressed on the apical membrane of enterocytes and effluxing substrates back into the lumen, it has been noted to play an important role as a detoxification efflux transporter and limiting drug absorption in the GIT (Zaher et al. 2006).

BCRP exhibits broad substrate specificity and accepts diverse chemical space, as do other ABC transporters. Substrates to BCRP include (Table 1): chemotherapy agents (mitoxantrone, camptothecins, tyrosine kinase inhibitors), antivirals (zidovudine, lamivudine), HMG-CoA reductase inhibitors (statins), benzimidazoles, and antibiotics (ciprofloxacin, rifampicin) (Bailey et al. ; Merino et al. 2005; Huang et al. 2006; Takano et al.

2006; Ando et al. 2007; Dauchy et al. 2009; Ieiri et al. 2009). Some of the BCRP substrates are also effectively effluxed by P-gp. For example, etoposide, irinotecan and tamoxifen are substrates for both BCRP and P-gp (Table 1). In a clinical study, Kruijtzer *et al.* showed an increase in bioavailability of topotecan from 40% to 97% in the presence of GF120918, a potent inhibitor of BCRP and P-gp (Kruijtzer et al. 2002). Yamasaki *et al.* investigated the impact of genetic polymorphisms of ABCG2 (421c>A) and NAT2 on the pharmacokinetics of sulfasalazine, in 37 healthy volunteers and suggested sulfasalazine as a useful probe substrate for evaluating the role of BCRP in the intestinal disposition (Yamasaki et al. 2008). BCRP polymorphism significantly affects the pharmacokinetics of several HMG-CoA reductase inhibitors, including atrovastatin, rosuvastatin, fluvastatin and simvastatin lactone, but has no significant effect on pravastatin or simvastatin acid (Bailey et al. ; Huang et al. 2006; Ieiri et al. 2009; Keskitalo et al. 2009; Keskitalo et al. 2009). For example, rosuvastatin AUC was 100% and 144% greater in the c.421AA genotype population than in those with c.421CA and the c.421CC genotypes, respectively. Although, few clinical studies have been reported on the role of BCRP in the intestinal absorption, several studies using BCRP knock-out mice suggest significant impact (Merino et al. 2006; Seamon et al. 2006; Zaher et al. 2006; Yamagata et al. 2007).

Due to general selectivity, substrates of BCRP can be either negatively or positively charged, hydrophobic or hydrophilic, and unconjugated or conjugated. Several attempts were made to establish SAR for BCRP interaction, however, many analysis methods were based on the datasets of inhibitors (Saito et al. 2006; Matsson et al. 2007; Matsson et al. 2009; Nicolle et al. 2009). Yoshikawa *et al.* studied BCRP substrate specificity of 14 camptothecin (CPT) analogues, and noted that CPT analogues that showed ATP-dependent transport in BCRP-overexpressing membrane vesicles possess one –hydroxy or –amino group (Yoshikawa et al. 2004). Also CPT analogues showed a good correlation between polarity and BCRP-association, where highly polar compounds showed substrate specificity. It is likely that the presence of hydroxyl and amino functional groups facilitate hydrogen bonding with the amino acid residues at the binding site of BCRP. Furthermore, presence of a negative electrostatic potential area at position 10 for SN-38 and SN-398, but not in SN-22, suggests that CPT analogues with this feature are potential substrates for BCRP (Nakagawa et al. 2006). BCRP substrate specificity of a set of pyrrolobenzodiazepine (PBD) derivatives showed a good correlation with the electrostatic potential and aromaticity (Kaliszczak et al. 2010). PBDs with a greater number of HBA and the electronegativity and aromaticity of the C2 substitution show affinity to BCRP. Evidently, BCRP-mediated efflux could be circumvented by limiting C2 aryl substituents and the number of aromatic rings. In general, BCRP substrates share a same set of molecular properties as that of substrates to P-gp and other efflux pumps (Begley 2004; Kunta and Sinko 2004; Takano et al. 2006).

Peptide transporter 1 (Pept1)

PepT1 (*SLC15A1*), an electrogenic, H^+-dependent transporter, was first cloned from the rabbit intestine and subsequently from both rat and human (Fei et al. 1994). The cloned human PepT1 cDNA sequence encodes a 708 amino acid protein (MW 79 kDa) with an isoelectric point of 8.6 and several putative glycosylation and phosphorylation sites. There are 12 putative α-helical TM domains and a large extracellular loop between the IX and X TM domains, which possess intacellularly localized N- and C- termini (Liang et al. 1995; Rubio-Aliaga and Daniel 2008). Herrera-Ruiz *et al.* reported that PepT1 appears to be localized predominantly in the duodenum, with decreasing expression in the jejunum and ileum (Herrera-Ruiz et al. 2001).

PepT1 has been shown to be independent of Na$^+$ and uses H$^+$-gradient and inside-negative membrane potential to provide the necessary driving force for substrate translocation. At the brush border membrane of enterocytes, an in-ward proton gradient is generated through the activity of an electroneutral proton/cation exchanger, Na$^+$/H$^+$ antiporter. This enables the uptake of PepT1 transporter substrates to be coupled with the influx of protons back into the enterocytes (Adibi 1997). The uptake of the PepT1 substrates is strongly dependent on the extracellular pH, where a pH of 4.5-6.5 (depending on the net charge of the substrate), is needed for optimal transport activity. Irie *et al.* investigated the transport mechanism of PepT1 for neutral and charged substrates by experimental studies and computational simulation (Irie et al. 2005). These uptake studies suggested that the K_m of glycylsarcosine (Gly-Sar), a neutral substrate, decreased as the pH dropped from 7.4 to 5.5, yet increased at a pH of 5.0. The K_m value of an anionic substrate, ceftibuten, declined steadily with a decreasing pH. Furthermore, the maximum transporter rate (V_{max}) values gradually increased with a fall in pH from 7.4 to 5.0, for both substrates. Consequently, the group hypothesized that unlike neutral and cationic substrates, negatively charged molecules not only require H$^+$ binding to H$^+$-binding site, but also to the substrate-binding site.

The 3D structure of the substrate binding site of PepT1 is not yet known, but its template has been proposed by the large variety of substrates (Foley et al. ; Meredith and Price 2006). It is interesting to note that the peptide bond is not required for substrate binding specificity of PepT1 transporter (Brandsch et al. 2004). Only the two oppositely charged free head groups (carboxylic carbon and amino nitrogen) separated by a 4 spacer carbon unit were identified as a minimal structural feature requirement (Doring et al. 1998). In the presence of a peptide bond, it is only the backbone carbonyl that is functional. This minimal configuration also explains the efficient transport of δ-aminolevulinic acid, which serves as a precursor for the endogenous porphyrin accumulation on which photodynamic therapy of tumors is based. In addition, the side chains provided in both di and tripeptides and in xenobiotics with charge polarity and conformation are pivotal in determining the binding affinities. It should also be emphasized that for the di and tripeptides, only the trans-configuration of the peptide bond is transported. Besides a preferred free N-terminal amino group, a high electron density around the terminal carboxylic group in dipeptide, or alternatively around the carbonyl group of the second amino acid in a tripeptide structure, is needed to ensure optimum binding affinity. Furthermore, high electron densities at the first and third side chains, as well as the presence of hydrophobic side chains, significantly contribute to overall binding affinity (Brandsch et al. 1999).

PepT1 is a low-affinity (K_m of 200 μM to 15 mM), high-capacity transporter and is known to play a pivotal role in the absorption and distribution of peptidomimetics that include β-lactam antibiotics such as cephalosporins and penicillins, angiotensin converting enzyme inhibitor such as zofenopril, fosinopril, benazepril, quinapril, trandolapril, spirapril, cilazapril, ramipril, moexipril, quinaprilat, and perindopril., selected rennin inhibitors, antitumor agents such as bestatin, and dopamine receptor antagonists such as sulpiride (Terada et al. 1997; Bretschneider et al. 1999; Watanabe et al. 2002; Watanabe et al. 2002; Watanabe et al. 2004; Knutter et al. 2008). Using PepT1 as an intestinal transporter to increase oral exposure of compounds with low oral bioavailability was shown to be an effective strategy (Kikuchi et al. 2009). For example, acyclovir is usually associated with suboptimal oral plasma exposure (oral bioavailability 15%) that can lead to resistant viral strains. To overcome this limitation, valacyclovir, a L-valine ester prodrug of acyclovir was effectively designed to increase the oral absorption and plasma exposure of acyclovir (Ganapathy et al. 1998).

Organic Anion-Transporting Polypeptides (OATPS)

OATPs (SLCO) are transmembrane solute carriers that mediate the proton-dependent transport of a wide range of amphipathic endogenous and exogenous organic compounds across the plasma membrane. Currently, 39 members of the OATP/SLCO superfamily have been identified in mammalian species (Hagenbuch and Meier 2004). The OATPs represent integral membrane proteins that contain 12 TM domains where amino and carboxy termini are oriented to the cytoplasmic spaces. There is limited information regarding the tertiary structures of OATPs, although more recent studies are beginning to address this aspect. In this book chapter , we focus on OATP2B1 (SLCO2B1) and OATP1A2 (SLCO1A2). OATP2B1 plays a key role in the uptake of various xenobiotics and was originally isolated from the human brain and named OATP-B (Tamai et al. 2000; Kullak-Ublick et al. 2001) or SLC21A9 (Hagenbuch and Meier 2003). OATP2B1 mRNA is expressed in the human small intestine (Tamai et al. 2000; Kullak-Ublick et al. 2001; Sai et al. 2006) and its protein is immunolocalised at the apical surface of human small intestine (Kobayashi et al. 2003) and Caco-2 cell monolayers (Sai et al. 2006).

Similar to other OATPs, transport via OATP2B1 is generally considered to occur in a bidirectional fashion driven by the solute concentration gradient across the membrane. Heterologous expression of OATP2B1 produces a Na^+-independent, pH-gradient dependent transporter with a relatively narrow substrate specificity compared to other OATPs (Nozawa et al. 2004). Extracellular acidification promoted solute uptake, a property of OATP2B1 that bears relevance to the small intestinal environment in which the transporter is expressed on the apical membrane of the enterocytes. Kobayashi et al. studied the impact of pH on the uptake of both estrone-3-sulfate and pravastatin in OATP-2B1 transfected HEK 293 cells. The group reported that the uptake of both compounds were pH dependent, where higher uptake at pH 5.5 relative to that at 7.4 pH was reported. It is interesting to note that an increase was only observed in V_{max} with a decrease of pH from 7.4 to 5.0 and a negligible change was observed in K_m at studied pH (Kobayashi et al. 2003). In a recent study, our group examined the role of OATP2B1 in the intestinal absorption and tissue uptake of 3-hydroxy-3-methylglutaryl-CoenzymeA (HMG-CoA) reductase inhibitors (statins) (Varma et al. Accepted). We first investigated impact of extracellular pH on the functional affinity of statins to the transporter using OATP2B1-transfeced HEK293 cells. The results indicated that OATP2B1-mediated transport is significant for rosuvastatin, fluvastatin and atorvastatin, at neutral pH. However, OATP2B1 showed broader substrate specificity as well as enhanced transporter activity at acidic pH consistent with other research groups' findings (Kobayashi et al. 2003). Furthermore, uptake at acidic pH was diminished in the presence of proton ionophore, suggesting proton-gradient as the driving force for OATP2B1 activity. Notably, passive transport rates are predominant or comparable to active transport rates for statins, except for rosuvastatin and fluvastatin. Second, we studied the effect of OATP modulators on statins uptake. At pH 6.0, OATP2B1-mediated transport of atorvastatin and cerivastatin was not inhibitable, while rosuvastatin transport was inhibited by E-3-S, rifamycin SV and cyclosporine with IC_{50} values of 19.7±3.3μM, 0.53±0.2μM and 2.2±0.4μM, respectively. Rifamycin SV inhibited OATP2B1-mediated transport of E-3-S and rosuvastatin with similar IC_{50} values at pH 6.0 and 7.4, suggesting that the inhibitor affinity is not pH-dependent. Finally, we noted that OATP2B1-mediated transport of E-3-S, but not rosuvastatin, is pH-sensitive in intestinal epithelial (Caco-2) cells. However, uptake of E-3-S and rosuvastatin by Caco-2 cells was diminished in the presence of proton ionophore (FCCP). The present results indicate that OATP2B1 may be involved in the tissue uptake of rosuvastatin and fluvastatin, while OATP2B1 may play a significant role in the intestinal absorption of several statins due to their transporter affinity at acidic pH.

The physiological and pharmacological role played by OATP2B1 in intestinal absorption may also vary between individuals. For example, a single nucleotide polymorphism (SNP) (found in 31% of the Japanese population investigated within the referenced study) leads to an amino acid change in the OATP2B1 protein (S486F), which is associated with a greater than 50% reduction in transport capacity (Nozawa et al. 2002).

Since the unavailability of crystal structures of OATPs and relative difficulties in validating their homology models, pharmacophore models have helped elucidate the key molecular features involved in the substrate/inhibitor and protein interactions. These models have demonstrated good structure and activity correlation within the studied chemical space. The proposed OATP2B1 pharmacophores may share the similar molecular features for the consideration of the substrate binding at the positively-charged region. Its substrates may have features such as a hydrophobic core to form the π-stacking interaction with the imidazole ring of H579, or a HBD to directly interact with the nitrogen atom of the imidazole ring, both of which should be oriented at the energetically favored position inside the pore. To model these interactions structurally using molecular docking and dynamics, the minimal requirement will be a validated homology model of OATP2B1. To date, the strategy to elucidate the SAR of OATP2B1 is the combination of QSAR, pharmacophore, and structure-based modeling with the support of *in vitro* and cell-based experimental data.

Another OATP transporter that plays a role in the intestinal absorption of xenobiotics is OATP1A2 (also known as human OATP-A or *SLCO1A2*). This transporter consists of 670 amino acids and is expressed in the brain, kidney and apical membrane of the enterocytes (Kullak-Ublick et al. 1995). Unlike other OATP transporters, OATP1A2 possesses perhaps the broadest spectrum of solutes in that compounds of acidic, basic, and neutral character are substrates. It has been reported to transport bile salts and bromosulfophtalein (BSP), steroid sulfates, thyroid hormones [triiodothyronine (T3), thyroxine (T4), and reverse T3], prostaglandin E2, fexofenadine, opioid peptides [e.g., deltorphin II and (*d*-penicillamine)enkephalin], rocuronium, *N*-methylquinine and *N*-methylquinidine, ouabain, the endothelin receptor antagonist BQ-123, talinolol, and the thrombin inhibitor CRC-220 (Ianculescu et al. ; Loubiere et al. ; Kullak-Ublick et al. 1995; Hsiang et al. 1999; Gao et al. 2000; Geyer et al. 2004; Schwarz et al. 2005; Shimizu et al. 2005; Kalliokoski and Niemi 2009). Similar to OATP2B1, genetic variations has been reported in *SLCO1A2*. For example, Lee *et al.* identified six non-synonymous SNPs in the coding region of SLCO1A2. The c.516A>C (p.Glu172Asp) variant had markedly reduced uptake capacity for the OATP1A2 substrates estrone 3-sulfate and the d-opioid receptor agonists, deltorphin II and [D-penicillamine2,5]-enkephalin *in vitro*. The group concluded that considering its substrate specificity and expression in organs such as the brain, kidney and intestine, genetic variations in *SLCO1A2* may be an important contributor to inter-individual variability in drug disposition and central nervous system entry of OATP1A2 substrate drugs (Lee et al. 2005).

In the clinic, the effect of grapefruit juice on the oral exposure of fexofendadine was evaluated. The oral plasma exposure of fexofenadine was decreased 63%. This seems likely to be mediated by inhibition of intestinal absorption via OATP1A2. (Dresser et al. 2005; Bailey et al. 2007). Similar findings were reported in a study that evaluated the effect of single and repeated grapefruit juice ingenstion on the oral plasma exposure of talinolol in humans. The decrease in the oral plasma exposure of talinolol (44%) was attributed to the inhibition of OATP1A2 (Shirasaka et al.; Schwarz et al. 2005). Overall, these findings identify OATP1A2 as a potential site for diet-drug interactions and clearly demonstrate the potential role of OATP1A2 in the absorption of xenobiotics.

Monocarboxylate transporter 1 (MCT1)

The bi-directional movement of monocarboxylic acids across the plasma membrane is catalyzed by a family of proton-linked monocarboxylate transporters (MCTs). MCTs are encoded by the *SLC16A* gene family, of which there are 14 known members that were identified through screening genomic and expressed sequence tag databases (Halestrap and Meredith 2004). Only MCTs 1-4 have been shown to catalyze the proton-coupled transport of metabolically important monocarboxylates such as lactate and pyruvate (Halestrap and Meredith 2004). This book chapter will focus on the first member of the MCT family, MCT1 (*SLC16A*1), which is well characterized and known to play a role in the intestinal drug absorption.

MCT1 consists of 12 TM α-helical domains with a large intracellular loop between TM segments VI and VII and intracellular C- and N- termini (Poole et al. 1996; Halestrap and Price 1999). MCT1 is expressed in most tissues and is especially prominent in the heart, red skeletal muscle, erythrocytes, and all cells under hypoxic conditions, where it can either be involved in the uptake or efflux of glycolytically produced lactic acid. MCT1 is also highly expressed in the small and large intestine (Gill et al. 2005), where it is responsible for the absorption of short chain fatty acids such as acetate, propionate and butyrate, produced from microbial fermentation of dietary fiber (Cummings and Macfarlane 1991).

MCT1 catalyses the facilitative diffusion of substrate across the plasma membrane, coupled with the translocation of a proton. The driving force for transport is provided by both the substrate and H^+-concentration gradients, with the pH gradient determining the extent of transport activity (Juel 1997; Halestrap and Price 1999). Based on the reported crystal structures of two members of the major facilitator superfamily, the Escherischia coli glycerol-3-phosphate transporter (G1pT) and lactose permease (Lac Y) (Abramson et al. 2003; Huang et al. 2003), the structure of MCT1 has been modelled (Manoharan et al. 2006). Futhermore, site-directed mutagenesis identifying key substrate-binding residues together with structural modeling has lead to the suggestion of a translocation cycle as the mechanism of transport for MCT1 (Wilson et al. 2009). This mechanism of transport is consistent with the "Rocker Switch" mechanism (Law et al. 2008). This model describes MCT1 existing in an open and closed conformation, with the N- and C-terminal halves tilting against each other along an axis that separates the two domains, allowing the substrate binding site alternating access to the either side of the membrane (Wilson et al. 2009). MCT1 also requires an ancillary protein, CD147, for correct trafficking to the plasma membrane as well as functional activity (Wilson et al. 2005). CD147 is a member of the immunoglobulin gene superfamily, and has been shown to closely interact with both MCT1 and MCT4 (Kirk et al. 2000).

MCT1 is a low affinity, high capacity transporter that has been shown to transport unbranched aliphatic monocarboxylates such as acetate and proprionate and substituted monocarboxylates pyruvate, lactate, acetoacetate and β-hydroxybutyrate, with the K_m values for pyruvate and lactate about 0.7 and 3-5 mM, respectively (Halestrap and Meredith 2004). Other MCT1 monocarboxylate substrates include the branched chain keto-acids (formed from the transamination of leucine, isoleucine and valine) and the ketone bodies acetoacetate, β-hydroxybutyrate and acetate (Poole and Halestrap 1993), and exogenous acids p-aminohippuric acid, benzoic acid, γ-hydroxy butyrate, foscarnet, mevolonic acid, and salicylic acid (Enerson and Drewes 2003; Lam et al. 2010). MCT1 is also thought to be responsible for the intestinal absorption of the β-lactam antibiotics such as carbenicillin indanyl sodium as well as phenethicillin and propicillin (Li et al. 1999). The targeting of MCT1 by pharmacologically active drugs has been shown to result in enhanced intestinal drug uptake. For example, XP13512 is rapidly absorbed along the length of the intestine via MCT1 (as well as the SMVT). XP13512 is an anionic compound produced by the reversible modification of the amine group of gabapentin (which has limited oral absorption), with an acyloxyalkylcarbamate promoeity (Cundy et al. 2004). Overall, prototypical substrates of MCT1 generally consist of weak organic acids with the carboxyl group attached to a relatively small R group containing lipophilic or hydrophilic properties (Enerson and Drewes 2003).

5.2 Physicochemical factors that impact oral drug absorption

Our group recently investigated the interrelation of physicochemical properties and individual parameters for a database comprised of Fa, Fg, Fh, and F values for 309 drugs in humans (Varma et al. 2010). The aim is to define the physicochemical space for optimum human oral bioavailability. The current data set suggested an even distribution of the bioavailability values, with about 17% of compounds showing F less than 0.2 and 34% of compounds showing F more than 0.8. However, the vast majority of compounds showed Fa (71%), Fg (70%), and Fh (73%) more than 0.8. The current data set indicated that bioavailability is mainly limited by absorption as evident from the subset of compounds showing bioavailability less than 0.2, where mean and median values suggest the rank-order of limiting parameters as Fa > Fg > Fh.

The distribution of the data set in physicochemical space is heterogeneous and thoroughly covered the range of conventional small molecule marketed drugs. Trend analysis clearly indicate that ionization state, molecular weight (MW), lipophilicity, polar descriptors, and free rotatable bonds (RB) influence bioavailability. For example, ionization state analysis of compounds studied indicate that although bases tend to have higher Fa, they are relatively less bioavailable as compared to acids and neutrals. MW trends suggest that increasing the size of molecules above 400 g/mol will on average lead to a steady decline in bioavailability, mainly due to the effect on Fa. Lipophilicity (cLog P and cLog D $_{pH7.4}$) trends indicate that very hydrophilic compounds have drastically reduced intestinal absorption. On the other hands, RB and polar descriptors such as PSA, hydrogen bonding count (HBA + HBD) showed inverse relationship with Fa, in particular for compounds with RB > 12, PSA greater than 125 A$^{\circ 2}$, and hydrogen bond count more than 9.

The scholarship outlined above is consistent with the finding of Lipinski et al, who introduced the rule of 5 (RO5), which is one of the most widely used concepts to qualitatively predict oral drug absorption. The group analyzed 2245 compounds from the World Drug Index (WDI) database that were either considered for, or entered into, Phase II clinical trials. Results indicate that good oral absorption is more likely with drug molecules that have less than 5 hydrogen bond donors (defined as NH or OH groups)/10 hydrogen bond acceptors (defined as oxygen or nitrogen atoms, including those that are part of hydrogen-bond donors), a molecular weight that is smaller than 500, and a calculated lipophilicity (cLog P) that is smaller than 5 (Lipinski 1995; Lipinski 2000; Lipinski et al. 2001). Poor bioavailability is more likely when the compounds violate two or more of the RO5. Using the current data set, we evaluated the relationships between number of violations and bioavailability and the individual processes. From Figure 1, it is evident that median bioavailability dropped considerably from 0.70 to 0.35 (p < 0.005) for the compound subsets with no violation and two violations, respectively. Compounds with three violations showed a further decline in median bioavailability (0.05). However, similar relationship was observed only with Fa but not with Fg and Fh, suggesting that relationship of rule-of-five and bioavailability is associated mainly with intestinal absorption.

5.3 Biopharmaceutical factors that impact oral drug absorption

5.3.1 Particle size

Drug dissolution rate is an important parameter that affects oral drug absorption (Chaumeil 1998; Boobis et al. 2002; Hilgers et al. 2003). A drug is defined as being poorly soluble when its dissolution rate is so slow that dissolution takes longer than the transit time past its absorptive sites, resulting in incomplete oral absorption. Based on the Noyes-Whitney equation, many factors can affect a drug's dissolution rate (Healy 1984; Frenning and Stromme 2003):

$$DR = \frac{A \cdot D}{h}(C_s - C) \tag{6}$$

Where DR is the dissolution rate, A is the surface area available for dissolution, D is the diffusion coefficient of the drug, h is the thickness of the boundary diffusion layer adjacent to the dissolving drug surface, C_s, is the saturation solubility of the drug in the diffusion layer, C is the concentration of the drug in the bulk solution at time t. As shown in the equation above, the drug dissolution rate is directly proportional to the surface area of the drug particle, which in turn is increased with decreasing particle size. This can be accomplished by micronization or by the use of nanosuspension to reduce the particle size of the drug and therefore increases drug dissolution rate, which usually is associated with an increase in the extent as well as rate of oral absorption (Chaumeil 1998; Li et al. 2005; Borm et al. 2006). Examples on a drug for which reducing its particle size had significant impact on its dissolution rate is griseofulvin. This molecule has a particularly low solubility and was thus studied as a micronized powder with a median particle size of 3 μM (Nystrom et al. 1985; Nystrom and Bisrat 1986). Measurement of the amount dissolved in water *versus* time using a micronized powder showed that the rate of dissolution depended on the area of contact, which is related to the particle size. Increasing this area was an effective way of increasing the rate of dissolution of this drug (Sjökvist et al. 1989).

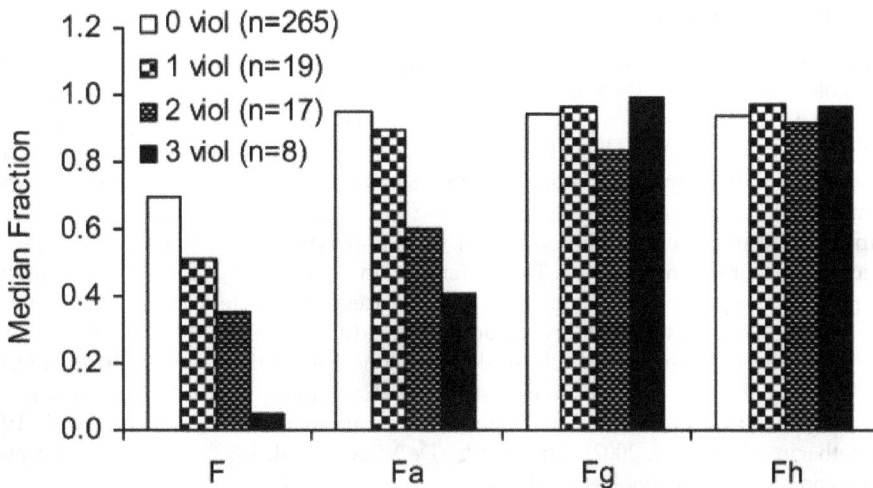

Fig. 1. Relationship between number of violations of rule-offive and bioavailability and individual processes. "n" is the number of compounds in each bin (Varma et al. 2010).

5.3.2 Salt form

As noted above, many drug molecules can be classified as either weak acids or bases that tend to form strong ionic interaction with an oppositely charged counter-ion and maintain that interaction through crystallization. The resulting solid comprises charged drug molecules and their associated oppositely charged counter-ions and is usually referred to as salt. The use of salt forms as active pharmaceutical ingredients is well established in the literature (Berge et al. 1977; Chowhan 1978). A salt form of a drug molecule changes the coulombic attraction between the drug molecule and its counterion and alters the potential energy of the solid state. This is usually associated with alteration of the pH of the diffusion layer at the surface of the dissolving solid, and therefore significantly increases the solubility of the parent drug molecule (C_s), in that layer over its inherent solubility at the pH of the dissolution medium (C). In general, these changes can result in a significant increase in the dissolution rates and higher apparent solubility of the drug molecules in physiologically relevant timescales. Overall, if other relevant factors such as chemical stability, permeability, intestinal and liver metabolism remain constant, the dissolution rate of a compound should determine the rate of build-up of blood levels with time and the maximal levels achieved (Nelson 1957; Chowhan 1978; Hendriksen et al. 2003; Huang and Tong 2004; Li et al. 2005).

In summary, the drug salt form usually alters the drug dissolution rate by modifying the diffusion layer pH at the surface of the dissolving solid (Nelson 1957). Nelson was the first to report this phenomenon in which the salts of acidic theophylline with high diffusion layer pH's had greater *in vitro* dissolution rates than those exhibiting a lower diffusion layer pH. In fact, the rank order of dissolution rates of theophylline was closely correlated with the clinical blood exposure. This report led many additional studies that demonstrated the influence of the salt form on drug dissolution and the benefit of changing nonionized drug to salts (Nelson 1957; Nelson 1958; Berge et al. 1977; Nang et al. 1977; Chowhan 1978; Chen et al. 2002; Hendriksen et al. 2003; Huang and Tong 2004; Strickley 2004; Li et al. 2005)

5.3.3 Polymorphism and drug amorphous form

Polymorphs of a drug substance are chemically identical. However, due to the differences in their molecular packing, they have different physical properties such as crystal shape, molecular density, melting temperature, hygroscopicity, and enthalpy of fusion (Huang and Tong 2004; Li et al. 2005). Albeit these differences, the various polymorphs tend to have comparable solubility profile. Pudipeddi and Serajuddin evaluated the effect of various polymorphs of drug molecules reported in the literature on their solubility profiles. The group reported that the solubility values of various polymorphs for these drug molecules did not differ more than two-folds. This difference in the solubility value is not expected to have profound impact on the compound biopharmaceutical profile depending on the doses used, particle sizes, and solubility values (Pudipeddi and Serajuddin 2005). However, polymorphism may influence the physical and chemical stability of various drug molecules by influencing the rate and mechanism of decay (Cohen and Green 1973; Matsuda et al. 1993; Singhal and Curatolo 2004). Examples are carbamezepine (Matsuda et al. 1993), indomethacin (Chen et al. 2002), furosemide (De Villiers et al. 1992), and enalapril maleate (Cohen and Green 1973; Eyjolfsson 2002).

There are significant differences between crystalline polymorphs and the amorphous form of a drug. In general, the amorphous form tends to have significantly higher dissolution rate and solubility compared to their crystalline forms, which may significantly increase their rate and extent of oral absorption. However, the amorphous form is generally less chemically stable due to the lack of a three dimensional crystalline lattice, higher free volume, and greater molecular mobility. The chemical stability of amorphous systems has been discussed in detail elsewhere (Craig et al. 1999; Doelker 2002; Kaushal et al. 2004; Singhal and Curatolo 2004).

5.3.4 Drug complexation

The drug complexes of interest are generally divided into two major categories based on the energy of attraction between the components of the complexes. They are (1) covalently linked complexes, (2) ionic/inclusion complexes. It is interesting to note that the energy of attraction of covalently linked complexes is about 100 kcal/mol. Whereas; the latter type of complexes is less than 10 kcal/mol. Examples on covalently linked complexes are prodrugs that are prepared by chemical modification of the drug through the addition of a labile moiety, such as ester group (Van Gelder et al. 2000). This approach is widely used to increase drug solubility/permeability and thus improving drug bioavailability. The labile groups are usually broken by enzymatic action, and the parent drug is freed to produce its pharmacological action. The prodrug approach has been widely used in the development of bacampicillin, chloramphenicol, pivampicillin, and enalapril (Van Gelder et al. 2000; van De Waterbeemd et al. 2001; Beaumont et al. 2003).

Inclusion compounds, which form the second category of complexes, result more from the architecture of molecules than from their chemical interaction. One of the constituents of the complex is trapped in the cage-like molecular structure of the other to yield a stable arrangement. Cyclodextrins have been most widely used for this purpose, since they can trap lipophilic drugs in their molecular envelope and form a complex having a comparatively more hydrophilic character (Shimpi et al. 2005). It is well established in the literature that a complex formation of a drug with cyclodextrin is known to improve drug solubility or dissolution rate, and thereby its oral bioavailability (Irie and Uekama 1997; Loftsson et al. 2002; Strickley 2004; Shimpi et al. 2005).

It should be stressed that the drug molecules can also form complexes that may adversely affect their oral bioavailability. One widely reported example is the complexation of tetracycline with aluminum, calcium, or magnesium ions to form an insoluble complex that cannot be absorbed (Kakemi et al. 1968; Kakemi et al. 1968). Before the complexation phenomenon was known, the administration of antacids with tetracycline was suggested to minimize the gastrointestinal disturbance (nausea and vomiting) caused by the antibiotic (Gugler and Allgayer 1990). As most antacids contain aluminum or magnesium hydroxide and/or calcium carbonate ions, such coadministration have reduced greatly the bioavailability of the antibiotic. However, complexation can also arise due to the calcium ions present in milk and other dairy products (Jung et al. 1997). For example, for democycline, only 13% was absorbed when administered with milk. Doxycycline has been reported to be less prone to complexation with dairy products, yet only 10% was absorbed when coadministered with aluminum hydroxide gel (Gugler and Allgayer 1990).

6. BCS and BDDCS

Solubility and permeability are the fundamental properties determining the bioavailability of an orally active drug. Based on these properties Amidon *et al.* proposed biopharmaceutic classification system (BCS), which in present times is serving as a guide for regulatory and industrial purposes (Amidon et al. 1995). This concept exploring dose number, dissolution number, and absorption number of an orally administered drug clearly dictate its systemic availability. These three numbers are associated with a number of multifaceted hurdles, which include (i) physicochemical properties of the molecule (solubility/dissolution) (ii) stability of drug in GI environment (acid degradation) (iii) enzymatic stability in GI lumen, epithelium and liver (iv) permeability (molecular weight, log P, H-bonding efficiency) and (v) substrates specificity to various uptake and efflux transporters. The US FDA, other regulatory agencies, and healthcare organizations have implemented the BCS to enable the use of in vitro solubility and permeability data to waive conducting expensive bioequivalence clinical studies (BE) of high solubility-high permeability (Class I) drugs. While the pharmaceutical industry has taken advantage of BCS-based biowaivers, its principles are used throughout the drug discovery and development to drive oral active programs. On the basis of the apparent correlation between intestinal permeability rate and extent of drug metabolism, Benet and coworkers proposed biopharmaceutics drug disposition classification system (BDDCS), and suggested that the extent of drug metabolism may be used for characterizing high intestinal permeability drugs (Wu and Benet 2005; Benet 2009).

7. Intestinal metabolism

Small intestine has an ability to metabolize drugs by several pathways involving both phase I and phase II reactions and may lead to limited oral bioavailability. CYP3A4, the most abundant cytochrome P450 present in human hepatocytes and intestinal enterocytes is implicated in the metabolic elimination of many drugs (Paine et al. 2006; Thummel 2007). It has also been proposed that drug interactions involving CYP3A inhibition and induction may be largely occurring at the level of the intestine (Hebert et al. 1992; van Waterschoot et al. 2009). In a recent analysis of 309 drugs with intravenous and oral clinical pharmacokinetic data, we noted that roughly 30% of the drugs in the data set show more than 20% intestinal extraction, underscoring the importance of considering intestinal metabolism in predicting bioavailability and dose projections in drug discovery and development settings (Varma et al. 2010). Although, the average human intestinal content of CYP3A has been estimated to be only about 1% of the average hepatic content (Paine et al. 2006), the data set indicated that intestinal metabolism may contribute to first-pass extraction more than the hepatic metabolism for certain drugs. This could be a result of better access to the enzymes in the enterocytes; a function of transcellular flux and the large absorptive area, and/or due to reduced access to hepatic enzymes because of potential plasma protein binding (Thummel 2007).

The intestinal first-pass metabolism in humans is indirectly estimated under certain assumption, by comparing the plasma AUCs following intravenous and oral dosing. Early studies in liver transplant patients during the anhepatic phase indicated the relative importance of the gut extraction to the first-pass metabolism for drugs such as midazolam and cyclosporine (Paine et al. 1996). Further clinical evidences were obtained in the grape-fruit juice interaction studies, where coadministration of grape-fruit juice result in the inhibition of gut CYP3A4 without significantly affecting the hepatic metabolism of drugs like felodipine (Gertz et al. 2008). However, assessment of the quantitative contribution of intestinal and hepatic extraction in first-pass metabolism is limited by ethical and technical challenges. There exist gaps in predicting the gut extraction before the clinical development stage due to shortcomings in the *in vitro-in vivo* extrapolation (Eg. utilizing human intestinal microsomal stability). Also species differences exist where rat and monkey typically under-predicts the fraction escaping gut extraction (Fg) in human (Cao et al. 2006; Nishimuta et al. 2010). Recently, transgenic mice model with constitutive expression of human CYP3A4 in liver or intestine that provides quantitative estimation of the contribution of hepatic and gut extraction to the first-pass metabolism has been generated (van Waterschoot et al. 2009). Overall, due to limited access to the sophisticated models and complexities with *in vitro in vivo* extrapolation and species differences, intestinal metabolic disposition is far from consistently predictable.

Recent studies demonstrated that efflux transporters present on the apical membrane of enterocytes, in particular Pgp, can affect the intestinal metabolism by prolonging the enterocytic transit time and consequent exposure to CYP3A enzymes (Wacher et al. 2001). A significant overlap has also been identified between substrates and inhibitors of CYP3A4 and Pgp, suggesting that these two proteins may act complementarily in further limiting Fg of CYP3A substrates. Due to the complexity in these biochemical processes and the lack of availability of extensive experimental models, application of physiologically-based pharmacokinetic (PBPK) models and systems biology seem to provide quantitative prediction of first-pass metabolism. These emerging tools aim towards appropriate reconstruction of the physicochemical, anatomical and biochemical complexities in mathematical terms.

8. Conclusions

Reliable delivery of drugs via oral administration is most sort after in drug industry. Consequently, the design and development of orally active drugs has to take into account a plethora of factors which may include the physicochemical, biopharmaceutical and physiological determinants. While, solubility and permeability, are fundamental biopharmaceutical parameters that determine the oral absorption, physicochemical and drug substance properties are directly or indirectly associated with these parameters. Lipophilicity, hydrogen bonding ability and number of rotatable bonds are generally identified as critical molecular properties of drugs influencing the rate of membrane transport and thus the intestinal absorption (Fa). However, for drugs with low membrane permeability, role of uptake and efflux transporters may become significant and thus need appropriate characterization. It is believed that targeting intestinal uptake transporter and circumventing efflux transporters may be an useful strategy to design drugs with oral activity. Understanding the contribution of intestinal metabolism to the oral bioavailability is also key in projecting clinical pharmacokinetics and doses. Modeling intestinal absorption and metabolism is complicated due to variability in the physiology and gradient enzyme and transporter localization. Nevertheless, better characterization of factors influencing intestinal absorption and metabolism might result in improved pharmacokinetic optimization in discovery and development settings.

9. References

Abrahamsson, B. & Lennernas, H. (2005). Application of the biopharmaceutic classification system now and in the future. Drug Bioavailability, Estimation of Solubility, Permeability, Absorption, and Bioavailability. Waterbeemd, H. v. d., Lennernas, H. & Artursson, P., WILEY-VCH. 18: 495-531.

Abramson, J., Smirnova, I., Kasho, V., Verner, G., Kaback, H., R & Iwata, S. (2003). Structure and mechanism of the lactose permease of *Escherichia coli*. *Science*, Vol.301, pp. 610-615.

Adibi, S. A. (1997). The oligopeptide transporter (Pept-1) in human intestine: biology and function. *Gastroenterology*, Vol.113, No.1, pp. 332-340.

Ambudkar, S. V., Dey, S., Hrycyna, C. A., Ramchandra, M., Pastan, I. & Gottesman, M. M. (1999). Biochemical, cellular, and pharmacological aspects of the multidrug transporter. *Annu. Rev. Pharmacol. Toxicol.*, Vol.39, pp. 361-398.

Amidon, G. L., Lennernas, H., Shah, V. P. & Crison, J. R. (1995). A theoretical basis for a biopharmaceutic drug classification: the correlation of in vitro drug product dissolution and in vivo bioavailability. *Pharm. Res.*, Vol.12, No.3, pp. 413-420.

Ando, T., Kusuhara, H., Merino, G., Alvarez, A. I., Schinkel, A. H. & Sugiyama, Y. (2007). Involvement of breast cancer resistance protein (ABCG2) in the biliary excretion mechanism of fluoroquinolones. *Drug Metab Dispos*, Vol.35, No.10, pp. 1873-1879.

Avdeef, A. (2001). Physicochemical profiling (solubility, permeability and charge state). *Curr. Top. Med. Chem.*, Vol.1, No.4, pp. 277-351.

Bailey, D. G., Dresser, G. K., Leake, B. F. & Kim, R. B. (2007). Naringin is a major and selective clinical inhibitor of organic anion-transporting polypeptide 1A2 (OATP1A2) in grapefruit juice. *Clin Pharmacol Ther*, Vol.81, No.4, pp. 495-502.

Bailey, K. M., Romaine, S. P., Jackson, B. M., Farrin, A. J., Efthymiou, M., Barth, J. H., Copeland, J., McCormack, T., Whitehead, A., Flather, M. D., Samani, N. J., Nixon, J., Hall, A. S. & Balmforth, A. J. Hepatic metabolism and transporter gene variants enhance response to rosuvastatin in patients with acute myocardial infarction: the GEOSTAT-1 Study. *Circ Cardiovasc Genet*, Vol.3, No.3, pp. 276-285.

Bardelmeijer, H. A., van Tellingen, O., Schellens, J. H. & Beijnen, J. H. (2000). The oral route for the administration of cytotoxic drugs: strategies to increase the efficiency and consistency of drug delivery. *Invest. New Drugs*, Vol.18, No.3, pp. 231-241.

Beaumont, K., Webster, R., Gardner, I. & Dack, K. (2003). Design of ester prodrugs to enhance oral absorption of poorly permeable compounds: challenges to the discovery scientist. *Curr. Drug Metab.*, Vol.4, No.6, pp. 461-485.

Begley, D. J. (2004). ABC transporters and the blood-brain barrier. *Curr Pharm Des*, Vol.10, No.12, pp. 1295-1312.

Beierle, I., Meibohm, B. & Derendorf, H. (1999). Gender differences in pharmacokinetics and pharmacodynamics. *Int. J. Clin. Pharmacol. Ther.*, Vol.37, No.11, pp. 529-547.

Benet, L. Z. (2009). The drug transporter-metabolism alliance: uncovering and defining the interplay. *Mol Pharm*, Vol.6, No.6, pp. 1631-1643.

Berge, S. M., Bighley, L. D. & Monkhouse, D. C. (1977). Pharmaceutical salts. *J. Pharm. Sci.*, Vol.66, No.1, pp. 1-19.

Blaut, M., Schoefer, L. & Braune, A. (2003). Transformation of flavonoids by intestinal microorganisms. *Int. J. Vitam. Nutr. Res.*, Vol.73, No.2, pp. 79-87.

Boobis, A., Gundert-Remy, U., Kremers, P., Macheras, P. & Pelkonen, O. (2002). In silico prediction of ADME and pharmacokinetics - Report of an expert meeting organised by COST B15. *European Journal of Pharmaceutical Sciences*, Vol.17, No.4-5, pp. 183-193.

Borm, P., Klaessig, F. C., Landry, T. D., Moudgil, B., Pauluhn, J., Thomas, K., Trottier, R. & Wood, S. (2006). Research strategies for safety evaluation of nanomaterials, part V: role of dissolution in biological fate and effects of nanoscale particles. *Toxicol. Sci.*, Vol.90, No.1, pp. 23-32.

Brandsch, M., Knutter, I. & Leibach, F. H. (2004). The intestinal H+/peptide symporter PEPT1: structure-affinity relationships. *Eur J Pharm Sci*, Vol.21, No.1, pp. 53-60.

Brandsch, M., Knutter, I., Thunecke, F., Hartrodt, B., Born, I., Borner, V., Hirche, F., Fischer, G. & Neubert, K. (1999). Decisive structural determinants for the interaction of proline derivatives with the intestinal H+/peptide symporter. *Eur J Biochem*, Vol.266, No.2, pp. 502-508.

Bretschneider, B., Brandsch, M. & Neubert, R. (1999). Intestinal transport of beta-lactam antibiotics: analysis of the affinity at the H+/peptide symporter (PEPT1), the uptake into Caco-2 cell monolayers and the transepithelial flux. *Pharm Res*, Vol.16, No.1, pp. 55-61.

Bruyere, A., Decleves, X., Bouzom, F., Ball, K., Marques, C., Treton, X., Pocard, M., Valleur, P., Bouhnik, Y., Panis, Y., Scherrmann, J. M. & Mouly, S. (2010). Effect of Variations in the Amounts of P-Glycoprotein (ABCB1), BCRP (ABCG2) and CYP3A4 along the Human Small Intestine on PBPK Models for Predicting Intestinal First Pass. *Mol Pharm*.

Cao, X., Gibbs, S. T., Fang, L., Miller, H. A., Landowski, C. P., Shin, H. C., Lennernas, H., Zhong, Y., Amidon, G. L., Yu, L. X. & Sun, D. (2006). Why is it challenging to predict intestinal drug absorption and oral bioavailability in human using rat model. *Pharm Res*, Vol.23, No.8, pp. 1675-1686.

Chaumeil, J. C. (1998). Micronization: a method of improving the bioavailability of poorly soluble drugs. *Methods Find Exp Clin Pharmacol*, Vol.20, No.3, pp. 211-215.

Chaumeil, J. C. (1998). Micronization: a method of improving the bioavailability of poorly soluble drugs. *Methods Find. Exp. Clin. Pharmacol.*, Vol.20, No.3, pp. 211-215.

Cheema, M., Palin, K. J. & Davis, S. S. (1987). Lipid vehicles for intestinal lymphatic drug absorption. *J. Pharm. Pharmacol.*, Vol.39, No.1, pp. 55-56.

Chen, X., Morris, K. R., Griesser, U. J., Byrn, S. R. & Stowell, J. G. (2002). Reactivity differences of indomethacin solid forms with ammonia gas. *J. Am. Chem. Soc.*, Vol.124, No.50, pp. 15012-15019.

Chiou, W. L. (1994). Effect of 'unstirred' water layer in the intestine on the rate and extent of absorption after oral administration. *Biopharm Drug Dispos*, Vol.15, No.8, pp. 709-717.

Chowhan, Z. T. (1978). pH-solubility profiles or organic carboxylic acids and their salts. *J. Pharm. Sci.*, Vol.67, No.9, pp. 1257-1260.

Cohen, M. D. & Green, B. S. (1973). Organic chemistry in the solid state. *Chem. Br.*, Vol.9, pp. 490-497.

Craig, D. Q., Royall, P. G., Kett, V. L. & Hopton, M. L. (1999). The relevance of the amorphous state to pharmaceutical dosage forms: glassy drugs and freeze dried systems. *Int. J. Pharm.*, Vol.179, No.2, pp. 179-207.

Cummings, J. H. & Macfarlane, G. T. (1991). The control and consequences of bacterial fermentation in the human colon., *J Appl Bacteriol*, Vol.70, No.6, pp. 443-459.

Cummings, J. H. & Macfarlane, G. T. (1997). Role of intestinal bacteria in nutrient metabolism. *J. Parenter. Enteral. Nutr.*, Vol.21, No.6, pp. 357-365.

Cundy, K. C., Branch, R., Chernov-Rogan, T., Dias, T., Estrada, T. o., Hold, K., Koller, K., Liu, X., Mann, A., Panuwat, M., Raillard, S. P., Upadhyay, S., Wu, Q. Q., Xiang, J.-N., Yan, H., et al. (2004). XP13512 [(±)-1-([(α-Isobutanoyloxyethoxy)carbonyl] aminomethyl)-1-cyclohexane Acetic Acid], A Novel Gabapentin Prodrug: I. Design, Synthesis, Enzymatic Conversion to Gabapentin, and Transport by Intestinal Solute Transporters *J Pharmacol Exp Ther*, Vol.311, No.1, pp. 315-323.

Dauchy, S., Miller, F., Couraud, P. O., Weaver, R. J., Weksler, B., Romero, I. A., Scherrmann, J. M., De Waziers, I. & Decleves, X. (2009). Expression and transcriptional regulation of ABC transporters and cytochromes P450 in hCMEC/D3 human cerebral microvascular endothelial cells. *Biochem Pharmacol*, Vol.77, No.5, pp. 897-909.

De Villiers, M. M., van der Watt, J. G. & Lotter, A. P. (1992). Kinetic study of the solid-state photolytic degradation of two polymorphic forms of furosemide. *Int. J. Pharm.* , Vol.88, pp. 275-283.

DeSesso, J. M. & Jacobson, C. F. (2001). Anatomical and physiological parameters affecting gastrointestinal absorption in humans and rats. *Food Chem. Toxicol.*, Vol.39, No.3, pp. 209-228.

Didziapetris, R., Japertas, P., Avdeef, A. & Petrauskas, A. (2003). Classification analysis of P-glycoprotein substrate specificity. *J Drug Target*, Vol.11, No.7, pp. 391-406.

Doelker, E. (2002). Crystalline modifications and polymorphism changes during drug manufacture. *Ann. Pharm. Fr.*, Vol.60, No.3, pp. 161-176.

Doring, F., Walter, J., Will, J., Focking, M., Boll, M., Amasheh, S., Clauss, W. & Daniel, H. (1998). Delta-aminolevulinic acid transport by intestinal and renal peptide transporters and its physiological and clinical implications. *J Clin Invest*, Vol.101, No.12, pp. 2761-2767.

Doyle, L. A. & Ross, D. D. (2003). Multidrug resistance mediated by the breast cancer resistance protein BCRP (ABCG2). *Oncogene*, Vol.22, No.47, pp. 7340-7358.

Dresser, G. K., Kim, R. B. & Bailey, D. G. (2005). Effect of grapefruit juice volume on the reduction of fexofenadine bioavailability: possible role of organic anion transporting polypeptides. *Clin Pharmacol Ther*, Vol.77, No.3, pp. 170-177.

Enerson, B. E. & Drewes, L. R. (2003). Molecular features, regulation, and function of monocarboxylate transporters: implications for drug delivery. *J Pharm Sci*, Vol.92, No.8, pp. 1531-1544.

Englund, G., Rorsman, F., Ronnblom, A., Karlbom, U., Lazorova, L., Grasjo, J., Kindmark, A. & Artursson, P. (2006). Regional levels of drug transporters along the human intestinal tract: co-expression of ABC and SLC transporters and comparison with Caco-2 cells. *Eur J Pharm Sci*, Vol.29, No.3-4, pp. 269-277.

Eyjolfsson, R. (2002). Enalapril maleate polymorphs: instability of form II in a tablet formulation. *Pharmazie*, Vol.57, No.5, pp. 347-348.

Fei, Y. J., Kanai, Y., Nussberger, S., Ganapathy, V., Leibach, F. H., Romero, M. F., Singh, S. K., Boron, W. F. & Hediger, M. A. (1994). Expression cloning of a mammalian proton-coupled oligopeptide transporter. *Nature*, Vol.368, No.6471, pp. 563-566.

Fenner, K. S., Troutman, M. D., Kempshall, S., Cook, J. A., Ware, J. A., Smith, D. A. & Lee, C. A. (2009). Drug-drug interactions mediated through P-glycoprotein: clinical relevance and in vitro-in vivo correlation using digoxin as a probe drug. *Clin Pharmacol Ther*, Vol.85, No.2, pp. 173-181.

Foley, D. W., Rajamanickam, J., Bailey, P. D. & Meredith, D. Bioavailability through PepT1: the role of computer modelling in intelligent drug design. *Curr Comput Aided Drug Des*, Vol.6, No.1, pp. 68-78.

Frenning, G. & Stromme, M. (2003). Drug release modeled by dissolution, diffusion, and immobilization. *Int. J. Pharm.*, Vol.250, No.1, pp. 137-145.

Ganapathy, M. E., Huang, W., Wang, H., Ganapathy, V. & Leibach, F. H. (1998). Valacyclovir: a substrate for the intestinal and renal peptide transporters PEPT1 and PEPT2. *Biochem. Biophys. Res. Commun.*, Vol.246, No.2, pp. 470-475.

Gao, B., Hagenbuch, B., Kullak-Ublick, G. A., Benke, D., Aguzzi, A. & Meier, P. J. (2000). Organic anion-transporting polypeptides mediate transport of opioid peptides across blood-brain barrier. *J Pharmacol Exp Ther*, Vol.294, No.1, pp. 73-79.

Garanero, G., Ramanathan, S. & Amidon, G. (2005). Gastrointestinal Dissolution and Absorption of Drugs. Drug Bioavailability: Estimation of Solubility, Permeability, Absorption and Bioavailability. Waterbeemd, H. v. d., Lennernas, H. & Artursson, P. Zurich, WILEY-VCH. 18: 191-210.

Gertz, M., Davis, J. D., Harrison, A., Houston, J. B. & Galetin, A. (2008). Grapefruit juice-drug interaction studies as a method to assess the extent of intestinal availability: utility and limitations. *Curr Drug Metab*, Vol.9, No.8, pp. 785-795.

Geyer, J., Doring, B., Failing, K. & Petzinger, E. (2004). Molecular cloning and functional characterization of the bovine (Bos taurus) organic anion transporting polypeptide Oatp1a2 (Slco1a2). *Comp Biochem Physiol B Biochem Mol Biol*, Vol.137, No.3, pp. 317-329.

Giacomini, K. M., Huang, S. M., Tweedie, D. J., Benet, L. Z., Brouwer, K. L., Chu, X., Dahlin, A., Evers, R., Fischer, V., Hillgren, K. M., Hoffmaster, K. A., Ishikawa, T., Keppler, D., Kim, R. B., Lee, C. A., et al. (2010). Membrane transporters in drug development. *Nat Rev Drug Discov*, Vol.9, No.3, pp. 215-236.

Gill, R. K., Saksena, S., Alrefai, W. A., Sarwar, Z., Goldstein, J. L., Carroll, R. E., Ramaswamy, K. & Dudeja, P. K. (2005). Expression and membrane localization of MCT isoforms along the length of the human intestine. *Am J Physiol Cell Physiol* Vol.289, No.4, pp. C846-852.

Graf, G. A., Yu, L., Li, W. P., Gerard, R., Tuma, P. L., Cohen, J. C. & Hobbs, H. H. (2003). ABCG5 and ABCG8 are obligate heterodimers for protein trafficking and biliary cholesterol excretion. *J Biol Chem*, Vol.278, No.48, pp. 48275-48282.

Gramatte, T., Oertel, R., Terhaag, B. & Kirch, W. (1996). Direct demonstration of small intestinal secretion and site-dependent absorption of the beta-blocker talinolol in humans. *Clin Pharmacol Ther*, Vol.59, No.5, pp. 541-549.

Greiner, B., Eichelbaum, M., Fritz, P., Kreichgauer, H. P., von Richter, O., Zundler, J. & Kroemer, H. K. (1999). The role of intestinal P-glycoprotein in the interaction of digoxin and rifampin., *J Clin Invest*, Vol.104, No.2, pp. 147-153.

Gugler, R. & Allgayer, H. (1990). Effects of antacids on the clinical pharmacokinetics of drugs. An update. *Clin. Pharmacokinet.*, Vol.18, No.3, pp. 210-219.

Hagenbuch, B. & Meier, P. J. (2003). The superfamily of organic anion transporting polypeptides. *Biochim Biophys Acta*, Vol.1609, No.1, pp. 1-18.

Hagenbuch, B. & Meier, P. J. (2004). Organic anion transporting polypeptides of the OATP/ SLC21 family: phylogenetic classification as OATP/ SLCO superfamily, new nomenclature and molecular/functional properties. *Pflugers Arch*, Vol.447, No.5, pp. 653-665.

Halestrap, A. P. & Meredith, D. (2004). The SLC16 gene family — from monocarboxylate transporters (MCTs) to aromatic amino acid transporters and beyond. *Pflügers Archiv Eur J Physiol*, Vol.447, No.5, pp. 619-628.

Halestrap, A. P. & Price, N. T. (1999). The proton-linked monocarboxylate transporter (MCT) family: structure, function and regulation. *Biochem J*, Vol.343, No.(Pt 2), pp. 281-299.

Hanano, M. (1993). Fat-soluble vitamins: Intestinal absorption. *Nippon Rinsho*, Vol.51, No.4, pp. 851-857.

Hayton, W. L. (1980). Rate-limiting barriers to intestinal drug absorption: a review. *J. Pharmacokinet. Biopharm.*, Vol.8, No.4, pp. 321-334.

Hazai, E. & Bikadi, Z. (2008). Homology modeling of breast cancer resistance protein (ABCG2). *J Struct Biol*, Vol.162, No.1, pp. 63-74.

Healy, M. A. (1984). Theoretical model of gastrointestinal absorption of lead. *J. Clin. Hosp. Pharm.*, Vol.9, No.3, pp. 257-261.

Hebert, M. F., Roberts, J. P., Prueksaritanont, T. & Benet, L. Z. (1992). Bioavailability of cyclosporine with concomitant rifampin administration is markedly less than predicted by hepatic enzyme induction. *Clin Pharmacol Ther*, Vol.52, No.5, pp. 453-457.

Hellriegel, E. T., Bjornsson, T. D. & Hauck, W. W. (1996). Interpatient variability in bioavailability is related to the extent of absorption: implications for bioavailability and bioequivalence studies. *Clin. Pharmacol. Ther.*, Vol.60, No.6, pp. 601-607.

Hendriksen, B. A., Felix, M. V. & Bolger, M. B. (2003). The composite solubility versus pH profile and its role in intestinal absorption prediction. *AAPS PharmSci*, Vol.5, No.1, pp. E4.

Herrera-Ruiz, D., Wang, Q., Gudmundsson, O. S., Cook, T. J., Smith, R. L., Faria, T. N. & Knipp, G. T. (2001). Spatial expression patterns of peptide transporters in the human and rat gastrointestinal tracts, Caco-2 in vitro cell culture model, and multiple human tissues. *AAPS PharmSci*, Vol.3, No.1, pp. E9.

Hilgers, A. R., Smith, D. P., Biermacher, J. J., Day, J. S., Jensen, J. L., Sims, S. M., Adams, W.
    J., Friis, J. M., Palandra, J., Hosley, J. D., Shobe, E. M. & Burton, P. S. (2003).
    Predicting oral absorption of drugs: A case study with a novel class of
    antimicrobial agents. *Pharmaceutical Research*, Vol.20, No.8, pp. 1149-1155.
Horter, D. & Dressman, J. B. (2001). Influence of physicochemical properties on dissolution
    of drugs in the gastrointestinal tract. *Adv. Drug Deliv. Rev.*, Vol.46, No.1-3, pp. 75-
    87.
Hsiang, B., Zhu, Y., Wang, Z., Wu, Y., Sasseville, V., Yang, W. P. & Kirchgessner, T. G.
    (1999). A novel human hepatic organic anion transporting polypeptide (OATP2).
    Identification of a liver-specific human organic anion transporting polypeptide and
    identification of rat and human hydroxymethylglutaryl-CoA reductase inhibitor
    transporters. *J Biol Chem*, Vol.274, No.52, pp. 37161-37168.
Huang, L., Wang, Y. & Grimm, S. (2006). ATP-dependent transport of rosuvastatin in
    membrane vesicles expressing breast cancer resistance protein. *Drug Metab Dispos*,
    Vol.34, No.5, pp. 738-742.
Huang, L. F. & Tong, W. Q. (2004). Impact of solid state properties on developability
    assessment of drug candidates. *Adv. Drug Deliv. Rev.*, Vol.56, No.3, pp. 321-334.
Huang, Y., Lemieux, M. J., Song, J., Auer, M. & Wang, D.-N. (2003). Structure and
    Mechanism of the Glycerol-3-Phosphate Transporter from Escherichia coli. *Science*,
    Vol.301, No.5633, pp. 616-620.
Hurst, S., Loi, C. M., Brodfuehrer, J. & El-Kattan, A. (2007). Impact of physiological,
    physicochemical and biopharmaceutical factors in absorption and metabolism
    mechanisms on the drug oral bioavailability of rats and humans. *Expert Opin. Drug
    Metab. Toxicol.*, Vol.3, No.4, pp. 469-489.
Hurst, S., Loi, C. M., Brodfuehrer, J. & El-Kattan, A. (2007). Impact of physiological,
    physicochemical and biopharmaceutical factors in absorption and metabolism
    mechanisms on the drug oral bioavailability of rats and humans. *Expert Opin Drug
    Metab Toxicol*, Vol.3, No.4, pp. 469-489.
Ianculescu, A. G., Friesema, E. C., Visser, T. J., Giacomini, K. M. & Scanlan, T. S. Transport of
    thyroid hormones is selectively inhibited by 3-iodothyronamine. *Mol Biosyst*, Vol.6,
    No.8, pp. 1403-1410.
Ieiri, I., Higuchi, S. & Sugiyama, Y. (2009). Genetic polymorphisms of uptake (OATP1B1,
    1B3) and efflux (MRP2, BCRP) transporters: implications for inter-individual
    differences in the pharmacokinetics and pharmacodynamics of statins and other
    clinically relevant drugs. *Expert Opin Drug Metab Toxicol*, Vol.5, No.7, pp. 703-729.
Irie, M., Terada, T., Katsura, T., Matsuoka, S. & Inui, K. (2005). Computational modelling of
    H+-coupled peptide transport via human PEPT1. *J Physiol*, Vol.565, No.Pt 2, pp.
    429-439.
Irie, T. & Uekama, K. (1997). Pharmaceutical applications of cyclodextrins. III. Toxicological
    issues and safety evaluation. *J. Pharm. Sci.*, Vol.86, No.2, pp. 147-162.
Juel, C. (1997). Lactate-proton cotransport in skeletal muscle. *Physiol Rev*, Vol.77, No.2, pp.
    321-358.
Juliano, R. L. & Ling, L. (1976). A surface glycoprotien on modulating drug permeability in
    chinease hamster overy cell mutants. *Biochim. Biophys. Acta*, Vol.555, pp. 152-162.
Jung, H., Peregrina, A. A., Rodriguez, J. M. & Moreno-Esparza, R. (1997). The influence of
    coffee with milk and tea with milk on the bioavailability of tetracycline. *Biopharm.
    Drug Dispos.*, Vol.18, No.5, pp. 459-463.

Kakemi, K., Sezaki, H., Hayashi, M. & Nadai, T. (1968). Absorption and excretion of drugs. XXXVII. Effect of Ca2+ on the absorption of tetracycline from the small intestine. (2). *Chem. Pharm. Bull. (Tokyo)*, Vol.16, No.11, pp. 2206-2212.

Kakemi, K., Sezaki, H., Ogata, H. & Nadai, T. (1968). Absorption and excretion of drugs. XXXVI. Effect of Ca2+ on the absorption of tetracycline from the small intestine. (1). *Chem. Pharm. Bull. (Tokyo)*, Vol.16, No.11, pp. 2200-2205.

Kaliszczak, M., Antonow, D., Patel, K. I., Howard, P., Jodrell, D. I., Thurston, D. E. & Guichard, S. M. (2010). Optimization of the Antitumor Activity of Sequence-specific Pyrrolobenzodiazepine Derivatives Based on their Affinity for ABC Transporters. *Aaps J*.

Kalliokoski, A. & Niemi, M. (2009). Impact of OATP transporters on pharmacokinetics. *Br J Pharmacol*, Vol.158, No.3, pp. 693-705.

Kararli, T. T. (1995). Comparison of the gastrointestinal anatomy, physiology, and biochemistry of humans and commonly used laboratory animals. *Biopharm. Drug Dispos.*, Vol.16, No.5, pp. 351-380.

Karlsson, J., Ungell, A., Grasjo, J. & Artursson, P. (1999). Paracellular drug transport across intestinal epithelia: influence of charge and induced water flux. *Eur. J. Pharm. Sci.*, Vol.9, No.1, pp. 47-56.

Katsura, T. & Inui, K. (2003). Intestinal absorption of drugs mediated by drug transporters: mechanisms and regulation. *Drug Metab. Pharmacokinet.*, Vol.18, No.1, pp. 1-15.

Kaushal, A. M., Gupta, P. & Bansal, A. K. (2004). Amorphous drug delivery systems: molecular aspects, design, and performance. *Crit. Rev. Ther. Drug Carrier Syst.*, Vol.21, No.3, pp. 133-193.

Keskitalo, J. E., Pasanen, M. K., Neuvonen, P. J. & Niemi, M. (2009). Different effects of the ABCG2 c.421C>A SNP on the pharmacokinetics of fluvastatin, pravastatin and simvastatin. *Pharmacogenomics*, Vol.10, No.10, pp. 1617-1624.

Keskitalo, J. E., Zolk, O., Fromm, M. F., Kurkinen, K. J., Neuvonen, P. J. & Niemi, M. (2009). ABCG2 polymorphism markedly affects the pharmacokinetics of atorvastatin and rosuvastatin. *Clin Pharmacol Ther*, Vol.86, No.2, pp. 197-203.

Kikuchi, A., Tomoyasu, T., Tanaka, M., Kanamitsu, K., Sasabe, H., Maeda, T., Odomi, M. & Tamai, I. (2009). Peptide derivation of poorly absorbable drug allows intestinal absorption via peptide transporter. *J Pharm Sci*, Vol.98, No.5, pp. 1775-1787.

Kimura, T. & Higaki, K. (2002). Gastrointestinal transit and drug absorption. *Biol. Pharm. Bull.*, Vol.25, No.2, pp. 149-164.

Kirilenko, V. N. & Gregoriadis, G. (1993). Fat soluble vitamins in liposomes: studies on incorporation efficiency and bile salt induced vesicle disintegration. *J Drug Target*, Vol.1, No.4, pp. 361-368.

Kirk, P., Wilson, M. C., Heddle, C., Brown, M. H., Barclay, A. N. & Halestrap, A. P. (2000). CD147 is tightly associated with lactate transporters MCT1 and MCT4 and facilitates their cell surface expression. *EMBO J*, No.15, pp. 3896-3904.

Klaassen, C. D. & Aleksunes, L. M. (2010). Xenobiotic, bile acid, and cholesterol transporters: function and regulation. *Pharmacol Rev*, Vol.62, No.1, pp. 1-96.

Knutter, I., Wollesky, C., Kottra, G., Hahn, M. G., Fischer, W., Zebisch, K., Neubert, R. H., Daniel, H. & Brandsch, M. (2008). Transport of angiotensin-converting enzyme inhibitors by H+/peptide transporters revisited. *J Pharmacol Exp Ther*, Vol.327, No.2, pp. 432-441.

Kobayashi, D., Nozawa, T., Imai, K., Nezu, J., Tsuji, A. & Tamai, I. (2003). Involvement of human organic anion transporting polypeptide OATP-B (SLC21A9) in pH-dependent transport across intestinal apical membrane. *J Pharmacol Exp Ther*, Vol.306, No.2, pp. 703-708.

Kramer, S. D. & Wunderli-Allenspach, H. (2001). Physicochemical properties in pharmacokinetic lead optimization. *Farmaco*, Vol.56, No.1-2, pp. 145-148.

Kruijtzer, C. M., Beijnen, J. H., Rosing, H., ten Bokkel Huinink, W. W., Schot, M., Jewell, R. C., Paul, E. M. & Schellens, J. H. (2002). Increased oral bioavailability of topotecan in combination with the breast cancer resistance protein and P-glycoprotein inhibitor GF120918. *J Clin Oncol*, Vol.20, No.13, pp. 2943-2950.

Kullak-Ublick, G. A., Hagenbuch, B., Stieger, B., Schteingart, C. D., Hofmann, A. F., Wolkoff, A. W. & Meier, P. J. (1995). Molecular and functional characterization of an organic anion transporting polypeptide cloned from human liver. *Gastroenterology*, Vol.109, No.4, pp. 1274-1282.

Kullak-Ublick, G. A., Ismair, M. G., Stieger, B., Landmann, L., Huber, R., Pizzagalli, F., Fattinger, K., Meier, P. J. & Hagenbuch, B. (2001). Organic anion-transporting polypeptide B (OATP-B) and its functional comparison with three other OATPs of human liver. *Gastroenterology*, Vol.120, No.2, pp. 525-533.

Kunta, J. R. & Sinko, P. J. (2004). Intestinal drug transporters: in vivo function and clinical importance. *Curr. Drug Metab.*, Vol.5, No.1, pp. 109-124.

Lam, W. K., Felmlee, M. A. & Morris, M. E. (2010). Monocarboxylate Transporter-Mediated Transport of $\mathrm{\hat{I}^3}$-Hydroxybutyric Acid in Human Intestinal Caco-2 Cells. *Drug Metab Disposition*, Vol.38, No.3, pp. 441-447.

Law, C. J., Maloney, P. C. & Wang, D.-N. (2008). Ins and Outs of Major Facilitator Superfamily Antiporters. *Annual Review of Microbiology* Vol.62, No.1, pp. 289-305.

Lee, W., Glaeser, H., Smith, L. H., Roberts, R. L., Moeckel, G. W., Gervasini, G., Leake, B. F. & Kim, R. B. (2005). Polymorphisms in human organic anion-transporting polypeptide 1A2 (OATP1A2): implications for altered drug disposition and central nervous system drug entry. *J Biol Chem*, Vol.280, No.10, pp. 9610-9617.

Lennernas, H. (1995). Does fluid flow across the intestinal mucosa affect quantitative oral drug absorption? Is it time for a reevaluation?, *Pharm. Res.*, Vol.12, No.11, pp. 1573-1582.

Li, S., He, H., Parthiban, L. J., Yin, H. & Serajuddin, A. T. (2005). IV-IVC considerations in the development of immediate-release oral dosage form. *J. Pharm. Sci.*, Vol.94, No.7, pp. 1396-1417.

Li, Y.-H., Ito, K., Tsuda, Y., Kohda, R., Yamada, H. & Itoh, T. (1999). Mechanism of Intestinal Absorption of an Orally Active $\mathrm{\hat{I}^2}$-Lactam Prodrug: Uptake and Transport of Carindacillin in Caco-2 Cells. *J Pharmacol Exp Ther* Vol.290, No.3, pp. 958-964.

Liang, R., Fei, Y. J., Prasad, P. D., Ramamoorthy, S., Han, H., Yang-Feng, T. L., Hediger, M. A., Ganapathy, V. & Leibach, F. H. (1995). Human intestinal H+/peptide cotransporter. Cloning, functional expression, and chromosomal localization. *J Biol Chem*, Vol.270, No.12, pp. 6456-6463.

Lichtenstein, A. H. (1990). Intestinal cholesterol metabolism. *Ann. Med.*, Vol.22, No.1, pp. 49-52.

Lipinski, C. A. (1995). Computational alerts for potential absorption problems: profiles of clinically tested drugs. In: Tools for Oral Absorption. Part Two. Predicting Human Absorption. AAPS Meeting. Miami, AAPS.

Lipinski, C. A. (2000). Drug-like properties and the causes of poor solubility and poor permeability. *J. Pharmacol. Tox. Methods*, Vol.44, No.1, pp. 235-249.

Lipinski, C. A. (2004). Solubility in water and DMSO: Issues and potential solutions. Pharmaceutical Profiling in Drug Discovery for Lead Selection. Borchardt, R. T., Kerns, E. H., Lipinski, C. A., Thakker, D. R. & Wang, B. W. Washington DC, AAPS Press.

Lipinski, C. A., Lombardo, F., Dominy, B. W. & Feeney, P. J. (2001). Experimental and computational approaches to estimate solubility and permeability in drug discovery and development settings. *Adv. Drug Deliv. Rev.*, Vol.46, No.1-3, pp. 3-26.

Loftsson, T., Masson, M. & Sigurdsson, H. H. (2002). Cyclodextrins and drug permeability through semi-permeable cellophane membranes. *Int. J. Pharm.*, Vol.232, No.1-2, pp. 35-43.

Loubiere, L. S., Vasilopoulou, E., Bulmer, J. N., Taylor, P. M., Stieger, B., Verrey, F., McCabe, C. J., Franklyn, J. A., Kilby, M. D. & Chan, S. Y. Expression of thyroid hormone transporters in the human placenta and changes associated with intrauterine growth restriction. *Placenta*, Vol.31, No.4, pp. 295-304.

Mahar Doan, K. M., Humphreys, J. E., Webster, L. O., Wring, S. A., Shampine, L. J., Serabjit-Singh, C. J., Adkison, K. K. & Polli, J. W. (2002). Passive permeability and P-glycoprotein-mediated efflux differentiate central nervous system (CNS) and non-CNS marketed drugs. *J Pharmacol Exp Ther*, Vol.303, No.3, pp. 1029-1037.

Manoharan, C., Wilson, M. C., Sessions, R. B. & Halestrap, A. P. (2006). The role of charged residues in the transmembrane helices of monocarboxylate transporter 1 and its ancillary protein basigin in determining plasma membrane expression and catalytic activity
Mol Membr Biol, Vol.23, No.486-498.

Martinez, M. N. & Amidon, G. L. (2002). A mechanistic approach to understanding the factors affecting drug absorption: a review of fundamentals. *J. Clin. Pharm.*, Vol.42, No.6, pp. 620-643.

Matsson, P., Englund, G., Ahlin, G., Bergstrom, C. A., Norinder, U. & Artursson, P. (2007). A global drug inhibition pattern for the human ATP-binding cassette transporter breast cancer resistance protein (ABCG2). *J Pharmacol Exp Ther*, Vol.323, No.1, pp. 19-30.

Matsson, P., Pedersen, J. M., Norinder, U., Bergstrom, C. A. & Artursson, P. (2009). Identification of novel specific and general inhibitors of the three major human ATP-binding cassette transporters P-gp, BCRP and MRP2 among registered drugs. *Pharm Res*, Vol.26, No.8, pp. 1816-1831.

Matsuda, Y., Akazawa, R., Teraoka, R. & Otsuka, M. (1993). Pharmaceutical evaluation of carbamazepine modifications: comparative study of photostability for carbamazepine polymorphs by using Fourier-transformed reflection-absorption infrared spectroscopy and calorimetric measurement. . *J. Pharm. Phamacol.*, Vol.46, pp. 162-167.

Meredith, D. & Price, R. A. (2006). Molecular modeling of PepT1--towards a structure. *J Membr Biol*, Vol.213, No.2, pp. 79-88.

Merino, G., Alvarez, A. I., Pulido, M. M., Molina, A. J., Schinkel, A. H. & Prieto, J. G. (2006). Breast cancer resistance protein (BCRP/ABCG2) transports fluoroquinolone antibiotics and affects their oral availability, pharmacokinetics, and milk secretion. *Drug Metab Dispos*, Vol.34, No.4, pp. 690-695.

Merino, G., Jonker, J. W., Wagenaar, E., Pulido, M. M., Molina, A. J., Alvarez, A. I. & Schinkel, A. H. (2005). Transport of anthelmintic benzimidazole drugs by breast cancer resistance protein (BCRP/ABCG2). *Drug Metab Dispos*, Vol.33, No.5, pp. 614-618.

Muenster, U., Grieshop, B., Ickenroth, K. & Gnoth, M. J. (2008). Characterization of substrates and inhibitors for the in vitro assessment of Bcrp mediated drug-drug interactions. *Pharm Res*, Vol.25, No.10, pp. 2320-2326.

Murakami, T. & Takano, M. (2008). Intestinal efflux transporters and drug absorption. *Expert Opin Drug Metab Toxicol*, Vol.4, No.7, pp. 923-939.

Nakagawa, H., Saito, H., Ikegami, Y., Aida-Hyugaji, S., Sawada, S. & Ishikawa, T. (2006). Molecular modeling of new camptothecin analogues to circumvent ABCG2-mediated drug resistance in cancer. *Cancer Lett*, Vol.234, No.1, pp. 81-89.

Nang, L. S., Cosnier, D., Terrie, G. & Moleyre, J. (1977). Consequence of solubility alteration by salt effect on dissolution enhancement and biological response of a solid dispersion of an experimental antianginal drug. *Pharmacol.*, Vol.15, No.6, pp. 545-550.

Nelson, E. (1957). Solution rate of theophylline salts and effects from oral administration. *J. Am. Pharm. Assoc. (Baltim)*, Vol.46, No.10, pp. 607-614.

Nelson, E. (1958). Comparative dissolution rates of weak acids and their sodium salts. *J. Am. Pharm. Assoc. (Baltim)*, Vol.47, No.4, pp. 297-299.

Nicolle, E., Boumendjel, A., Macalou, S., Genoux, E., Ahmed-Belkacem, A., Carrupt, P. A. & Di Pietro, A. (2009). QSAR analysis and molecular modeling of ABCG2-specific inhibitors. *Adv Drug Deliv Rev*, Vol.61, No.1, pp. 34-46.

Nishimuta, H., Sato, K., Mizuki, Y., Yabuki, M. & Komuro, S. (2010). Prediction of the intestinal first-pass metabolism of CYP3A substrates in humans using cynomolgus monkeys. *Drug Metab Dispos*, Vol.38, No.11, pp. 1967-1975.

Nozawa, T., Imai, K., Nezu, J., Tsuji, A. & Tamai, I. (2004). Functional characterization of pH-sensitive organic anion transporting polypeptide OATP-B in human. *J Pharmacol Exp Ther*, Vol.308, No.2, pp. 438-445.

Nozawa, T., Nakajima, M., Tamai, I., Noda, K., Nezu, J., Sai, Y., Tsuji, A. & Yokoi, T. (2002). Genetic polymorphisms of human organic anion transporters OATP-C (SLC21A6) and OATP-B (SLC21A9): allele frequencies in the Japanese population and functional analysis. *J Pharmacol Exp Ther*, Vol.302, No.2, pp. 804-813.

Nystrom, C. & Bisrat, M. (1986). Coulter Counter measurements of solubility and dissolution rate of sparingly soluble compounds using micellar solutions. *J Pharm Pharmacol*, Vol.38, No.6, pp. 420-425.

Nystrom, C., Mazur, J., Barnett, M. I. & Glazer, M. (1985). Dissolution rate measurements of sparingly soluble compounds with the Coulter Counter model TAII. *J Pharm Pharmacol*, Vol.37, No.4, pp. 217-221.

Paine, M. F., Hart, H. L., Ludington, S. S., Haining, R. L., Rettie, A. E. & Zeldin, D. C. (2006). The human intestinal cytochrome P450 "pie". *Drug Metab Dispos*, Vol.34, No.5, pp. 880-886.

Paine, M. F., Shen, D. D., Kunze, K. L., Perkins, J. D., Marsh, C. L., McVicar, J. P., Barr, D. M., Gillies, B. S. & Thummel, K. E. (1996). First-pass metabolism of midazolam by the human intestine. *Clin Pharmacol Ther*, Vol.60, No.1, pp. 14-24.

Polli, J. W., Wring, S. A., Humphreys, J. E., Huang, L., Morgan, J. B., Webster, L. O. & Serabjit-Singh, C. S. (2001). Rational use of in vitro P-glycoprotein assays in drug discovery. *J Pharmacol Exp Ther*, Vol.299, No.2, pp. 620-628.

Poole, R. C. & Halestrap, A. P. (1993). Transport of lactate and other monocarboxylates across mammalian plasma membranes. *Am J Physiol* Vol.264, No.4, pp. C761-C782.

Poole, R. C., Sansom, C. E. & Halestrap, A. P. (1996). Studies of the membrane topology of the rat erythrocyte H+/lactate cotransporter (MCT1). *Biochemical Journal,* Vol.320, pp. 817-824.

Pouton, C. W. (2006). Formulation of poorly water-soluble drugs for oral administration: Physicochemical and physiological issues and the lipid formulation classification system. *Eur. J. Pharm. Sci.,* Vol.29, No.3-4, pp. 278-287.

Pudipeddi, M. & Serajuddin, A. T. (2005). Trends in solubility of polymorphs. *J. Pharm. Sci.,* Vol.94, No.5, pp. 929-939.

Rubio-Aliaga, I. & Daniel, H. (2008). Peptide transporters and their roles in physiological processes and drug disposition. *Xenobiotica,* Vol.38, No.7-8, pp. 1022-1042.

Sabnis, S. (1999). Factors influencing the bioavailability of peroral formulations of drugs for dogs. *Vet. Res. Commun.,* Vol.23, No.7, pp. 425-447.

Sai, Y., Kaneko, Y., Ito, S., Mitsuoka, K., Kato, Y., Tamai, I., Artursson, P. & Tsuji, A. (2006). Predominant contribution of organic anion transporting polypeptide OATP-B (OATP2B1) to apical uptake of estrone-3-sulfate by human intestinal Caco-2 cells. *Drug Metab Dispos,* Vol.34, No.8, pp. 1423-1431.

Saito, H., Hirano, H., Nakagawa, H., Fukami, T., Oosumi, K., Murakami, K., Kimura, H., Kouchi, T., Konomi, M., Tao, E., Tsujikawa, N., Tarui, S., Nagakura, M., Osumi, M. & Ishikawa, T. (2006). A new strategy of high-speed screening and quantitative structure-activity relationship analysis to evaluate human ATP-binding cassette transporter ABCG2-drug interactions. *J Pharmacol Exp Ther,* Vol.317, No.3, pp. 1114-1124.

Schinkel, A. H., Kemp, S., Dolle, M., Rudenco, G. & Wagenaar, E. (1993). N-glycosylation and deletion mutants of the human *MDR1* P-glycoprotein. *J. Biol. Chem,* Vol.268, pp. 7474-7481.

Schwarz, U. I., Seemann, D., Oertel, R., Miehlke, S., Kuhlisch, E., Fromm, M. F., Kim, R. B., Bailey, D. G. & Kirch, W. (2005). Grapefruit juice ingestion significantly reduces talinolol bioavailability. *Clin Pharmacol Ther,* Vol.77, No.4, pp. 291-301.

Seamon, J. A., Rugg, C. A., Emanuel, S., Calcagno, A. M., Ambudkar, S. V., Middleton, S. A., Butler, J., Borowski, V. & Greenberger, L. M. (2006). Role of the ABCG2 drug transporter in the resistance and oral bioavailability of a potent cyclin-dependent kinase/Aurora kinase inhibitor. *Mol Cancer Ther,* Vol.5, No.10, pp. 2459-2467.

Seelig, A. (1998). A general pattern for substrate recognition by P-glycoprotein. *Eur J Biochem,* Vol.251, No.1-2, pp. 252-261.

Seelig, A. (1998). How does P-glycoprotein recognize its substrates?, *Int J Clin Pharmacol Ther,* Vol.36, No.1, pp. 50-54.

Seelig, A. & Landwojtowicz, E. (2000). Structure-activity relationship of P-glycoprotein substrates and modifiers. *Eur J Pharm Sci,* Vol.12, No.1, pp. 31-40.

Seithel, A., Karlsson, J., Hilgendorf, C., Bjorquist, A. & Ungell, A. L. (2006). Variability in mRNA expression of ABC- and SLC-transporters in human intestinal cells: comparison between human segments and Caco-2 cells. *Eur J Pharm Sci,* Vol.28, No.4, pp. 291-299.

Shargel, L. & Yu, A. B. C. (1999). *Applied Biopharmaceutics and Pharmacokinetics.* Appleton and Lange, Stamford.

Shimizu, M., Fuse, K., Okudaira, K., Nishigaki, R., Maeda, K., Kusuhara, H. & Sugiyama, Y. (2005). Contribution of OATP (organic anion-transporting polypeptide) family transporters to the hepatic uptake of fexofenadine in humans. *Drug Metab Dispos,* Vol.33, No.10, pp. 1477-1481.

Shimpi, S., Chauhan, B. & Shimpi, P. (2005). Cyclodextrins: application in different routes of drug administration. *Acta. Pharm.*, Vol.55, No.2, pp. 139-156.

Shirasaka, Y., Kuraoka, E., Spahn-Langguth, H., Nakanishi, T., Langguth, P. & Tamai, I. Species difference in the effect of grapefruit juice on intestinal absorption of talinolol between human and rat. *J Pharmacol Exp Ther*, Vol.332, No.1, pp. 181-189.

Singhal, D. & Curatolo, W. (2004). Drug polymorphism and dosage form design: a practical perspective. *Adv. Drug Deliv. Rev.*, Vol.56, No.3, pp. 335-347.

Sjökvist, E., Nyström, C. & Aldén, M. (1989). Physicochemical aspects of drug release. IX. Investigation of some factors that impair dissolution of drugs from solid particulate dispersion systems *Int. J. Pharm.*, Vol.54, No.2, pp. 161-170

Staud, F. & Pavek, P. (2005). Breast cancer resistance protein (BCRP/ABCG2). *Int J Biochem Cell Biol*, Vol.37, No.4, pp. 720-725.

Stouch, T. R. & Gudmundsson, O. (2002). Progress in understanding the structure-activity relationships of P-glycoprotein. *Adv Drug Deliv Rev*, Vol.54, No.3, pp. 315-328.

Strickley, R. G. (2004). Solubilizing excipients in oral and injectable formulations. *Pharm. Res.*, Vol.21, No.2, pp. 201-230.

Strocchi, A., Corazza, G., Furne, J., Fine, C., Di Sario, A., Gasbarrini, G. & Levitt, M. D. (1996). Measurements of the jejunal unstirred layer in normal subjects and patients with celiac disease. *Am J Physiol*, Vol.270, No.3 Pt 1, pp. G487-491.

Taipalensuu, J., Tornblom, H., Lindberg, G., Einarsson, C., Sjoqvist, F., Melhus, H., Garberg, P., Sjostrom, B., Lundgren, B. & Artursson, P. (2001). Correlation of gene expression of ten drug efflux proteins of the ATP-binding cassette transporter family in normal human jejunum and in human intestinal epithelial Caco-2 cell monolayers. *J Pharmacol Exp Ther*, Vol.299, No.1, pp. 164-170.

Takano, M., Yumoto, R. & Murakami, T. (2006). Expression and function of efflux drug transporters in the intestine. *Pharmacol Ther*, Vol.109, No.1-2, pp. 137-161.

Tamai, I., Nezu, J., Uchino, H., Sai, Y., Oku, A., Shimane, M. & Tsuji, A. (2000). Molecular identification and characterization of novel members of the human organic anion transporter (OATP) family. *Biochem Biophys Res Commun*, Vol.273, No.1, pp. 251-260.

Terada, T., Saito, H., Mukai, M. & Inui, K. (1997). Characterization of stably transfected kidney epithelial cell line expressing rat H+/peptide cotransporter PEPT1: localization of PEPT1 and transport of beta-lactam antibiotics. *J Pharmacol Exp Ther*, Vol.281, No.3, pp. 1415-1421.

Thiebut, F., Tsuruo, T., Hamada, H., Gottesman, M. M. & Pastan, I. (1987). Celluar localisation of the multidrug resistance gene product P-glycoprotien in normal human tissues. *Proc. National. Acad. Sci. USA*, Vol.84, pp. 7735-7738.

Thomas, V. H., Bhattachar, S., Hitchingham, L., Zocharski, P., Naath, M., Surendran, N., Stoner, C. L. & El-Kattan, A. (2006). The road map to oral bioavailability: an industrial perspective. *Expert Opin Drug Metab Toxicol*, Vol.2, No.4, pp. 591-608.

Thomas, V. H., Bhattachar, S., Hitchingham, L., Zocharski, P., Naath, M., Surendran, N., Stoner, C. L. & El-Kattan, A. (2006). The road map to oral bioavailability: An industrial perspective. *Expert Opin. Drug Metab. Toxicol.*, Vol.2, No.4, pp. 591-608.

Thummel, K. E. (2007). Gut instincts: CYP3A4 and intestinal drug metabolism. *J Clin Invest*, Vol.117, No.11, pp. 3173-3176.

Trevaskis, N. L., Lo, C. M., Ma, L. Y., Tso, P., Irving, H. R., Porter, C. J. & Charman, W. N. (2006). An acute and coincident increase in FABP expression and lymphatic lipid and drug transport occurs during intestinal infusion of lipid-based drug formulations to rats. *Pharm. Res.*, Vol.23, No.8, pp. 1786-1796.

Trevaskis, N. L., Porter, C. J. & Charman, W. N. (2005). Bile increases intestinal lymphatic drug transport in the fasted rat. *Pharm. Res.*, Vol.22, No.11, pp. 1863-1870.

Trevaskis, N. L., Porter, C. J. & Charman, W. N. (2006). The lymph lipid precursor pool is a key determinant of intestinal lymphatic drug transport. *J. Pharmacol. Exp. Ther.*, Vol.316, No.2, pp. 881-891.

Tsuji, A. & Tamai, I. (1996). Carrier-mediated intestinal transport of drugs. *Pharm Res*, Vol.13, No.7, pp. 963-977.

van De Waterbeemd, H., Smith, D. A., Beaumont, K. & Walker, D. K. (2001). Property-based design: optimization of drug absorption and pharmacokinetics. *J. Med. Chem.*, Vol.44, No.9, pp. 1313-1333.

Van Gelder, J., Shafiee, M., De Clercq, E., Penninckx, F., Van den Mooter, G., Kinget, R. & Augustijns, P. (2000). Species-dependent and site-specific intestinal metabolism of ester prodrugs. *Int. J. Pharm.*, Vol.205, No.1-2, pp. 93-100.

van Waterschoot, R. A., Rooswinkel, R. W., Sparidans, R. W., van Herwaarden, A. E., Beijnen, J. H. & Schinkel, A. H. (2009). Inhibition and stimulation of intestinal and hepatic CYP3A activity: studies in humanized CYP3A4 transgenic mice using triazolam. *Drug Metab Dispos*, Vol.37, No.12, pp. 2305-2313.

Varma, M. V., Ambler, C. M., Ullah, M., Rotter, C. J., Sun, H., Litchfield, J., Fenner, K. S. & El-Kattan, A. F. (2010). Targeting intestinal transporters for optimizing oral drug absorption. *Curr Drug Metab*, Vol.11, No.9, pp. 730-742.

Varma, M. V., Obach, R. S., Rotter, C., Miller, H. R., Chang, G., Steyn, S. J., El-Kattan, A. & Troutman, M. D. (2010). Physicochemical space for optimum oral bioavailability: contribution of human intestinal absorption and first-pass elimination. *J Med Chem*, Vol.53, No.3, pp. 1098-1108.

Varma, M. V., Rotter, C. J., Chupka, J., Whalen, K. M., Duignan, D. B., Feng, B., Litchfield, J., Goosen, T. C. & El-Kattan, A. (Accepted). pH-Sensitive Interaction of HMG CoA Reductase Inhibitors (Statins) With Organic Anion Transporting Polypeptide 2B1. *Molecular Pharmaceutics*.

Varma, M. V. S., Ashokraj, Y., Dey, C. S. & Panchagnula, R. (2003). P-glycoprotein inhibitors and their screening: a perspective from bioavailability enhancement. *Pharmacol Res*, Vol.48, pp. 347-359.

Varma, M. V. S., Khandavilli, S., Ashokraj, Y., Jain, A., Dhanikula, A., Sood, A., Thomas, N. S., Pillai, O. P., Sharma, P., Gandhi, R., Agrawal, S., Nair, V. & Panchagnula, R. (2004a). Biopharmaceutic classification system:A scientific framework for pharmacokinetic optimization in drug research. *Curr Drug Metab*, Vol.5, pp. 375-388.

Wacher, V. J., Salphati, L. & Benet, L. Z. (2001). Active secretion and enterocytic drug metabolism barriers to drug absorption. *Adv Drug Deliv Rev*, Vol.46, No.1-3, pp. 89-102.

Watanabe, K., Sawano, T., Endo, T., Sakata, M. & Sato, J. (2002). Studies on intestinal absorption of sulpiride (2): transepithelial transport of sulpiride across the human intestinal cell line Caco-2. *Biol Pharm Bull*, Vol.25, No.10, pp. 1345-1350.

Watanabe, K., Sawano, T., Jinriki, T. & Sato, J. (2004). Studies on intestinal absorption of sulpiride (3): intestinal absorption of sulpiride in rats. *Biol Pharm Bull*, Vol.27, No.1, pp. 77-81.

Watanabe, K., Sawano, T., Terada, K., Endo, T., Sakata, M. & Sato, J. (2002). Studies on intestinal absorption of sulpiride (1): carrier-mediated uptake of sulpiride in the human intestinal cell line Caco-2. *Biol Pharm Bull*, Vol.25, No.7, pp. 885-890.

Westphal, K., Weinbrenner, A., Zschiesche, M., Franke, G., Knoke, M., Oertel, R., Fritz, P., von Richter, O., Warzok, R., Hachenberg, T., Kauffmann, H. M., Schrenk, D., Terhaag, B., Kroemer, H. K. & Siegmund, W. (2000). Induction of P-glycoprotein by rifampin increases intestinal secretion of talinolol in human beings: a new type of drug/drug interaction. *Clin Pharmacol Ther*, Vol.68, No.4, pp. 345-355.

Wilson, M. C., Meredith, D., Bunnun, C., Sessions, R. B. & Halestrap, A. P. (2009). Studies on the DIDS-binding Site of Monocarboxylate Transporter 1 Suggest a Homology Model of the Open Conformation and a Plausible Translocation Cycle. *Journal of Biological Chemistry*, Vol.284, No.30, pp. 20011-20021.

Wilson, M. C., Meredith, D., Fox, J. E. M., Manoharan, C., Davies, A. J. & Halestrap, A. P. (2005). Basigin (CD147) Is the Target for Organomercurial Inhibition of Monocarboxylate Transporter Isoforms 1 and 4: The ancillary protein for the pCMBS insensitive MCT2 is embigin (gp70). *J Biol Chem*, Vol.280, No.29, pp. 27213-27221.

Winne, D. (1976). Unstirred layer thickness in perfused rat jejunum in vivo. *Experientia*, Vol.32, No.10, pp. 1278-1279.

Wu, C. Y. & Benet, L. Z. (2005). Predicting drug disposition via application of BCS: transport/absorption/ elimination interplay and development of a biopharmaceutics drug disposition classification system. *Pharm. Res.*, Vol.22, No.1, pp. 11-23.

Yamagata, T., Kusuhara, H., Morishita, M., Takayama, K., Benameur, H. & Sugiyama, Y. (2007). Improvement of the oral drug absorption of topotecan through the inhibition of intestinal xenobiotic efflux transporter, breast cancer resistance protein, by excipients. *Drug Metab Dispos*, Vol.35, No.7, pp. 1142-1148.

Yamasaki, Y., Ieiri, I., Kusuhara, H., Sasaki, T., Kimura, M., Tabuchi, H., Ando, Y., Irie, S., Ware, J., Nakai, Y., Higuchi, S. & Sugiyama, Y. (2008). Pharmacogenetic characterization of sulfasalazine disposition based on NAT2 and ABCG2 (BCRP) gene polymorphisms in humans. *Clin Pharmacol Ther*, Vol.84, No.1, pp. 95-103.

Yoshikawa, M., Ikegami, Y., Hayasaka, S., Ishii, K., Ito, A., Sano, K., Suzuki, T., Togawa, T., Yoshida, H., Soda, H., Oka, M., Kohno, S., Sawada, S., Ishikawa, T. & Tanabe, S. (2004). Novel camptothecin analogues that circumvent ABCG2-associated drug resistance in human tumor cells. *Int J Cancer*, Vol.110, No.6, pp. 921-927.

Zaher, H., Khan, A. A., Palandra, J., Brayman, T. G., Yu, L. & Ware, J. A. (2006). Breast cancer resistance protein (Bcrp/abcg2) is a major determinant of sulfasalazine absorption and elimination in the mouse. *Mol Pharm*, Vol.3, No.1, pp. 55-61.

Zaher, H., Khan, A. A., Palandra, J., Brayman, T. G., Yu, L. & Ware, J. A. (2006). Breast cancer resistance protein (Bcrp/abcg2) is a major determinant of sulfasalazine absorption and elimination in the mouse. *Mol. Pharm.*, Vol.3, No.1, pp. 55-61.

Zhou, H. (2003). Pharmacokinetic strategies in deciphering atypical drug absorption profiles. *J. Clin. Pharmacol.*, Vol.43, No.3, pp. 211-227.

3

Phase II Drug Metabolism

Petra Jančová[1] and Michal Šiller[2]
[1]*Department of Environmental Protection Engineering, Faculty of Technology,*
Tomas Bata University, Zlin,
[2]*Department of Pharmacology and Institute of Molecular and Translational Medicine,*
Faculty of Medicine and Dentistry, Palacky University, Olomouc,
Czech Republic

1. Introduction

All organisms are constantly and unavoidably exposed to xenobiotics including both man-made and natural chemicals such as drugs, plant alkaloids, microorganism toxins, pollutants, pesticides, and other industrial chemicals. Formally, biotransformation of xenobiotics as well as endogenous compounds is subdivided into phase I and phase II reactions. This chapter focuses on phase II biotransformation reactions (also called ´conjugation reactions´) which generally serve as a detoxifying step in metabolism of drugs and other xenobiotics as well as endogenous substrates. On the other hand, these conjugations also play an essential role in the toxicity of many chemicals due to the metabolic formation of toxic metabolites such as reactive electrophiles. Gene polymorphism of biotransformation enzymes may often play a role in various pathophysiological processes. Conjugation reactions usually involve metabolite activation by a high-energy intermediate and have been classified into two general types: type I (e.g., glucuronidation and sulfonation), in which an activated conjugating agent combines with substrate to yield the conjugated product, and type II (e.g., amino acid conjugation), in which the substrate is activated and then combined with an amino acid to yield a conjugated product (Hodgson, 2004). In this chapter, we will concentrate on the most important conjugation reactions, namely glucuronide conjugation, sulfoconjugation, acetylation, amino acid conjugation, glutathione conjugation and methylation.

2. Phase II reactions

2.1 Glucuronidation

UDP-glucuronosyltransferases (UGTs) belong among the key enzymes of metabolism of various exogenous as well as endogenous compounds. Conjugation reactions catalyzed by the superfamily of these enzymes serve as the most important detoxification pathway for broad spectrum of drugs, dietary chemicals, carcinogens and their oxidized metabolites, and other various environmental chemicals in all vertebrates. Furthermore, UGTs are involved in the regulation of several active endogenous compounds such as bile acids or hydroxysteroids due to their inactivation via glucuronidation (Miners & McMackenzie, 1991; Kiang et al., 2005). In humans, almost 40-70% of clinically used drugs are subjected to glucuronidation (Wells et al., 2004). In general, UGTs mediate the addition of UDP-hexose to nucleophilic atom (O-, N-, S- or C- atom) in the acceptor molecule (Mackenzie et al., 2008). The UDP–glucuronic acid is the most important co-substrate involved in the conjugation reactions (called glucuronidation) carried out by UGTs. Newly formed β–D–glucuronides exhibit increased water-solubility and are easily eliminated from the body in urine or bile. The scheme of typical glucuronidation reactions is shown in Figure 1. Glucuronidation O–linked moieties (acyl, phenolic, hydroxy) predominates the diversity in substrate recognition, and all of the UGTs are capable of forming O–linked glucuronides, albeit with different efficiencies and turn–over rates (Tukey & Strassburg, 2000). UGTs are membrane–bound enzymes similarly to cytochromes P450 with subcellular localization in the endoplasmic reticulum (ER). In contrast to cytochromes P450, the active site of these enzymes is embedded in the lumenal part of ER.

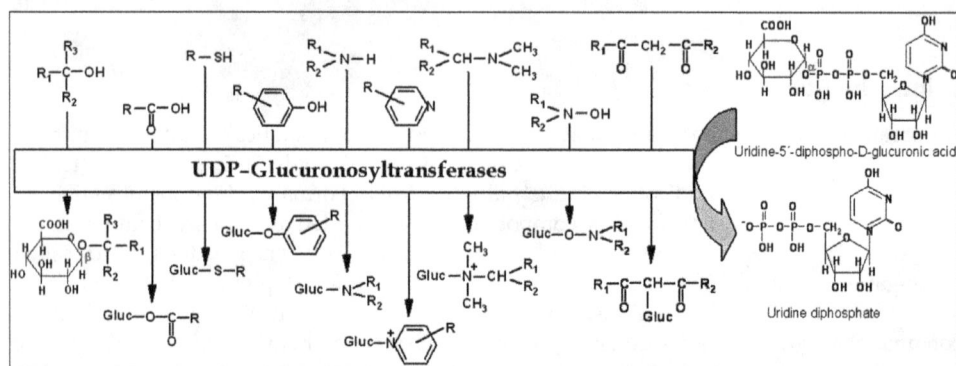

Fig. 1. Glucuronides formation. The summary of chemical structures commonly subjected to glucuronidation.

2.1.1 Human forms of UGTs and their tissue distribution

To date, the mammalian *UGT* gene superfamily comprises of 117 members. Four UGT families have been identified in humans: UGT1, UGT2 involving UGT2A and UGT2B subfamily, UGT3 and UGT8. Enzymes included in the UGT1 and UGT2 subfamily are responsible for the glucuronidation of exo– and endogenous compounds, whereas members of the UGT3 and UGT8 subfamilies have their distinct functions (See section *Substrates of UGTs, inhibition, induction*) (Mackenzie et al., 2008). The members of the UGT1A subfamily have been found to be identical in their terminal carboxyl 245 amino acids, which are encoded by exons 2–5. Only the uniqueness of first exon in the *UGT1A* subfamily genes differentiates one enzyme from each other. In contrast to the UGT1A subfamily, the members of the *UGT2* gene subfamily contain a different set of exons (Tukey & Strassburg, 2000). The UGT enzymes of each family share at least 40% homology in DNA sequence, whereas members of UGT subfamilies exert at least 60% identity in DNA sequence (Burchell et al., 1995). As of the time of writing, 22 human UGT proteins can be distinguished: UGT1A1, UGT1A3, UGT1A4, UGT1A5, UGT1A6, UGT1A7, UGT1A8, UGT1A9, UGT1A10, UGT2A1, UGT2A2, UGT2A3, UGT2B4, UGT2B7, UGT2B10, UGT2B11, UGT2B15, UGT2B17, UGT2B28, UGT3A1, UGT3A2, and UGT8A1 (Mackenzie et al., 2008; Miners et al., 2006; Court et al., 2004; Patten, 2006; Sneitz et al., 2009). In general, human UGT enzymes apparently exhibit a broad tissue distribution, although the liver is the major site of expression for many UGTs. The UGT1A1, UGT1A3, UGT1A4, UGT1A6, UGT1A9, UGT2B7, and UGT2B15 belong among the main liver xenobiotic–conjugating enzymes, whereas UGT1A7, UGT1A8, and UGT1A10 are predominantly extrahepatic UGT forms. Moreover, glucuronidation activity was also detected in other tissues such as kidney (Sutherland et al., 1993), brain (King et al.,1999), or placenta (Collier et al., 2002).

2.1.2 UGTs substrates. Inhibition and induction of UGTs

First of all, the fact that most xenobiotic metabolising UGTs show overlapping substrate specificities should be noted. Two UGTs, namely UGT8A1 and UGT3A1, stand apart from other UGT enzymes since they possess specific functions in the body. UGT8A1 takes part in the biosynthesis of glycosphingolipids, cerebrosides, and sulfatides of nerve cells (Bosio et al., 1996). Recently, the UGT3A1 enzyme has been shown to have a certain role in the metabolism of ursodeoxycholic acid used in therapy of cholestasis or gallstones (Mackenzie et al., 2008). Although many substrates (therapeutic drugs, environmental chemicals) are glucuronidated by multiple UGTs, several compounds exhibit a relative specificity towards individual UGT enzymes. Bilirubin is exclusively metabolised by UGT1A1 (Wang et al., 2006). Conjugation reactions by the UGT2B7 enzyme constitute an important step in the metabolism of opioids (Coffman et al., 1998). Carboxylic acids including several non-steroidal anti–inflammatory agents are conjugated mainly by UGT1A3, UGT1A4, UGT1A9, and UGT2B7 (Tukey & Strassburg, 2000). Acetaminophen (paracetamol) is glucuronidated predominantly by UGTs of the UGT1A subfamily (UGT1A1, UGT1A6, and UGT1A9) (Court et al., 2001). Despite the fact that in most cases UGTs are responsible for O–glucuronidation of their substrates, members of the UGT1A subfamily have been found to catalyze N–glucuronidation of several amine–containing substrates (chlorpromazine, amitryptyline) (Tukey & Strassburg, 2000). The intestinal UGT1A8 and UGT1A10 enzymes were suggested to have a negative impact on the bioavailability of orally administered therapeutic drugs (Mizuma, 2009). For example, raloxifene, a selective estrogen receptor modulator used in therapy of osteoporosis, naturally has a low bioavailability and has also been shown to be extensively metabolised by UGT1A8 and UGT1A10 (Kemp et al., 2002). UGTs might also play a significant role in the inactivation of carcinogens from diet or cigarette smoke (Dellinger et al., 2006). Hanioka et al. (2008) proposed that the glucuronidation of bisphenol A (an environmental endocrine disruptor) by UGT2B15 serves as a major detoxification pathway of this molecule. UGTs are notably inhibited by various compounds. Analgesics, non–steroidal anti–inflammatory drugs (NSAIDs), anxiolytics, anticonvulsants, or antiviral agents have been shown to have possible inhibitory effect on the enzymatic activities of various UGTs (thoroughly reviewed by Kiang et al., 2005). Recently, non–steroidal anti-inflammatory drugs have been shown to partially impair an equilibrium between biological functioning and degradation of aldosterone due to involvement of renal UGT2B7 in both the glucuronidation of aldosterone (deactivation) and the glucuronidation of NSAIDs (Knights et al., 2009). Similarly to other drug metabolising enzymes, UGTs are subject to induction by various xenobiotics or biologically active endogenous compounds (hormones) via nuclear receptors and transcription factors. For example, the aryl hydrocarbon receptor plays role in induction of UGT1A1 while the activation of pregnane X receptor and the constitutive androstane receptor leads to induction of UGT1A6 and UGT1A9 (Lin & Wong, 2002; Mackenzie et al., 2003; Xie et al., 2003). Several classes of drugs including analgesics, antivirals, or anticonvulsants are suspected to act as human UGTs inducers.

2.1.3 Genetic polymorphism in UGTs

Many human UGT enzymes were found to be genetically polymorphic. The mutations in *UGT1A1* gene result in several syndromes connected with decreased bilirubin detoxification capacity of UGT1A1. Kadakol et al. (2000) summed up data about more than 50 mutations of UGT1A1 causing Crigler–Najjar syndrome type I and type II. Patients suffering from type I, also called congenital familial nonhemolytic jaundice with kernicterus, completely lack the UGT1A1 enzymatic activity resulting in toxic effects of bilirubin on the central nervous system. The most common deficiency of UGT1A1 enzyme is Gilbert's syndrome. 2–12% of the population suffer from this benign disorder characterized by intermittent unconjugated hyperbilirubinemia. In most cases, this syndrome is caused by a mutation in the promotor region of *UGT1A1* gene (Monaghan et al., 1996). Increased toxicity of a pharmacologically active metabolite of irinotecan (SN-38) has been described in patients suffering from Gilbert's syndrome as UGT1A1 is the main enzyme responsible for the formation of the inactive SN–38 glucuronide (Wasserman et al., 1997). The genetic variability in the *UGT1* or *UGT2* gene families was also suggested to alter risk of cancer either as a result of decreased inactivation of hormones such as estrogens or due to reduced detoxification of environmental carcinogens and their reactive metabolites (Guillemette, 2003).

2.2 Sulfoconjugation

Sulfoconjugation (or sulfonation) constitutes an important pathway in the metabolism of numerous both exogenous and endogenous compounds. The sulfonation reaction was first recognized by Baumann in 1876. Baumann detected phenyl sulfate in the urine of a patient who had been administered phenol. The sulfonation reactions are mediated by a supergene family of enzymes called sulfotransferases (SULTs). In general, these enzymes catalyze the transfer of sulfonate (SO_3^-) from the universal sulfonate donor 3'–phosphoadenosine 5'–phosphosulfate (PAPS) to the hydroxyl or amino group of an acceptor molecule, Fig. 2. The incorrect term sulfation is sometimes used since sulfated products are formed in this type of reactions. PAPS is a universal donor of sulfonate moiety in sulfonation reactions and has been shown to by synthesized by almost all tissues in mammals from inorganic sulfate (Klaassen & Boles, 1997). Depletion of PAPS due to lack of inorganic sulfate or due to genetic defects of enzymes participating in PAPS synthesis may lead to reducing of sulfonation capacity which could affect the metabolism of xenobiotics or disrupt the equilibrium between synthesis and degradation of active endogenous compounds.

To date, two large groups of SULTs have been identified. The first group includes membrane–bound enzymes with no demonstrated xenobiotic–metabolising activity. These enzymes are localized in the Golgi apparatus and they are involved in metabolism of endogenous peptides, proteins, glycosaminoglycans, and lipids (Habuchi, 2000). Cytosolic SULTs constitute the second group of sulfotransferases and play a major role in conjugation of a broad spectrum of xenobiotics including environmental chemicals, natural compounds, drugs (Gamage et al., 2006) as well as endogenous compounds such as steroid hormones, iodothyronines, catecholamines, eicosanoids, retinol or vitamin D (Glatt & Meinl, 2004). Moreover, cytosolic SULTs are presumed to play a crucial role in the detoxification processes occurring in the developing human fetus since no UGTs transcripts have been detected in fetal liver at 20 weeks of gestation (Strassburg et al., 2002). Sulfonation is generally described as a detoxification pathway for many xenobiotics. Addition of the sulfonate moiety to the molecule of a parent compound or most often to the molecule of its metabolite originating in the oxidative phase of drug metabolism leads to formation of a water–soluble compound which is then easily eliminated from the body. However, in several cases the sulfonation reaction can lead to formation of a more active metabolite compared to the parent compound as is the case for the hair follicle stimulant minoxidil (Buhl et al., 1990) or the diuretic agent triamterene (Mutschler et al., 1983). Furthermore, the role of sulfotransferases in the activation of various procarcinogens and promutagens was confirmed (Gilissen et al., 1994).

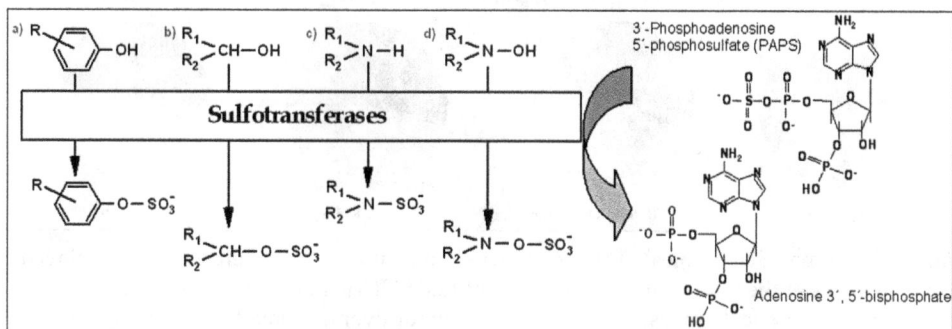

Fig. 2. The formation of sulfates (R–O–SO$_3^-$) and sulfamates (R$_1$–NR$_2$–SO$_3^-$). These reactions are catalyzed by 3'–phosphoadenosine 5'–phosphosulfate (PAPS)–dependent sulfotransferases.

2.2.1 Human forms of cytosolic SULTs and tissue distribution

In the following text we will focus only on cytosolic sulfotransferases, since this enzyme superfamily plays a key role in the biotransformation of multiple xenobiotics as well as endogenous substrates. Recently, a nomenclature system for the superfamily of cytosolic SULTs has been established analogously to those of other drug metabolising enzymes such as cytochromes P450 or UDP-glucuronosyltranferases (Blanchard et al., 2004). The superfamily of cytosolic sulfotransferases is subsequently divided into families and subfamilies according to the amino acid sequence identity among individual SULTs. In detail, members of one SULTs family share at least 45% amino acid sequence identity, whereas SULTs subfamily involves individual members with at least 60% identity. To date, four human SULT families, SULT1, SULT2, SULT4 and SULT6, have been identified. These SULT families include at least 13 different members. The SULT1 family comprises of 9 members divided into 4 subfamilies (1A1, 1A2, 1A3, 1A4, 1B1, 1C1, 1C2, 1C3 and 1E1). SULT2A (SULT2A1) and SULT2B (SULT2B1a and SULT2B1b) belong to SULT2 family. The SULT4A1 and SULT6B1 are the only members of the SULT4 and SULT6 family, respectively (Lindsay et al., 2008). Cytosolic sulfotransferases exert relatively broad tissue distribution. The members of SULT1A family were found in liver, brain, breast, intestine, jejunum, lung, adrenal gland, endometrium, placenta, kidney and in blood platelets. Figure 3 displays SULT expression "pies" of the most important human cytosolic transferases in human tissues. SULT1A1 is predominantly expressed in the liver (Hempel et al., 2007). In contrast to SULT1A1, the SULT1A3 enzyme was not detected in human adult liver. SULT1B1 has been found in liver, small intestine, colon, and leukocytes (Wang et al., 1998). Members of

SULT1C subfamily were identified in fetal human tissues such as liver (Hehonah et al., 1999) or lung and kidney (Sakakibara et al., 1998) as well as in adult human stomach (Her et al., 1997). The predominant expression of SULT1E1 was found in human liver and jejunum (Riches et al., 2009). Major sites of SULT2A1 expression are the liver, adrenal gland, ovary, and duodenum (Javitt et al., 2001). Members of SULT2B subfamily are localized in human prostate, placenta, adrenal gland, ovary, lung, kidney, and colon (Glatt & Meinl, 2004). Recently, an exclusive localization of human SULT4A1 in the brain was confirmed (Falany et al., 2000).

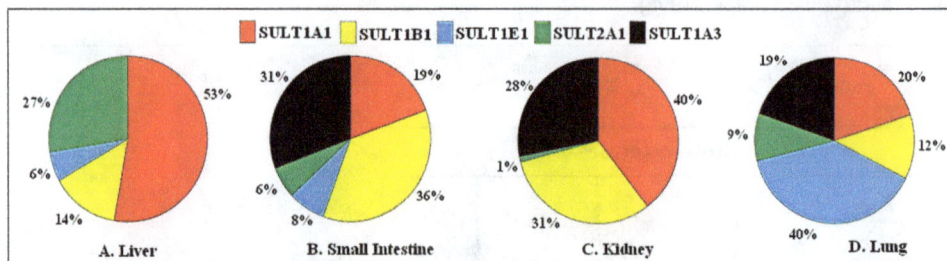

Fig. 3. The human SULT "pies". The mean expression values for each enzyme are displayed as percentages of the total sum of immunoquantified SULTs (maximum five enzymes) present in each tissue. Expression values are shown for liver (A), small intestine (B), kidney (C), and lung (D) (Riches et al., 2009).

2.2.2 Substrates of SULTs

SULT1A1 has been shown to be one of the most important sulfotransferases participating in metabolism of xenobiotics in humans. It has also been termed phenol sulfotransferase (P-PST) or thermostable phenol sulfotransferase (TS PST1). In general, SULT1A1 is responsible for sulfoconjugation of phenolic compounds such as monocyclic phenols, naphtols, benzylic alcohols, aromatic amines or hydroxylamines (Glatt & Meinl, 2004). Acetaminophen, minoxidil as well as dopamine or iodothyronines undergo sulfonation by SULT1A1. SULT1A1 also takes part in transformation of hydroxymethyl polycyclic aromatic hydrocarbons, N–hydroxyderivatives of arylamines, allylic alcohols and heterocyclic amines to their reactive intermediates which are able to bind to nucleophilic structures such as DNA and consequently act as mutagens and carcinogens (Glatt et al., 2001). SULT1A2 also plays an important role in the toxification of several aromatic hydroxylamines (Meinl et al., 2002). SULT1A3, formerly known as thermolabile phenol SULT (TL PST) or monoamine sulfotransferase, exhibits high affinity for catecholamines (dopamine) and contributes to the regulation of the rapidly fluctuating levels of neurotransmitters. The human SULT1B1 was isolated and described by Fujita et al. (1997) and was shown to be the most important sulfotransferase in thyroid hormone metabolism. SULT1E1 plays a key role in estrogen homeostasis. This enzyme conjugates 17β–estradiol and other estrogens in a step leading to their inactivation. Since 17β–estradiol and relative compounds regulate various processes occurring in humans, inactivation of these compounds by the SULT1E1 enzyme constitute an important step in the prevention and development of certain diseases. Down regulation or loss of SULT1E1 could be to a certain extent responsible for growth of tumor in hormone sensitive cancers such as breast or endometrial cancer (Cole et al., 2010). SULT2A and SULT2B subfamilies include the hydroxysteroid sulfotransferases with partially overlapping substrate specifities. SULT2A1 is also termed as dehydroepiandrosterone sulfotransferase (DHEA ST) and conjugates various hydroxysteroids such as DHEA, androgens, bile acids and oestrone (Comer et al., 1993). Recently, a role of SULT2A1 in metabolism of quinolone drugs in humans was confirmed (Senggunprai et al., 2009). Clinically relevant substrates for other cytosolic sulfotransferases have not been identified yet.

2.2.3 Genetic polymorphisms in SULTs

Genetic polymorphism was detected in many SULT forms such as the SULT1A1, SULT1A3, SULT1C2, SULT2A1, SULT2A3 and SULT2B1 enzyme (Lindsay et al., 2008). Single nucleotide polymorphism in the *SULT1A1* gene leading to an $Arg_{213} \rightarrow$ His amino acid substitution is relatively frequent in the Caucasian population (25.4–36.5%) (Glatt & Meinl, 2004). This mutation results in a variation of SULT1A1 thermal stability and enzymatic activity. Several authors have claimed that SULT1A1 polymorphism might play a role in the pathophysiology of lung cancer (Arslan et al., 2009), urothelial carcinoma (Huang, 2009), and meningiomal brain tumors (Bardakci, 2008).

2.3 Glutathione S–conjugation

Since the first detection of glutathione transferase activity in rat liver cytosol by Booth in the early 1960s, the family of glutathione transferases (synonymously glutathione S–transferases; GSTs) has been studied in detail. Undoubtedly, the members of glutathione transferase family play an important role in metabolism of certain therapeutics, detoxification of environmental carcinogens and reactive intermediates formed from various chemicals by other xenobiotic–metabolising enzymes. Furthermore, GSTs constitute an important intracellular defence against oxidative stress and they appear to be involved in synthesis and metabolism of several derivatives of arachidonic acid and steroids (van Bladeren, 2000). On the other hand, various chemicals have been shown to be activated into potentially dangerous compounds by these enzymes (Sherratt et al., 1997). In general, these enzymes catalyze a nucleophilic attack of reduced glutathione on lipophilic compounds containing an electrophilic atom (C–, N– or S–). In addition to nucleophilic substitutions, these transferases also account for Michael additions, isomerations, and hydroxyperoxide reductions. In most cases, more polar glutathione conjugates are eliminated into the bile or are subsequently subjected to other metabolic steps eventually leading to formation of mercapturic acids. Figure 4 shows the sequential steps in the synthesis of mercapturic acids. Mercapturic acids are excreted from the body in urine (Commandeur et al., 1995). For instance, industrial chemicals such as acrylamide or trichloroethylene are detoxified via mercapturic acids (Boettcher et al., 2005; Popp et al., 1994).

2.3.1 Differentiation of GSTs, their cellular localization and tissue distribution

Up to now, two different superfamilies of GSTs have been described. The first one includes soluble dimeric enzymes localized mainly in cytosole but certain members of this superfamily have been also identified in mitochondria (Robinson et al., 2004) or in peroxisomes (Morel et al., 2004). The superfamily of human soluble GSTs is further divided into eight separate classes: Alpha (A1–A4), Kappa (K1), Mu (M1–M5), Pi (P1), Sigma (S1), Theta (T1–T2), Zeta (Z1) and Omega (O1–O2) (Hayes et al., 2005). Microsomal GSTs designated as the membrane associated proteins in eicosanoid and glutathione metabolism

(MAPEG) consitute the second family of human GSTs. The human MAPEG superfamily includes six members: 5–lipoxygenase activating protein (FLAP), leukotriene C_4 synthase (both involved in leukotriene synthesis), MGST1, MGST2, MGST3 (GSTs as well as glutathione dependent peroxidases) and prostaglandin E synthase (PGES) (Bresell et al., 2005). Both the soluble GSTs and MAPEG exhibit a broad tissue distribution; being found in liver, kidney, brain, lung, heart, pancreas, small intestine, prostate, spleen, and skeletal muscles (Hayes & Strange, 2000).

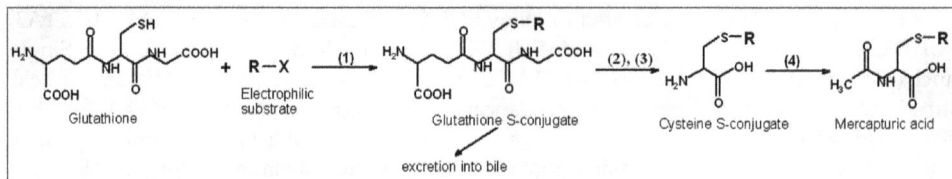

Fig. 4. Formation of mercapturic acid. Glutathione S–transferase (1) catalyzes the conjugation between glutathione and various endogenous or xenobiotic electrophilic compounds. Subsequently, the resulting glutathione S–conjugate is broken down to a cysteine S–conjugate by γ-glutamyltranspeptidase (2) and dipeptidases (3). Finally, cysteine S–conjugate N–acetyltransferase (4) catalyses formation of mercapturic acid.

2.3.2 Substrates of human GSTs

Various electrophilic compounds act as substrates for GSTs. They include a broad spectrum of ketones, quinones, sulfoxides, esters, peroxides, and ozonides (van Bladeren et al., 2000). Chemotherapeutics (such as busulfan, cis–platin, ethacrynic acid, cyclophosphamide, thiotepa); industrial chemicals, herbicides, pesticides (acrolein, lindane, malathion, tridiphane) are detoxified by GSTs (Hayes et al., 2005). Epoxides and other reactive intermediates formed from environmental procarcinogens mostly as a result of metabolism by cytochromes P450 (aflatoxin B_1, polycyclic aromatic hydrocarbons, styrene, benzopyrene, heterocyclic amines) also undergo detoxification by soluble GSTs. Besides their enzymatic activity, cytosolic GSTs (such as class Alpha) exhibit an ability to bind various hydrophobic ligands (xenobiotics as well as hormones) and thus contribute to their intracellular transport and disposition. GSTs play an essential role in the fight against products of oxidative stress which unavoidably damage cell membrane lipids, DNA, or proteins. Reactive intermediates resulting from lipid peroxidation (4–hydroxynonenal), nucleotide peroxidation (adenine propenal) or catecholamine peroxidation (aminochrome, dopachrome, adrenochrome) are particularly inactivated by GSTs (Dagnino–Subiabre et al., 2000). Several specific substrates for GSTs have been identified. For instance, ethacrynic acid has been found to be predominantly metabolised by GSTP1, whereas trans–stilbene oxide is a specific substrate for GSTM1 (van Bladeren, 2000). The GSTT1 enzyme is responsible for conjugation of halogenated organic compounds such as dichlormethane or ethylene–dibromide (Landi, 2000). This step leads to activation of these compounds to their reactive electrophilic metabolites with potential mutagenic and cancerogenic effect. Ethylene–dibromide, a gasoline additive and a fumigant, is presumed to be potential human carcinogen because it is transformed by GSTs to DNA–reacting episulfonium ion (van Bladeren, 2000). The glucocorticoid response element and the xenobiotic response element activated by glucocorticoids and planar aromatic hydrocarbons respectively might play a role in the induction of expression of GSTs (Talalay et al., 1988).

2.3.3 Genetic polymorphism in GSTs

Most members of both glutathione transferase superfamilies have been found to be genetically polymorphic. Several genetic variants of particular GSTs are supposed to contribute to the development of certain cancers or other diseases. Furthermore, genetic polymorphism in GSTs is pressumed to influence metabolism and disposition of various anticancerogenic drugs (Crettol et al., 2010). GSTP1 is responsible for metabolism of alkylating agents, topoisomerase inhibitors, antimetabolites, or tubulin inhibitors used in treatment of cancer. The common allele GSTP1*A is cytoprotective against the toxic effects of chemotherapeutics, whereas the functionally less competent allele GSTP1*B is thought to increase the toxicity of anticancerogenic drugs in patients with this gene variant due to decreased metabolic activity of impaired enzyme. Cyclophosphamide is biotransformed by GSTA1. Defective GSTA1*B allele was associated with increased survival in breast cancer patients treated with cyclophosphamide (Sweeney et al., 2003). On the other hand, several drugs activated by GSTs require a well–functioning enzyme. Patients with the active GSTM1 gene treated for acute myeloid leukemia with doxorubicin had a superior survival rate compared to patients with at least one null allele (Autrup et al., 2002). Individuals with lacking functional GSTM1, GSTT1, and GSTP1 have been shown to have a higher incidence of bladder, breast, colorectal, head/neck, and lung cancer. Genetically–based defects of these enzymes are also noteworthy because of their partial responsibility for increased risk of asthma, allergies, atherosclerosis, and rheumatoid arthritis (van Bladeren, 2000; Hayes et al., 2005).

2.4 Acetylation

Compared to sulfonations and glucuronidations, acetylations are modest in terms of the number and variety of substrates, but remain significant in a toxicological perspective. Drugs and other foreign compounds that are acetylated in intact animals are either aromatic amines or hydrazines, which are converted to aromatic amides and aromatic hydrazides (Parkinson, 2001). Acetylation reactions are characterized by the transfer of an acetyl moiety, the donor generally being acetyl coenzyme A, while the accepting chemical group is a primary amino function. As far as xenobiotic metabolism is concerned, three general reactions of acetylation have been documented, namely N- (Fig. 5a, b), O- (Fig. 5c), and N,O-acetylations (Fig. 5d). N-acetylation of aromatic amine is recognized as a major detoxification pathway in arylamine metabolism in experimental animals and humans (Hein et al., 2000). However, O- and N,O-acetylations occur in alternative metabolic pathways following activation by N-hydroxylation. The resulting N-acetoxyarylamines are highly unstable, spontaneously forming arylnitrenium ions that bind to DNA (Bland & Kadlubar, 1985) and ultimately lead to mutagenesis and carcinogenesis (Kerdar et al., 1993).

2.4.1 N–Acetyltransferases

In humans, acetylation reactions are catalyzed by two N-acetyltransferase isoenzymes (NATs), N-acetyltransferase 1 (NAT1) and 2 (NAT2). NATs are cytosolic enzymes found in many tissues of various species. The human NAT1 and NAT2 genes are located on chromosome 8 pter-q11, and share 87% coding sequence homology (Blum et al., 1990). NAT1 and NAT2 have distinct substrate specificities and differ markedly in terms of organ and tissue distribution. NAT2 protein is present mainly in the liver (Grant et al., 1990) and intestine (Hickman et al., 1998). NAT1 appears to be ubiquitous. Expression of human NAT1

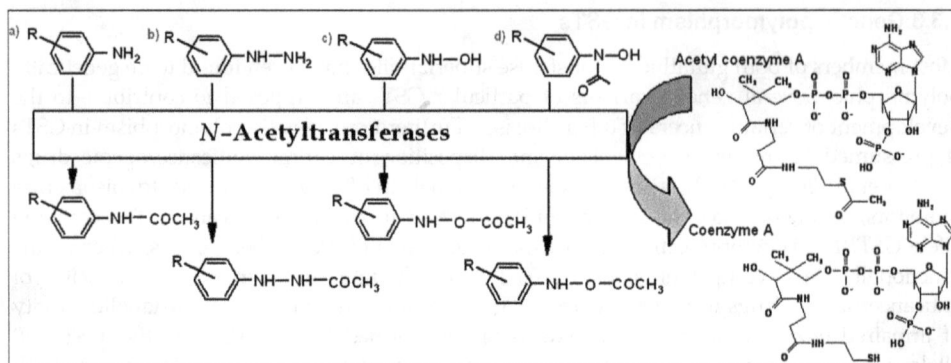

Fig. 5. Reactions catalysed by *N*–acetyltransferases. (a,b) *N*–acetylation of arylamine and arylhydrazine, (c) *O*–acetylation of *N*–arylhydroxylamine, (d) *N*, *O*–acetyltransfer of an *N*–hydroxamic acid. These reactions use acetyl–coenzyme A as acetyl donor.

has been detected in adult liver, bladder, digestive system, blood cells, placenta, skin, skeletal muscles, gingiva (Dupret & Lima, 2005), mammary tissue, prostate, and lung by a number of methods (Sim et al., 2008). A notable difference between the two isoenzymes is the presence of NAT1 activity in fetal and neonatal tissue, such as lungs, kidneys, and adrenal glands (Pacifici et al., 1986). By contrast, NAT2 is not evident until about 12 months after birth (Pariente-Khayat et al., 1991). NAT1 has also been detected in cancer cells, in which it may not only play a role in the development of cancers through enhanced mutagenesis but may also contribute to the resistance of some cancers to cytotoxic drugs (Adam et al., 2003). NATs are involved in the metabolism of a variety of different compounds to which we are exposed on a daily basis. In humans, acetylation is a major route of biotransformation for many arylamine and hydrazine drugs, as well as for a number of known carcinogens present in diet, cigarette smoke, car exhaust fumes, and environment in general. Human NAT1 and human NAT2 have distinct but overlapping substrate profiles and also have specific substrates which can be used as "probe" substrates for each particular isoenzyme. Substrates of NAT1 include *p*-aminobenzoic acid, *p*-aminosalicylic acid, the bacteriostatic antibiotics sulfamethoxazole and sulfanilamide, 2–aminofluorene and caffeine (Ginsberg et al., 2009). Moreover, it has been proposed by Minchin that human NAT1 plays a role in folate metabolism through the acetylation of the folate metabolite *p*-aminobenzoylglutamate (Minchin, 1995). Human NAT2 is a xenobiotic-metabolising enzyme that provides a major route of detoxification of drugs such as isoniazid (an anti-tuberculotic drug), hydralazine and endralazine (anti-hypertensive drugs), a number of sulphonamides (anti-bacterial drugs) (Kawamura et al., 2005), procainamide (anti-arrhythmic drug), aminoglutethimide (an inhibitor of adrenocortical steroid synthesis), nitrazepam (a benzodiazepine) and the anti-inflammatory drug dapsone (Ginsberg et al., 2009; Butcher at al., 2002). Both NAT1 and NAT2 are polymorphic enzymes, with 28 *NAT1* and 64 *NAT2* alleles having been identified to date (see http://louisville.edu/medschool/pharmacology/NAT.html for details of alleles; last update May 24, 2011). *N*-acetylation polymorphism represents one of the oldest and most intensively studied pharmacogenetic traits and refers to hereditary differences concerning the acetylation of drugs and toxicants. The genetic polymorphism in NAT activity was first recognised in tuberculosis patients treated with isoniazid, which is metabolised principally by N-acetylation. The polymorphism causes individual differences in the rate of metabolism of this drug. Individuals with a faster rate are called rapid acetylators and individuals with a slower rate are called slow acetylators. Rapid acetylators were competent in isoniazid acetylation but the drug was cleared less efficiently in the slow acetylator group, which resulted in elevated serum concentration and led to adverse neurologic side effects due to an accumulation of unmetabolized drug (Brockton et al., 2000). Consistent with the toxicity of isoniazid in slow acetylators, there is an increased incidence of other drug toxicities in subjects carrying defective *NAT2* alleles, such as lupus erythematosus in patients treated with hydralazine or procainamide (Sim et al., 1988), and haemolytic anemia and inflammatory bowel disease after treatment with sulfasalazine (Chen et al., 2007). The high frequency of the NAT2 and also NAT1 acetylation polymorphism in human population together with ubiquitous exposure to aromatic and heterocyclic amines suggest that *NAT1* and *NAT2* acetylator genotypes are important modifiers of human cancer susceptibility. Many studies suggested a relationship between acetylation phenotypes (in particular, arising from NAT2 genotypes) and the risk of various cancer including colorectal, liver, breast, prostate, head and neck (Agúndez, 2008) and other disease conditions such as birth defects (Lammer et al., 2004) or neurodegenerative and autoimmune diseases (Ladero, 2008).

2.5 Methylation

Methylation is a common but generally minor pathway of xenobiotic biotransformation. Unlike most other conjugative reactions, methylation often does not dramatically alter the solubility of substrates and results either in inactive or active compounds. Methylation reactions are primarily involved in the metabolism of small endogenous compounds such as neurotransmitters but also play a role in the metabolism of macromolecules for example nucleic acids and in the biotransformation of certain drugs. A large number of both endogenous and exogenous compounds can undergo N- (Fig. 6a), O- (Fig. 6b), S- (Fig. 6c) and arsenic-methylation during their metabolism (Feng et al., 2010). The co-factor required to form methyl conjugates is S-adenosylmethionine (SAM), which is primarily formed by the condensation of ATP and L-methionine.

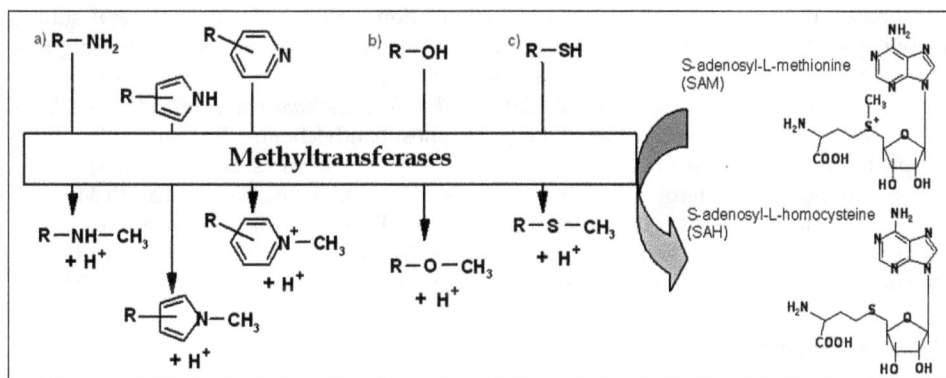

Fig. 6. Methylation reactions catalyzed by methyltransferases.

2.5.1 *N*–methylation

Several *N*–methyltransferases have been described in humans and other mammals; including *indolethylamine N–methyltransferase (INMT)*, which catalyzes the *N*–methylation of tryptamine and structurally related compounds. The INMT exhibits wide tissue distribution. Human INMT was expressed in the lung, thyroid, adrenal gland, heart, and muscle but not in the brain (Thompson et al., 1999). Since INMT is predominantly present in peripheral tissues, its main physiological function is presumably non–neural. *Nicotinamide N–methyltransferase (NNMT)* is a SAM–dependent cytosolic enzyme that catalyzes the *N*–methylation of nicotinamide, pyridines, and other structural analogues. NNMT is predominantly expressed in the liver; expression has been also reported in other tissues such as the kidney, lung, placenta, and heart (Zhang et al., 2010). Several *N*–methylated pyridines are well–established dopaminergic toxins and the NNMT can convert pyridines into toxic compounds (such as 4–phenylpyridine into *N*–methyl–4– phenylpyridinium ion [MPP+]). NNMT has been shown to be present in the human brain, a necessity for neurotoxicity, because charged compounds cannot cross the blood–brain barrier (Williams & Ramsden, 2005). NNMT was one of the potential tumor biomarkers identified in a wide range of tumors such as thyroid, gastric, colorectal, renal, and lung cancer (Zhang et al., 2010). *Histamine N–methyltransferase (HNMT)*, the second most important histamine inactivating enzyme, is a cytosolic enzyme specifically methylating the imidazole ring of histamine and closely related compounds in the intracellular space of cells. Levels of HNMT activity in humans are regulated genetically. HNMT is widely expressed in human tissues; the greatest expression is in the liver and kidney, but also in the spleen, colon, prostate, ovary, brain, bronchi, and trachea (Maintz & Novak, 2007). Common genetic polymorphisms for HNMT might be related to a possible role for individual variation in histamine metabolism in the pathophysiology of diseases such as allergy, asthma, peptic ulcer disease, and some neuropsychiatric illnesses (Preuss et al., 1998). *Phenylethanolamine N–methyltransferase (PNMT)* plays a role in neuroendocrine and blood pressure regulation in the central nervous system. PNMT, the terminal enzyme of the catecholamine biosynthesis pathway, catalyzes the *N*–methylation of the neurotransmitter norepinephrine to form epinephrine (Ji et al., 2005). PNMT is a cytosolic enzyme that is present in many tissues throughout the body, with particularly high concentration in the adrenal medulla, adrenergic neurons in the amygdala and retina and the left atrium of the heart (Haavik et al., 2008). Its activity increases after stress in response to glucocorticoids and neuronal stimulation (Saito et al., 2001). Several studies have suggested that two common *PNMT* promoter single nucleotide polymorphisms might be associated with risk of diseases such as essential hypertension, early–onset Alzheimer's disease, or multiple sclerosis (Ji et al., 2008). *Phosphatidylethanolamine N–methyltransferase (PEMT)* converts phosphatidylethanolamine to phosphatidylcholine in mammalian liver. Phosphatidylcholine is nutrient critical to many cellular processes such as phospholipid biosynthesis, lipid–cholesterol transport, or transmembrane signaling. The human *PEMT* gene encodes for two isoforms of the enzyme, namely PEMT1, which is localized in the endoplasmic reticulum and generating most of the PEMT activity, and PEMT2, a liver specific isoform exclusively localized in mitochondria–associated membranes (Tessitore et al., 2003).

2.5.2 *O*–methylation

The process of *O*–methylation of phenols and catechols is catalyzed by two different enzymes known as phenol *O*–methyltransferase and catechol *O*–methyltransferase. *Phenol*

O–methyltransferase (POMT) is an enzyme that transfers the methyl group of SAM to phenol to form anisole. POMT is a localized in the microsomes of the liver and lungs of mammals but is also present in other tissues. *Catechol O–methyltransferase (COMT)* is a magnesium–dependent enzyme which was first described by Axelrod in 1957. It is an enzyme that plays a key role in the modulation of catechol–dependent functions such as cognition, cardiovascular function, and pain processing. COMT is involved in the inactivation of catecholamine neurotransmitters such as epinephrine, norepinephrine, and dopamine, but also catecholestrogens and catechol drugs such as the anti-Parkinson´s disease agent L–DOPA and the anti–hypertensive methyldopa (Weinshilboum et al., 1999). Two forms of human COMT have been identified, a cytoplasmic soluble form (S–COMT) and a membrane–bound form (MB–COMT) located in the cytosolic side of the rough endoplasmic reticulum The S–COMT is predominantly expressed in the human liver, intestine and kidney (Taskinen et al., 2003), whereas the membrane–bound form is more highly expressed in all regions of the human central nervous system (Tunbridge et al., 2006). A common functional polymorphism at codons 108 and 158 in the genes coding for S–COMT and MB–COMT (COMT Val 108/158 Met), respectively, has been examined in relationship to a number of neurological disorders involving the noradrenergic or dopaminergic systems, such as schizophrenia (Park et al., 2002) or Parkinson's disease (Kunugi et al., 1997). It has also been suggested that a common functional genetic polymorphism in the *COMT* gene may contribute to the etiology of alcoholism (Wang et al., 2001).

2.5.3 *S*–methylation

Thiol methylation is important in the metabolism of many sulfhydryl drugs. Human tissues contain two separate genetically regulated enzymes that can catalyze thiol *S*–methylation. *Thiol methyltransferase (TMT)* is a membrane–bound enzyme that preferentially catalyzes the *S*–methylation of aliphatic sulfhydryl compounds such as captopril and D–penicillamine, whereas *thiopurine S–methyltransferase (TPMT)* is a cytoplasmic enzyme that preferentially catalyzes the *S*–methylation of aromatic and heterocyclic sulfhydryl compounds including anticancer and immunosuppressive thiopurines such as 6–mercaptopurine, 6–thioguanine, and azathioprine. Thiopurine drugs have a relatively narrow therapeutic index and are capable of causing life–threatening toxicity, most often myelosuppression (Sahasranaman et al., 2008). TPMT genetic polymorphism represents a striking example of the clinical importance of pharmacogenetics. In 2010, 29 different variant *TPMT* alleles have been described (Ford & Berg, 2010) and this may be associated with large interindividual variations in thiopurine drug toxicity and therapeutic efficacy. Allele frequencies for genetic polymorphism are such that ~1 in 300 Caucasians is homozygous for a defective allele or alleles for the trait of very low activity, ~11% of people are heterozygous and have intermediate activity. Subjects homozygous for low TPMT activity have a high risk of myelosuppression after treatment with standard dose of azathioprine. Generally, TPMT–deficient patients (homozygous mutant) can be treated with 6–10% of the standard dose of thiopurines (Zhou, 2006). TPMT shows the highest level of expression in liver and kidney and the physiological role of this enzyme, despite extensive investigation, remains unclear.

2.5.4 *As*–methylation

Arsenic is a well–known naturally occurring metaloid which is considered as a multiorgan human carcinogen. Occupational exposure to arsenic occurs in the smelting industry and during the manufacture of pesticides, herbicides, and other agricultural products. Arsenic plays a dual role as environmental carcinogenic pollutant and as a successful anticancer drug against promyelocytic leukemia (Wood et al., 2006). Its metabolism proceeds via a complicated enzymatic pathway, acting both as detoxification and producing more toxic intermediates. Methylation is an important reaction in the biotransformation of arsenic. Liver is considered to be the primary site for the methylation of inorganic arsenic (iAs) and *arsenic (+3 oxidation state) methyltransferase (AS3MT)* is shown to be critical specifically for the arsenic metabolism, and thus may be pharmacologically important as well. Methylated and dimethylated arsenic are the major urinary metabolites in human and many other species (Li et al., 2005). Two reaction schemes (Fig. 7) have been developed to describe the individual steps in the enzymatically catalysed conversion of iAs to methylated metabolites (Thomas, 2007). Although pentavalent methylated arsenicals (MAs^V, DMAs^V, TMAs^V) are less toxic than inorganic ones (iAs^V, iAs^{III}), the trivalent intermediated formed during the methylation process (MAs^{III}, DMAs^{III}) are much more cytotoxic and genotoxic (Hughes, 2009).

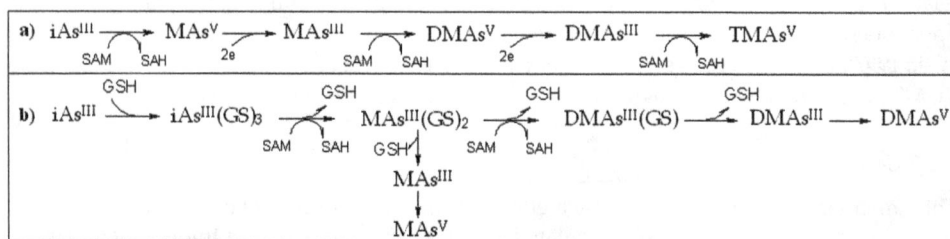

Fig. 7. Alternative schemes for the conversion of inorganic arsenic (iAs) into methylated metabolites. (a) Scheme for the oxidative methylation of arsenicals in which reduction of oxidized arsenicals is interposed between each methylation reaction. (b) Scheme for methylation of arsenic involving formation of arsenic–glutathione (GSH) complex. SAM, *S*–adenosylmethionine; SAH, *S*–adenosylhomocysteine (According to Thomas, 2007).

Several single nucleotide polymorphisms in exons and introns in this gene are reported to be related to inter–individual variation in the arsenic metabolism (Fujihara et al., 2010). Polymorphism in AS3MT may influence arsenic metabolism and potentially susceptibility to its toxic and carcinogenic effects.

2.6 Amino acid conjugation reactions

The first description of glycine conjugation was published in 1842 by Keller. Xenobiotics containing a carboxyl group (–COOH) are widely used as drugs (for example simvastatin, valproic acid, or acetylsalicylic acid), herbicides, insecticides, and food preservatives. In addition, many xenobiotics are readily metabolized to carboxylic acids which may then be conjugated with amino acids. The ability of xenobiotics to undergo amino acid conjugation depends on the steric hindrance around the carboxylic acid group, and on substituents of the aromatic ring or aliphatic side chain. Amino acid conjugation is the most important route of detoxification, not only for many xenobiotic carboxylic acids but also for endogenous acids. It is known that amino acid conjugation of exogenous carboxylic acids occurs in a two–step process (Reilly et al., 2007). Amino acids conjugation of carboxylic acids is a special form of acetylation and leads to amide bond formation. The most common amino acid in such reactions is glycine, and its prototypical substrate is benzoic acid, more precisely its benzoyl–CoA cofactor (Fig. 8). Bile acids are also conjugated by a similar sequence of reactions involving a microsomal cholyl–CoA synthetase and a cytosolic enzyme bile acid–CoA: amino acid N–acyltransferase (Falany et al., 1994). In relation to xenobiotic carboxylic acids, amino acid conjugation involves enzymes located principally in the mitochondria of liver and kidney while conjugation of bile acids is extramitochondrial, involving enzymes located in the endoplasmic reticulum and peroxisomes (Reilly et al., 2007; Knights et al., 2007).

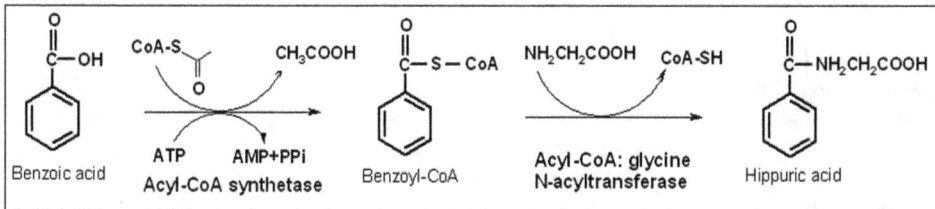

Fig. 8. Conjugation of a xenobiotic with amino acid, formation of hippuric acid.

Glycine and glutamate appear to be the most common acceptors of amino acids in mammals. In humans, more than 95% of bile acids are N–acyl amidates with glycine or taurine. Although products of amino acid conjugation are considered to be metabolically stable and nontoxic, it has been suggested that the first reaction of amino acid conjugation leads in some cases to formation of potentially toxic intermediates. This toxification pathway involves conjugation of N–hydroxy aromatic amines with the carboxylic acid group of serine and proline. Amino acid activated by aminoacyl–tRNA–synthetase (Fig. 9) subsequently reacts with an aromatic hydroxylamine to form N–ester that can degrade to produce a reactive nitrenium ion (Parkinson, 2001). In general, the toxicity of nitrenium ions is clinically relevant since these electrophiles possesing DNA–binding ability are responsible for carcinogenicity of aromatic amines.

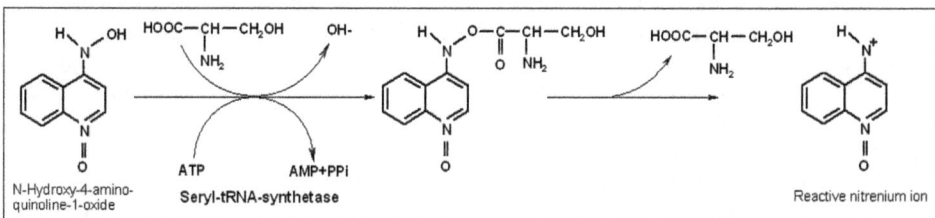

Fig. 9. Conjugation of a xenobiotic with amino acid, formation of electrophilic nitrenium ion.

3. Conclusion

Xenobiotic biotransformation is a key mechanism for maintaining homeostasis during exposure to various xenobiotics, such as drugs, industrial chemicals, or food procarcinogens. In humans and other mammals, the liver is the major site of expression of xenobiotic–metabolising enzymes, but extrahepatically localized enzymes also appear to be of great importance. In the intestine for example, several drug metabolising enzymes are presumed to decrease the bioavailability of orally administered drugs or to activate environmental carcinogens. Phase II of metabolism may or may not be preceded by Phase I reactions. Phase II enzymes undoubtedly play an important role in the detoxification of various xenobiotics. Furthermore, they significantly contribute to maintaining of homeostasis by binding, transport or inactivation of biologically active compounds such as hormones, bile acids, or other mediators. In contrast to their beneficial effects, these enzymes also participate in formation of reactive intermediates of various compounds. The most-discussed example of toxification reactions is the conjugation of N–hydroxy aromatic amines. These compounds undergo activation to toxic metabolites by numerous reactions, including N–glucuronidation by UGTs, O–acetylation by NATs, O–sulfonation by SULTs, and conjugation with amino acids by aminoacyl–tRNA–synthetase. The newly formed reactive electrophilic nitrenium and carbonium ions can act as carcinogens and mutagens due to covalent binding to DNA or to other biomolecules. Genetic polymorphisms of Phase II enzymes is another noteworthy issue. Impaired metabolism of drugs due to genetically based dysfunction of competent enzymes may lead to manifestation of toxic effects of clinically used drugs. Moreover, it is evident that genetic polymorphisms in these enzymes are responsible for the developement of a number of neurological disorders or cancers. In conclusion, Phase II enzymes are an interesting research field since they play an essential role in the metabolism of hundreds of foreign compounds as well as in regulation of metabolism and disposition of various endogenous biologically active substances and thus maintaining homeostasis in the human body.

4. Acknowledgment

Infrastructural part of this project has been supported by CZ.1.05/2.1.00/01.0030 (Biomedreg).

5. References

Adam, P.J.; Berry, J.; Loader, J.A.; Tyson, K.L.; Craggs, G.; Smith, P.; De Belin, J.; Steers, G.; Pezzella, F.; Sachsenmeir, K.F.; Stamps, A.C.; Herath, A.; Sim, E.; O'Hare, M.J.; Harris, A.L. & Terrett, J.A. (2003). Arylamine N–acetyltransferase-1 is highly expressed in breast cancers and conveys enhanced growth and resistance to etoposide in vitro. *Molecular Cancer Research*, Vol.1, No.11, (September 2003), pp.826–835, ISSN 1541–7786

Agúndez, J.A. (2008). Polymorphisms of human N–acetyltransferases and cancer risk. *Current Drug Metabolism*, Vol.9, No.6, (Jully 2008), pp.520–531, ISSN 1389–2002

Arslan, S.; Silig, Y. & Pinarbasi, H. (2009). An investigation of the relationship between SULT1A1 Arg(213)His polymorphism and lung cancer susceptibility in a Turkish population. *Cell Biochemistry and Function*, Vol.27, No.4, (June 2009), pp.211–215, ISSN 0263–6484

Autrup, J.L.; Hokland, P.; Pedersen, L. & Autrup, H. (2002). Effect of glutathione S–transferases on the survival of patients with acute myeloid leukaemia. *European Journal of Pharmacology*, Vol.438, No.1–2, (March 2002), pp.15–18, ISSN 0014–2999

Bardakci, F.; Arslan, S.; Bardakci, S.; Binatli, A.O. & Budak, M. (2008). Sulfotransferase 1A1 (SULT1A1) polymorphism and susceptibility to primary brain tumors. *Journal of*

Cancer Research and Clinical Oncology, Vol.134, No.1, (January 2008), pp.109–114, ISSN 0171–5216

Beland, F.A. & Kadlubar, F.F. (1985). Formation and persistence of arylamine DNA adducts in vivo. *Environmental Health Perspectives*, Vol.62, (October 1985), pp. 19–30, ISSN 0091–6765

Blanchard, R.L.; Freimuth, R.R.; Buck, J.; Weinshilboum, R.M. & Coughtrie, M.W. (2004). A proposed nomenclature system for the cytosolic sulfotransferase (SULT) superfamily. *Pharmacogenetics*, Vol.14, No.3, (March 2004), pp.199–211, ISSN 0960–314X

Blum, M.; Grant, D.M.; McBride, W.; Heim, M. & Meyer, U.A. (1990). Human arylamine N-acetyltransferase genes: isolation, chromosomal localization, and functional expression. DNA and Cell Biology, Vol.9, No.3, (April 1990), pp.193–203, ISSN 1044–5498

Boettcher, M.I.; Schettgen, T.; Kütting, B.; Pischetsrieder, M. & Angerer, J. (2005). Mercapturic acids of acrylamide and glycidamide as biomarkers of the internal exposure to acrylamide in the general population. *Mutation Research*, Vol.580, No.1–2, (February 2005), pp.167–176, ISSN 0027–5107

Bosio, A.; Binczek, E.; Le Beau, M.M.; Fernald, A.A. & Stoffel, W. (1996). The human gene CGT encoding the UDP–galactose ceramide galactosyl transferase (cerebroside synthase): cloning, characterization, and assignment to human chromosome 4, band q26. *Genomics*, Vol.34, No.1, (May 1996), pp.69–75, ISSN 0888–7543

Bresell A, Weinander R, Lundqvist G, Raza H, Shimoji M, Sun TH, Balk L, Wiklund R, Eriksson J, Jansson C, Persson B, Jakobsson PJ, Morgenstern R. (2005). Bioinformatic and enzymatic characterization of the MAPEG superfamily. *The FEBS Journal*, Vol.272, No.7, (April 2005), pp.1688–1703, ISSN 1742–464X

Brockton, N.; Little, J.; Sharp, L. & Cotton, S.C. (2000). N–acetyltransferase polymorphisms and colorectal cancer: a HuGE review. *American Journal of* Epidemiology, Vol.151, No.9, (May 2000), pp.846–861, ISSN 0002–9262

Buhl, A.E.; Waldon, D.J.; Baker, C.A. & Johnson, G.A. (1990). Minoxidil sulfate is the active metabolite that stimulates hair follicles. *The Journal of Investigative Dermatology*, Vol.95, No.5, (November 1990), pp.553–557, ISSN 0022–202X

Burchell, B.; Brierley, C.H. & Rance, D. (1995). Specificity of human UDP-glucuronosyltransferases and xenobiotic glucuronidation. *Life Sciences*, Vol.57, No.20, (1995), pp.1819–1831, ISSN 0024–3205

Butcher, N.J.; Boukouvala, S.; Sim, E. & Minchin R.F. (2002). Pharmacogenetics of the arylamine N-acetyltransferases. *The Pharmacogenomics Journal*, Vol.2, No.1, (2002), pp.30–42, ISSN 1470–269X

Chen, M.; Xia, B.; Chen, B.; Guo, Q.; Li, J.; Ye, M. & Hu, Z. (2007). N–acetyltransferase 2 slow acetylator genotype associated with adverse effects of sulphasalazine in the treatment of inflammatory bowel disease. *Canadian Journal of Gastroenterology*, Vol.21, No.3, (March 2007), pp.155–158, ISSN 0835–7900

Coffman, B.L.; King, C.D.; Rios, G.R. & Tephly, T.R. (1998). The glucuronidation of opioids, other xenobiotics, and androgens by human UGT2B7Y(268) and UGT2B7H(268). *Drug Metabolism and Disposition*, Vol.26, No.1, (January 1998), pp.73–77, ISSN 0090–9556

Cole, G.B.; Keum, G.; Liu, J.; Small, G.W.; Satyamurthy, N.; Kepe, V. & Barrio, J.R. (2010). Specific estrogen sulfotransferase (SULT1E1) substrates and molecular imaging probe candidates. *Proceedings of the National Academy of Sciences of the United States of America*, Vol.107, No.14, (April 2010), pp.6222–6227, ISSN 0027–8424

Collier, A.C.; Ganley, N.A.; Tingle, M.D.; Blumenstein, M.; Marvin, K.W.; Paxton, J.W.; Mitchell, M.D. & Keelan, J.A. (2002). UDP–glucuronosyltransferase activity, expression and cellular localization in human placenta at term. *Biochemical Pharmacology*, Vol.63, No.3, (February 2002), pp.409–419, ISSN 0006–2952

Comer, K.A.; Falany, J.L. & Falany, C.N. (1993). Cloning and expression of human liver dehydroepiandrosterone sulphotransferase. *The Biochemical Journal*, Vol.289, No. Pt 1, (January 1993), pp.233–240, ISSN 0264–6021

Commandeur, J.N.; Stijntjes, G.J. & Vermeulen, N.P. (1995). Enzymes and transport systems involved in the formation and disposition of glutathione S–conjugates. Role in bioactivation and detoxication mechanisms of xenobiotics. *Pharmacological Reviews*, Vol.47, No.2, (June 1995), pp. 271–330, ISSN 0031–6997

Court, M.H.; Duan, S.X.; von Moltke, L.L.; Greenblatt, D.J.; Patten, C.J.; Miners, J.O. & Mackenzie PI. (2001). Interindividual variability in acetaminophen glucuronidation by human liver microsomes: identification of relevant acetaminophen UDP–glucuronosyltransferase isoforms. *The Journal of Pharmacology and Experimental Therapeutics*, Vol.299, No.3, (December 2001), pp.998–1006, ISSN 0022–3565

Court, M.H.; Hao, Q.; Krishnaswamy, S.; Bekaii-Saab, T.; Al-Rohaimi, A.; von Moltke, L.L. & Greenblatt, D.J. (2004). UDP–glucuronosyltransferase (UGT) 2B15 pharmacogenetics: UGT2B15 D85Y genotype and gender are major determinants of oxazepam glucuronidation by human liver. *The Journal of Pharmacology and Experimental Therapeutics*, Vol.310, No.2, (August 2004), pp.656–665, ISSN 0022–3565

Crettol, S.; Petrovic, N. & Murray, M. (2010). Pharmacogenetics of phase I and phase II drug metabolism. *Current Pharmaceutical Design*, Vol.16, No.2, (2010), pp.204–219, ISSN 1381–6128

Dagnino–Subiabre, A.; Cassels, B.K.; Baez, S.; Johansson, A.S.; Mannervik, B. & Segura–Aguilar, J. (2000). Glutathione transferase M2-2 catalyzes conjugation of dopamine and dopa o–quinones. *Biochemical and Biophysical Research Communications*, Vol.274, No.1, (July 2000), pp.32–36, ISSN 0006–291X

Dellinger, R.W.; Fang, J.L.; Chen, G.; Weinberg, R. & Lazarus, P. (2006). Importance of UDP–glucuronosyltransferase 1A10 (UGT1A10) in the detoxification of polycyclic aromatic hydrocarbons: decreased glucuronidative activity of the UGT1A10139Lys isoform. *Drug Metabolism and Disposition*, Vol.34, No.6, (January 2006), pp.943–949, ISSN 0090–9556

Dupret, J.M. & Rodrigues–Lima F. (2005). Structure and regulation of the drug–metabolizing enzymes arylamine N–acetyltransferases. *Current Medicinal Chemistry*, Vol.12, No.3, (2005), pp.311–318, ISSN 0929–8673

Falany, C.N.; Johnson, M.R.; Barnes, S. & Diasio, R.B. (1994). Glycine and taurine conjugation of bile acids by a single enzyme. Molecular cloning and expression of human liver bile acid CoA:amino acid N–acyltransferase. *The Journal of Biological Chemistry*, Vol.269, No.30, (July 1994), pp.19375–19379, ISSN 0021–9258

Falany, C.N.; Xie, X.; Wang, J.; Ferrer, J. & Falany, J.L. (2000). Molecular cloning and expression of novel sulphotransferase–like cDNAs from human and rat brain. *The Biochemical Journal*, Vol.346, No.Pt 3, (March 2000), pp.857–864, ISSN 0264–6021

Feng, J.; Sun, J.; Wang, M.Z.; Zhang, Z.; Kim, S.T.; Zhu, Y.; Sun, J. & Xu, J. (2010). Compilation of a comprehensive gene panel for systematic assessment of genes that govern an individual's drug responses. *Pharmacogenomics*, Vol.11, No.10, (October 2010), pp.1403–1425, ISSN 1462–2416

Ford, L.T. & Berg, J.D. (2010). Thiopurine S–methyltransferase (TPMT) assessment prior to starting thiopurine drug treatment; a pharmacogenomic test whose time has come. *Journal of Clinical Pathology*, Vol.63, No.4, (April 2010), pp.288–295, ISSN 0021–9746

Fujihara, J.; Soejima, M.; Yasuda, T.; Koda, Y.; Agusa, T.; Kunito, T.; Tongu, M.; Yamada, T. & Takeshita, H. (2010). Global analysis of genetic variation in human arsenic (+3 oxidation state) methyltransferase (AS3MT). *Toxicology and Applied Pharmacology*, Vol.243, No.3, (March 2010), pp.292–299, ISSN 0041–008X

Fujita, K.; Nagata, K.; Ozawa, S.; Sasano, H. & Yamazoe, Y. (1997). Molecular cloning and characterization of rat ST1B1 and human ST1B2 cDNAs, encoding thyroid hormone sulfotransferases. *Journal of Biochemistry*, Vol.122, No.5, (November 1997), pp.1052–1061, ISSN 0021–924X

Gamage, N.; Barnett, A.; Hempel, N.; Duggleby, R.G.; Windmill, K.F.; Martin, J.L. & McManus, M.E. (2006). Human sulfotransferases and their role in chemical metabolism. *Toxicological Sciences*, Vol.90, No.1, (March 2006), pp.5–22, ISSN 1096–0929

Gilissen, R.A.; Bamforth, K.J.; Stavenuiter, J.F.; Coughtrie, M.W. & Meerman, J.H. (1994). Sulfation of aromatic hydroxamic acids and hydroxylamines by multiple forms of human liver sulfotransferases. *Carcinogenesis*, Vol.15, No.1, (January 1994), pp.39–45, ISSN 0143–3334

Ginsberg, G.; Smolenski, S.; Neafsey, P.; Hattis, D.; Walker, K.; Guyton, K.Z.; Johns, D.O. & Sonawane, B. (2009). The influence of genetic polymorphisms on population variability in six xenobiotic–metabolizing enzymes. *Journal of Toxicology and Environmental Health Part B: Critical Reviews*, Vol.12, No.5-6, (2009), pp.307–333, ISSN 1093–7404

Glatt, H.; Boeing, H.; Engelke, C.E.; Ma, L.; Kuhlow, A.; Pabel, U.; Pomplun, D.; Teubner, W. & Meinl, W. (2001). Human cytosolic sulphotransferases: genetics, characteristics, toxicological aspects. *Mutation Research*, Vol.482, No.1-2, (October 2001), pp.27–40, ISSN 0027–5107

Glatt, H. & Meinl, W. (2004). Pharmacogenetics of soluble sulfotransferases (SULTs). *Naunyn-Schmiedeberg's Archives of Pharmacology*, Vol.369, No.1, (January 2004), pp.55–68, ISSN 0028–1298

Grant, D.M.; Mörike, K.; Eichelbaum, M. & Meyer, U.A. (1990). Acetylation pharmacogenetics. The slow acetylator phenotype is caused by decreased or absent arylamine N–acetyltransferase in human liver. *The Journal of Clinical Investigation*, Vol.85, No.3, (March 1990), pp.968–972, ISSN 0021–9738

Guillemette, C. (2003). Pharmacogenomics of human UDP-glucuronosyltransferase enzymes. *The Pharmacogenomics Journal*, Vol.3, No.3, (2003), pp.136–158, ISSN 1470–269X

Haavik, J.; Blau, N. & Thöny, B. (2008). Mutations in human monoamine-related neurotransmitter pathway genes. *Human Mutation*, Vol.29, No.7, (July 2008), pp.891–902, ISSN 1059-7794

Habuchi, O. (2000). Diversity and functions of glycosaminoglycan sulfotransferases. *Biochimica et Biophysica Acta*, Vol.1474, No.2, (April 2000), pp.115–127, ISSN 0006-3002

Hanioka, N.; Naito, T. & Narimatsu, S. (2008). Human UDP-glucuronosyltransferase isoforms involved in bisphenol A glucuronidation. *Chemosphere*, Vol.74, No.1, (December 2008), pp.33–36, ISSN 0045-6535

Hayes, J.D. & Strange, R.C. (2000). Glutathione S-transferase polymorphisms and their biological consequences. *Pharmacology*, Vol.61, No.3, (September 2000), pp.154–166, ISSN 0031-7012

Hayes, J.D.; Flanagan, J.U. & Jowsey, I.R. (2005). Glutathione transferases. *Annual Review of Pharmacology and Toxicology*, Vol.45, (2005), pp.51–88, ISSN 0362-1642

Hehonah, N.; Zhu, X.; Brix, L.; Bolton-Grob, R.; Barnett, A.; Windmill, K. & McManus, M. (1999). Molecular cloning, expression, localisation and functional characterisation of a rabbit SULT1C2 sulfotransferase. *The International Journal of Biochemistry & Cell Biology*, Vol.31, No.8, (August 1999), pp.869–882, ISSN 1357-2725

Hein, D.W.; McQueen, C.A.; Grant, D.M.; Goodfellow, G.H.; Kadlubar, F.F. & Weber, W.W. (2000). Pharmacogenetics of the arylamine N-acetyltransferases: a symposium in honor of Wendell W. Weber. *Drug Metabolism and Disposition*, Vol.28, No.12, (December 2000), pp.1425–1432, ISSN 0090-9556

Hempel, N.; Gamage, N.; Martin, J.L. & McManus, M.E. (2007). Human cytosolic sulfotransferase SULT1A1. *The International Journal of Biochemistry & Cell Biology*, Vol.39, No.4, (October 2006), pp.685–689, ISSN 1357-2725

Her, C.; Kaur, G.P.; Athwal, R.S. & Weinshilboum, R.M. (1997). Human sulfotransferase SULT1C1: cDNA cloning, tissue-specific expression, and chromosomal localization. *Genomics*, Vol.41, No.3, (May 1997), pp.467–470, ISSN 0888-7543

Hickman, D.; Pope, J.; Patil, S.D.; Fakis, G.; Smelt, V.; Stanley, L.A.; Payton, M.; Unadkat, J.D. & Sim, E. (1998). Expression of arylamine N-acetyltransferase in human intestine. *Gut*, Vol.42, No.3, (March 1998), pp.402–409, ISSN 0017-5749

Hodgson, E. (2004). *A textbook of modern toxicology*, John Wiley & Sons, Inc., Retrieved from http://faculty.ksu.edu.sa/73069/Documents/Toxicology.pdf

Huang, S.K.; Chiu, A.W.; Pu, Y.S.; Huang, Y.K.; Chung, C.J.; Tsai, H.J.; Yang, M.H.; Chen, C.J. & Hsueh, Y.M. (2009). Arsenic methylation capability, myeloperoxidase and sulfotransferase genetic polymorphisms, and the stage and grade of urothelial carcinoma. *Urologia Internationalis*, Vol.82, No.2, (March 2009), pp.227–234, ISSN 0042-1138

Hughes, M.F. (2009). Arsenic methylation, oxidative stress and cancer--is there a link? *The Journal of the National Cancer Institute*, Vol.101, No.24, (December 2009), pp.1660–1661, ISSN 0027-8874

Javitt, N.B.; Lee, Y.C.; Shimizu, C.; Fuda, H. & Strott, C.A. (2001). Cholesterol and hydroxycholesterol sulfotransferases: identification, distinction from dehydroepiandrosterone sulfotransferase, and differential tissue expression. *Endocrinology*, Vol.142, No.7, (July 2001), pp.2978–2984, ISSN 0013-7227

Ji, Y.; Salavaggione, O.E.; Wang, L.; Adjei, A.A.; Eckloff, B.; Wieben, E.D. & Weinshilboum, R.M. (2005). Human phenylethanolamine N-methyltransferase pharmacogenomics: gene re-sequencing and functional genomics. *Journal of Neurochemistry*, Vol.95, No.6, (December 2005), pp.1766-1776, ISSN 0022-3042

Ji, Y.; Snyder, E.M.; Fridley, B.L.; Salavaggione, O.E.; Moon, I.; Batzler, A.; Yee, V.C.; Schaid, D.J.; Joyner, M.J.; Johnson, B.D. & Weinshilboum, R.M. (2008). Human phenylethanolamine N-methyltransferase genetic polymorphisms and exercise-induced epinephrine release. *Physiological Genomics*, Vol.33, No.3, (May 2008), pp.323-332, ISSN 1094-8341

Kadakol, A.; Ghosh, S.S.; Sappal, B.S.; Sharma, G.; Chowdhury, J.R. & Chowdhury, N.R. (2000). Genetic lesions of bilirubin uridine-diphosphoglucuronate glucuronosyltransferase (UGT1A1) causing Crigler–Najjar and Gilbert syndromes: correlation of genotype to phenotype. *Human Mutation*, Vol.16, No.4, (October 2000), pp.297-306, ISSN 1059-7794

Kawamura, A.; Graham, J.; Mushtaq, A.; Tsiftsoglou, S.A.; Vath, G.M.; Hanna, P.E.; Wagner, C.R. & Sim, E. (2005). Eukaryotic arylamine N-acetyltransferase. Investigation of substrate specificity by highthroughput screening. *Biochemical Pharmacology*, Vol.69, No.2, (January 2005), pp.347-359, ISSN 0006-2952

Kemp, D.C.; Fan, P.W. & Stevens, J.C. (2002). Characterization of raloxifene glucuronidation in vitro: contribution of intestinal metabolism to presystemic clearance. *Drug Metabolism and Disposition*, Vol.30, No.6, (June 2002), pp.694-700, ISSN 0090-9556

Kerdar, R.S.; Dehner, D. & Wild, D. (1993). Reactivity and genotoxicity of arylnitrenium ions in bacterial and mammalian cells. *Toxicology Letters*, Vol.67, No.1-3, (April 1993), pp.73-85, ISSN 0378-4274

Kiang, T.K.; Ensom, M.H. & Chang, T.K. (2005). UDP-glucuronosyltransferases and clinical drug-drug interactions. *Pharmacology & Therapeutics*, Vol.106, No.1, (April 2005), pp.97-132, ISSN 0163-7258

King, C.D.; Rios, G.R.; Assouline, J.A. & Tephly, T.R. (1999). Expression of UDPglucuronosyltransferases (UGTs) 2B7 and 1A6 in the human brain and identification of 5-hydroxytryptamine as a substrate. *Archives of Biochemistry and Biophysics*, Vol.365, No.1, (May1999), pp.156-162, ISSN 0003-9861

Klaassen, C.D. & Boles, J.W. (1997). Sulfation and sulfotransferases 5: the importance of 3'-phosphoadenosine 5'-phosphosulfate (PAPS) in the regulation of sulfation. *The FASEB Journal*, Vol.11, No.6, (May 1997), pp.404-418, ISSN 0892-6638

Knights, K.M.; Sykes, M.J. & Miners, J.O. (2007). Amino acid conjugation: contribution to the metabolism and toxicity of xenobiotic carboxylic acids. *Expert Opinion on Drug Metabolism & Toxicology*, Vol.3, No.2, (April 2007), pp.159-168, ISSN 1742-5255

Knights, K.M.; Winner, L.K.; Elliot, D.J.; Bowalgaha, K. & Miners, J.O. (2009). Aldosterone glucuronidation by human liver and kidney microsomes and recombinant UDP-glucuronosyltransferases: inhibition by NSAIDs. *British Journal of Clinical Pharmacology*, Vol.68, No.3, (September 2009), pp.402-412, ISSN 0306-5251

Kunugi, H.; Nanko, S.; Ueki, A.; Otsuka, E.; Hattori, M.; Hoda, F.; Vallada, H.P.; Arranz, M.J. & Collier, D.A. (1997). High and low activity alleles of catechol-O-methyltransferase gene: ethnic difference and possible association with Parkinson's disease. *Neuroscience Letters*, Vol.221, No.2-3, (January 1997), pp.202-204, ISSN 0304-3940

Ladero, J.M. (2008). Influence of polymorphic N–acetyltransferases on non–malignant spontaneous disorders and on response to drugs. *Current Drug Metabolism*, Vol.9, No.6, (July 2008), pp.532–537, ISSN 1389–2002

Lammer, E.J.; Shaw, G.M.; Iovannisci, D.M. & Finnell, R.H. (2004). Periconceptional multivitamin intake during early pregnancy, genetic variation of acetyl–N–transferase 1 (NAT1), and risk for orofacial clefts. *Birth Defects Research. Part A, Clinical and Molecular Teratology*, Vol.70, No.11, (November 2004), pp.846–852, ISSN 1542–0752

Landi, S. (2000). Mammalian class theta GST and differential susceptibility to carcinogens: a review. *Mutation Research*, Vol.463, No.3, (October 2000), pp.247–283, ISSN 0027–5107

Li, J.; Waters, S.B.; Drobna, Z.; Devesa, V.; Styblo, M. & Thomas, D.J. (2005). Arsenic (+3 oxidation state) methyltransferase and the inorganic arsenic methylation phenotype. *Toxicology and Applied Pharmacology*, Vol.204, No.2, (April 2005), pp.164–169, ISSN 0041–008X

Lin, J.H. & Wong, B.K. (2002). Complexities of glucuronidation affecting in vitro in vivo extrapolation. *Current Drug Metabolism*, Vol.3, No.6, (December 2002), pp.623–646, ISSN 1389–2002

Lindsay, J.; Wang, L.L.; Li, Y. & Zhou, S.F. (2008). Structure, function and polymorphism of human cytosolic sulfotransferases. *Current Drug Metabolism*, Vol.9, No.2, (February 2008), pp.99–105, ISSN 1389–2002

Mackenzie, P.I.; Gregory, P.A.; Gardner-Stephen, D.A.; Lewinsky, R.H.; Jorgensen, B.R.; Nishiyama, T.; Xie, W. & Radominska–Pandya, A. (2003). Regulation of UDP glucuronosyltransferase genes. *Current Drug Metabolism*, Vol.4, No.3, (June 2003), pp.249–257, ISSN 1389–2002

Mackenzie, P.I.; Rogers, A.; Treloar, J.; Jorgensen, B.R.; Miners, J.O. & Meech, R. (2008). Identification of UDP glycosyltransferase 3A1 as a UDP N–acetylglucosaminyltransferase. *The Journal of Biological Chemistry*, Vol.283, No.52, (December 2008), pp.36205–36210, ISSN 0021–9258

Maintz, L. & Novak, N. (2007). Histamine and histamine intolerance. *The American Journal of Clinical Nutrition*, Vol.85, No.5, (May 2007), pp.1185–1196, ISSN 0002–9165

Meinl, W.; Meerman, J.H. & Glatt, H. (2002). Differential activation of promutagens by alloenzymes of human sulfotransferase 1A2 expressed in Salmonella typhimurium. *Pharmacogenetics*, Vol.12, No.9, (December 2002), pp.677–689, ISSN 0960–314X

Minchin, R.F. (1995). Acetylation of p–aminobenzoylglutamate, a folic acid catabolite, by recombinant human arylamine N–acetyltransferase and U937 cells. *The Biochemical Journal*, Vol.307, No.Pt 1, (April 1995), pp.1–3, ISSN 0264–6021

Miners, J.O. & Mackenzie, P.I. (1991). Drug glucuronidation in humans. *Pharmacology & Therapeutics*, Vol.51, No.3, (1991), pp.347–369, ISSN 0163–7258

Miners, J.O.; Knights, K.M.; Houston, J.B. & Mackenzie, P.I. (2006). In vitro–in vivo correlation for drugs and other compounds eliminated by glucuronidation in humans: pitfalls and promises. *Biochemical Pharmacology*, Vol.71, No.11, (May 2006), pp.1531–1539, ISSN 0006–2952

Mizuma, T. (2009). Intestinal glucuronidation metabolism may have a greater impact on oral bioavailability than hepatic glucuronidation metabolism in humans: a study with raloxifene, substrate for UGT1A1, 1A8, 1A9, and 1A10. *International Journal of Pharmaceutics*, Vol.378, No.1–2, (August 2009), pp.140–141, ISSN 0378–5173

Monaghan, G.; Ryan, M.; Seddon, R.; Hume, R. & Burchell, B. (1996). Genetic variation in bilirubin UPD–glucuronosyltransferase gene promoter and Gilbert's syndrome. *Lancet*, Vol.347, No.9001, (March 1996), pp.578–581, ISSN 0140–6736

Morel, F.; Rauch, C.; Petit, E.; Piton, A.; Theret, N.; Coles, B. & Guillouzo, A. (2004). Gene and protein characterization of the human glutathione S–transferase kappa and evidence for a peroxisomal localization. *The Journal of Biological Chemistry*, Vol.279, No.16. (April 2004), pp.16246–16253, ISSN 0021–9258

Mutschler, E.; Gilfrich, H.J.; Knauf, H.; Möhrke, W. & Völger, K.D. (1983). Pharmacokinetics of triamterene. *Clinical and Experimental Hypertension. Part A, Theory and Practice*, Vol.5, No.2, (1983), pp.249–269, ISSN 0730–0077

Pacifici, G.M.; Bencini, C. & Rane, A. (1986). Acetyltransferase in humans: development and tissue distribution. *Pharmacology*, Vol.32, No.5, (1986), pp.283–91, ISSN 0031–7012

Pariente-Khayat, A.; Pons, G.; Rey, E.; Richard, M.O.; D'Athis, P.; Moran, C.; Badoual, J. & Olive, G. (1991). Caffeine acetylator phenotyping during maturation in infants. *Pediatric Research*, Vol.29, No.5, (May 1991), pp.492–495, ISSN 0031–3998

Park, T.W.; Yoon, K.S.; Kim, J.H.; Park, W.Y.; Hirvonen, A. & Kang, D. (2002). Functional catechol–O–methyltransferase gene polymorphism and susceptibility to schizophrenia. *European Neuropsychopharmacology*, Vol.12, No.4, (August 2002), pp.299–303, ISSN 0924–977X

Parkinson, A. (2001). *Casarett and Doull's Toxicology–the Basic Science of Poisons (6th Edition)*, McGraw–Hill, Retrieved from http://www.knovel.com/web/portal/basic_search/display?_EXT_KNOVEL_DIS PLAY_bookid=956

Patten, C.J. (2006). New technologies for assessing UDP–glucuronosyltransferase (UGT) metabolism in drug discovery and development. *Drug Discovery Today: Technologies*, Vol.3, No.1, (Spring 2006), pp.73–78, ISSN 1740–6749

Popp, W.; Vahrenholz, C.; Przygoda, H.; Brauksiepe, A.; Goch, S.; Müller, G.; Schell, C. & Norpoth, K. (1994). DNA–protein cross–links and sister chromatid exchange frequencies in lymphocytes and hydroxyethyl mercapturic acid in urine of ethylene oxide–exposed hospital workers. *International Archives of Occupational and Environmental Health*, Vol.66, No.5, (1994), pp.325–332, ISSN 0340–0131

Preuss, C.V.; Wood, T.C.; Szumlanski, C.L.; Raftogianis, R.B.; Otterness, D.M.; Girard, B., Scott, M.C. & Weinshilboum, R.M. (1998). Human histamine N–methyltransferase pharmacogenetics: common genetic polymorphisms that alter activity. *Molecular Pharmacology*, Vol.53, No.4, (April 1998), pp.708–717, ISSN 0026–895X

Reilly, S.J.; O'Shea, E.M.; Andersson, U.; O'Byrne, J.; Alexson, S.E. & Hunt, M.C. (2006). A peroxisomal acyltransferase in mouse identifies a novel pathway for taurine conjugation of fatty acids. *The FASEB Journal*, Vol.21, No.1, (January 2007), pp.99–107, ISSN 0892–6638

Riches, Z.; Stanley, E.L.; Bloomer, J.C. & Coughtrie, M.W. (2009). Quantitative evaluation of the expression and activity of five major sulfotransferases (SULTs) in human tissues: the SULT "pie". *Drug Metabolism and Disposition*, Vol.37, No.11, (November 2009), pp.2255–2261, ISSN 0142–2782

Robinson, A.; Huttley, G.A.; Booth, H.S. & Board, P.G. (2004). Modelling and bioinformatics studies of the human Kappa-class glutathione transferase predict a novel third glutathione transferase family with similarity to prokaryotic 2-hydroxychromene-2-carboxylate isomerases. *The Biochemical Journal*, Vol.379, No.Pt 3, (May 2004), pp.541-552, ISSN 0264-6021

Sahasranaman, S.; Howard, D. & Roy, S. (2008). Clinical pharmacology and pharmacogenetics of thiopurines. *European Journal of Clinical Pharmacology*, Vol.64, No.8, (August 2008), pp.753-767, ISNN 0031-6970

Saito, S.; Iida, A.; Sekine, A.; Miura, Y.; Sakamoto, T.; Ogawa, C.; Kawauchi, S.; Higuchi, S. & Nakamura, Y. (2001). Identification of 197 genetic variations in six human methyltranferase genes in the Japanese population. *Journal of Human Genetics*, Vol.46. No.9, (2001), pp.529-537, ISSN 1434-5161

Sakakibara, Y.; Yanagisawa, K.; Katafuchi, J.; Ringer, D.P.; Takami, Y.; Nakayama, T.; Suiko, M. & Liu, M.C. (1998). Molecular cloning, expression, and characterization of novel human SULT1C sulfotransferases that catalyze the sulfonation of N-hydroxy-2-acetylaminofluorene. *The Journal of Biological Chemistry*, Vol.273, No.51, (December 1998), pp.33929-33935, ISSN 0021-9258

Senggunprai, L.; Yoshinari, K. & Yamazoe, Y. (2009). Selective role of sulfotransferase 2A1 (SULT2A1) in the N-sulfoconjugation of quinolone drugs in humans. *Drug Metabolism and Disposition*, Vol.37, No.8, (August 2009), pp.1711-1717, ISSN 0090-9556

Sherratt, P.J.; Pulford, D.J.; Harrison, D.J.; Green, T. & Hayes, J.D. (1997). Evidence that human class Theta glutathione S-transferase T1-1 can catalyse the activation of dichloromethane, a liver and lung carcinogen in the mouse. Comparison of the tissue distribution of GST T1-1 with that of classes Alpha, Mu and Pi GST in human. *The Biochemical Journal*, Vol.326, No.Pt 3, (September 1997), pp.837-846, ISSN 0264-6021

Sim, E.; Stanley, L.; Gill, E.W. & Jones, A. (1988). Metabolites of procainamide and practolol inhibit complement components C3 and C4. *The Biochemical Journal*, Vol.251, No.2, (April 1988), pp.323-326, ISSN 0264-6021

Sim, E.; Walters, K. & Boukouvala, S. (2008). Arylamine N-acetyltransferases: from structure to function. *Drug Metabolism Reviews*, Vol.40, No.3, (2008), pp.479-510, ISSN 0360-2532

Sneitz, N.; Court, M.H.; Zhang, X.; Laajanen, K.; Yee, K.K.; Dalton. P.; Ding, X. & Finel, M. (2009). Human UDP-glucuronosyltransferase UGT2A2: cDNA construction, expression, and functional characterization in comparison with UGT2A1 and UGT2A3. *Pharmacogenetics and Genomics*, [Epub ahead of print], (October 2009), ISSN 1744-6872

Strassburg, C.P.; Strassburg, A.; Kneip, S.; Barut, A.; Tukey, R.H.; Rodeck, B. & Manns, M.P. (2002). Developmental aspects of human hepatic drug glucuronidation in young children and adults. *Gut*, Vol.50, No.2, (February 2002), pp.259-265, ISSN 0017-5749

Sutherland, L.; Ebner, T. & Burchell, B. (1993). The expression of UDPglucuronosyltransferases of the UGT1 family in human liver and kidney and in response to drugs. *Biochemical Pharmacology*, Vol.45, No.2, (January 1993), pp.295-301, ISSN 0006-2952

Sweeney, C.; Ambrosone, C.B.; Joseph, L.; Stone, A.; Hutchins, L.F.; Kadlubar, F.F. & Coles, B.F. (2003). Association between a glutathione S-transferase A1 promoter polymorphism and survival after breast cancer treatment. *International Journal of Cancer*, Vol.103, No.6, (March 2003), pp.810-814, ISSN 0020-7136

Talalay, P.; De Long, M.J. & Prochaska, H.J. (1988). Identification of a common chemical signal regulating the induction of enzymes that protect against chemical carcinogenesis. *Proceedings of the National Academy of Sciences of the United States of America*, Vol.85, No.21, (November 1988), pp.8261-8265, ISSN 0027-8424

Taskinen, J.; Ethell, B.T.; Pihlavisto, P.; Hood, A.M.; Burchell, B. & Coughtrie, M.W. (2003). Conjugation of catechols by recombinant human sulfotransferases, UDP-glucuronosyltransferases, and soluble catechol O-methyltransferase: structure-conjugation relationships and predictive models. *Drug Metaboslism and Disposition*, Vol.31, No.9, (September 2003), pp.1187-1197, ISSN 0090-9556

Tessitore, L.; Marengo, B.; Vance, D.E.; Papotti, M.; Mussa, A.; Daidone, M.G. & Costa, A. (2003). Expression of phosphatidylethanolamine N-methyltransferase in human hepatocellular carcinomas. *Oncology*, Vol.65, No.2, (2003), pp.152-158, ISSN 0030-2414

Thomas, D.J. (2007). Molecular processes in cellular arsenic metabolism. *Toxicology and Applied Pharmacology*, Vol.222, No.3, (August 2007), pp.365-373, ISSN 0041-008X

Thompson, M.A.; Moon, E.; Kim, U.J.; Xu, J.; Siciliano, M.J. & Weinshilboum, R.M. (1999). Human indolethylamine N-methyltransferase: cDNA cloning and expression, gene cloning, and chromosomal localization. *Genomics*, Vol.61, No.3, (November 1999), pp.285-297, ISSN 0888-7543

Tukey, R.H. & Strassburg, C.P. (2000). Human UDP-glucuronosyltransferases: metabolism, expression, and disease. *Annual Review of Pharmacology and Toxicology*, Vol.40, (2000), pp.581-616, ISSN 0362-1642

Tunbridge, E.M.; Harrison, P.J. & Weinberger, D.R. (2006). Catechol-o-methyltransferase, cognition, and psychosis: Val158Met and beyond. *Biological Psychiatry*, Vol.60, No.2, (July 2006), pp.141-151, ISSN 0006-3223

van Bladeren, P.J. (2000). Glutathione conjugation as a bioactivation reaction. *Chemico-biological Interactions*, Vol.129, No.1-2, (December 2000), pp.61-76, ISSN 0009-2797

Wang, J.; Falany, J.L. & Falany, C.N. (1998). Expression and characterization of a novel thyroid hormone-sulfating form of cytosolic sulfotransferase from human liver. *Molecular Pharmacology*, Vol.53, No.2, (February 1998), pp.274-282, ISSN 0026-895X

Wang, T.; Franke, P.; Neidt, H.; Cichon, S.; Knapp, M.; Lichtermann, D.; Maier, W.; Propping, P. & Nothen M.M. (2001). Association study of the lowactivity allele of catechol-O-methyltransferase and alcoholism using a family-based approach. *Molecular Psychiatry*, Vol.6, No.1, (January 2001), pp.109-111, ISSN 1359-4184

Wang, X.; Chowdhury, J.R. & Chowdhury, N.R. (2006). Bilirubin Metabolism: Applied physiology. *Current Paediatrcis*, Vol.16, No.1, (February 2006), pp.70-74, ISSN 0957-5839

Wasserman, E.; Myara, A.; Lokiec, F.; Goldwasser, F.; Trivin, F.; Mahjoubi, M.; Misset, J.L. & Cvitkovic, E. (1997). Severe CPT-11 toxicity in patients with Gilbert's syndrome: two case reports. *Annals of Oncology*, Vol.8, No.10, (October 1997), pp.1049-1051, ISSN 0923-7534

Weinshilboum, R.M.; Otterness, D.M. & Szumlanski, C.L. (1999). Methylation pharmacogenetics: catechol O–methyltransferase, thiopurine methyltransferase, and histamine N–methyltransferase. *Annual Review of Pharmacology and Toxicology*, Vol.39, (1999), pp.19–52, ISSN 0362–1642

Wells, P.G.; Mackenzie, P.I.; Chowdhury, J.R.; Guillemette, C.; Gregory, P.A.; Ishii, Y.; Hansen, A.J.; Kessler, F.K.; Kim, P.M.; Chowdhury, N.R. & Ritter, J.K. (2004). Glucuronidation and the UDP–glucuronosyltransferases in health and disease. *Drug Metabolism and Disposition*, Vol.32, No.3, (March 2004), pp.281–290, ISSN 0090–9556

Williams, A.C. & Ramsden, D.B. (2005). Autotoxicity, methylation and a road to the prevention of Parkinson's disease. *Journal of Clinical Neuroscience*, Vol.12, No.1, (January 2005), pp.6–11, ISSN 0967–5868

Wood, T.C.; Salavagionne, O.E.; Mukherjee, B.; Wang, L.; Klumpp, A.F.; Thomae, B.A.; Eckloff, B.W.; Schaid, D.J.; Wieben, E.D. & Weinshilboum RM. (2006). Human arsenic methyltransferase (AS3MT) pharmacogenetics: gene resequencing and functional genomics studies. *The Journal of Biological Chemistry*, Vol.281, No.11, (March 2006), pp.7364–7373, ISSN 0021–9258

Xie, W.; Yeuh, M.F.; Radominska–Pandya, A.; Saini, S.P.; Negishi, Y.; Bottroff, B.S.; Cabrera, G.Y.; Tukey, R.H. & Evans, R.M. (2003). Control of steroid, heme, and carcinogen metabolism by nuclear pregnane X receptor and constitutive androstane receptor. *Proceedings of the National Academy of Sciences of the United States of America*, Vol.100, No.7, (April 2003), pp.4150–4155, ISSN 0027–8424

Zhang, J.; Xie, X.Y.; Yang, S.W.; Wang, J. & He, C. (2010). Nicotinamide N–methyltransferase protein expression in renal cell cancer. *Journal of Zhejiang University. Science. B*, Vol.11, No.2, (February 2010), pp.136–143, ISSN 1673–1581

Zhou, S. (2006) Clinical pharmacogenomics of thiopurine S-methyltransferase. *Current Clinical Pharmacology*, Vol.1, No.1, (January 2006), pp.119–128, ISSN 1574–8847

4

Altered Drug Metabolism and Transport in Pathophysiological Conditions

Adarsh Gandhi and Romi Ghose
Department of Pharmacological and Pharmaceutical Sciences, University of Houston,
United States of America

1. Introduction

1.1 Overview of Drug Metabolizing Enzymes (DMEs) and transporters

Drug metabolism can either lead to detoxification, bio-inactivation and/or elimination of the drug from the body. Metabolism can be broadly categorized into phases I and II. Phase I drug metabolizing enzymes (DMEs) primarily comprise of the Cytochrome (CYP) 450 family of enzymes. CYP3A4 is the most common isoform expressed in human liver and intestine accounting for ~30-60% of CYPs (Nebert & Russell, 2002) More than 50% of the currently marketed drugs are metabolized by CYP3A4 in humans (Guengerich, 1999). Phase II metabolism consists of conjugation reactions forming polar metabolites leading to enhanced excretion. Phase II reactions include glucuronidation (Uridine 5'-diphospho-glucuronosyltransferase, UGT) sulfation (Sulfotransferase, SULT), methylation (Methyltransferase), glutathione conjugation (Glutathione S-transferase, GST), etc. (Jancova *et al.*, 2010; Meyer, 1996).

Drug transporters play a central role in the absorption, distribution, metabolism and elimination (ADME) processes of xenobiotics across the cellular barriers. They are broadly classified into uptake and efflux transporters which facilitate drug disposition in or out of the cells (Mizuno *et al.*, 2003). Major transporters include, but are not limited to: multidrug resistant gene/P-glycoprotein (MDR/P-gp), multidrug resistance associated protein (MRP1-3), breast cancer resistance protein (BCRP), organic anion transporting peptides (OATPs) and organic cationic transporters (OCTs) (Mizuno *et al.*, 2003; Mizuno & Sugiyama, 2002).

1.2 Altered drug metabolism and transport in pathophysiological conditions

Several studies have shown that drug metabolism and transport is disrupted during diseases and altered pathophysiological conditions primarily due to reductions in gene expression of these enzymes and transporters (Aitken *et al.*, 2006; Kato, 1977). The transcription factors such as nuclear factor-κB (NF-κB), CAAT enhancer-binding protein (C/EBP) or nuclear transcription factor E2-related factor 2 (Nrf2) have been shown to regulate DME and transporter gene expression *in vivo* and *in vitro* (Gonzalez & Lee, 1996; Shen & Kong, 2009; Zordoky & El-Kadi, 2009). In addition to basal transcription factors, the xenobiotic nuclear receptors, pregnane X receptor (PXR), constitutive androstane receptor (CAR) heterodimerize with the central nuclear receptor, retinoid X receptor (RXR) α to regulate the expression of DME and transporter genes (Chen *et al.*, 2004; Goodwin *et al.*, 2002; Kast *et al.*, 2002; Xie, 2008). Furthermore, nuclear receptors such as peroxisome proliferator activated receptor (PPAR), liver X receptor (LXR) or farsenoid X receptor (FXR) can also regulate DME and transporter gene expression (Xie, 2008). The orphan nuclear receptor, hepatocyte nuclear factor (HNF) 4α can regulate the gene expression of PXR and CAR mediated xenobiotic induction of CYP3A4 (Tirona *et al.*, 2003).

Altered drug metabolism can lead to adverse drug reactions which account for ~10% of hospitalized cases (Deng *et al.*, 2009; Maddox *et al.*, 2010). However, due to underreporting, the actual incidences may be much higher (Lazarou *et al.*, 1998., Pirmohamed *et al.*, 2004). As early as 1960s, variations in drug metabolism were observed in patients or animals with diabetes (Dixon *et al.*, 1961), cancer (Kato *et al.*, 1963), hepatitis (Klotz *et al.*, 1974; McHorse *et al.*, 1974) or influenza (Kraemer *et al.*, 1982). Changes in drug metabolism were also associated with a corresponding change in the pharmacodynamics (PD) of drugs (Dixon *et al.*, 1961; Kato *et al.*, 1968). These early studies prompted the researchers to study the alterations in DME and transporter gene expression and activity in pathophysiological conditions such as cancer, diabetes/obesity, rheumatoid arthritis (RA), non-alcoholic fatty liver disease (NAFLD) and cardiovascular diseases (CVDs) such as hypertension, heart failure, or stroke, etc. (Alkayed *et al.*, 2002; Charles *et al.*, 2006; Fisher *et al.*, 2008; 2009a; 2009b; Thum & Borlak, 2002). Overall, the readers of this chapter will benefit from the discussions of the changes in expression of DMEs and transporters, and pharmacokinetics/pharmacodynamics (PK/PD) of clinically relevant medications in different pathophysiological conditions.

2. Infection and inflammation

2.1 Bacterial infections

2.1.1 Drug metabolizing enzymes

Most of the studies on regulation on DMEs have been documented with gram-negative bacteria. Of clinical relevance, sepsis induced by cecal ligation and puncture (CLP) is the most frequently used model owing to its close resemblance in the progression and characteristics of human sepsis (Wichterman *et al.*, 1980). In a CLP rat model, total hepatic microsomal CYP content and activities were significantly reduced (Godellas *et al.*, 1995). Infection of pigs with the gram-negative respiratory pathogen, *Actinobacillus pleuropneumoniae,* led to decreased clearances of antipyrine, caffeine, and acetaminophen 24 h after inoculation. This was further supported by decreased microsomal metabolism of several CYP-dependent substrates (Monshouwer *et al.*, 1995). Another widely studied gram-negative pathogen, *Citrobacter rodentium,* is a natural murine pathogen which produces similar colonic pathology on the intestinal cells of the host as seen after enteropathogenic *Escherichia coli* infections in humans (Higgins *et al.*, 1999). The mRNA and protein levels of CYP4F18 and 2D9 were induced in a live mouse model of inflammatory bowel disease induced by *C. rodentium* (Chaluvadi *et al.*, 2009). The rapid down-regulation of CYP2Cs and CYP3As after intraperitoneal (i.p) injection and CYP4As after oral injection of *C. rodentium* were quantitatively and qualitatively different, suggesting that the effects of oral infection are not due to bacterial translocation to the liver (Chaluvadi *et al.*, 2009).

Although, gram-positive infections account for more than 50% of the total community acquired infections (Martin *et al.*, 2003), very few studies have linked the effects of gram-positive bacteria on regulation of DMEs. It was shown that in patients suffering from gram-positive bacteremia such as *Pseudomonas* or *Staphylococcus* infections, an increase in volume of distribution (V_d) and dilution of antimicrobial agents in plasma and extracellular fluids may occur, which needs careful monitoring of the dosage regimen (Pinder *et al.*, 2002). Listeriosis, caused by *Listeria monocytogenes*, is one of the most critical food-borne diseases in humans. *L. monocytogenes* induced CNS infection in rodents significantly down-regulated mRNA, protein and activity of hepatic CYPs (Garcia Del Busto Cano & Renton, 2003).

The gram-negative bacterial component, lipopolysaccharide (LPS), and the gram-positive bacterial component, lipoteichoic acid (LTA), serve as sterile infection models by inducing inflammatory responses in animals (Ginsburg, 2002; Leemans *et al.*, 2002). LPS can down-regulate the expression and activity of key hepatic, intestinal and renal DMEs in several animal species such as mice, rats or rabbits (Ghose *et al.*, 2008; Sewer *et al.*, 1996). Interestingly, studies have that changes in CYP expression and activity is dependent on the route of administrate at same dose of LPS (Shimamoto *et al.*, 1998). We recently showed that LTA significantly down-regulated the gene expression of several phase I and phase II DMEs in mice (Ghose *et al.*, 2009).

2.1.2 Drug transporters

Changes in expression of drug transporters can have significant impact on the safety and efficacy of the drugs. LPS treatment of mice significantly down-regulated P-gp and Mrp2, major transporters involved in disposition of clinically relevant drugs such as colchicine, verapamil, daunorubicin, cyclosporin A and the abundant food-derived carcinogen 2-amino-1-methyl-6-phenylimidazo[4,5-*b*]pyridine (PhIP) (Dietrich *et al.*, 2001; Petrovic *et al.*, 2007). LPS-treated mice had significantly lower hepatic P-gp (30% of control) and increased P-gp expression in the kidney (140% controls) (Hartmann *et al.*, 2001; 2005).

2.1.3 PK/PD studies

As early as 1980's, it was shown that vaccination with the bacillus Calmette-Guerin (BCG) decreased clearance of theophylline in human volunteers (Gray *et al.*, 1983). Altered PK was observed in other bacterial infections induced by *Streptococcus pneumoniae* (decreased antipyrine clearance) or *Mycoplasma pulmonis* (increased Tilmicosin plasma levels) (Modric *et al.*, 1998; Sonne *et al.*, 1985). LPS injections in animals and humans altered PK parameters such as maximum plasma concentration (C_{max}, increase), area under the curve (AUC, increase), half-life ($T_{1/2}$), V_d and clearance (CL, decrease) of several widely prescribed medications such as cisplatin, antipyrine, theophylline, hexobarbital, gentamicin and vancomycin (Gous *et al.*, 1995; Hasegawa *et al.*, 1994; Ishikawa *et al.*, 1990; Shedlofsky *et al.*, 1994). PK changes of drugs during bacterial infection or inflammation can profoundly affect the PD as well. E.g. turpentine oil-injected mice had very high anti-tumor activity of gimatecan compared to the controls (Frapolli *et al.*, 2010). On the other hand, several studies have shown that inflammation does not affect the PD of drugs. E.g. despite of very high plasma concentrations of the calcium channel blocker, verapmil, or potassium channel antagonists, sotalol or propranolol; no change in the PD was seen in inflamed animals (Guirguis & Jamali, 2003; Kulmatycki *et al.*, 2001; Mayo *et al.*, 2000). The authors concluded this to be due to altered receptor-functioning or receptor-ligand binding exhibited by inflammation. Nevertheless, the above studies need further evaluations to delineate the disparities in altered drug metabolism caused by different bacterial infections or inflammation which has significant clinical implications for drug therapy in disease states.

2.2 Viral infections

2.2.1 Drug metabolizing enzymes

Viral infections can also stimulate the immune system releasing various inflammatory mediators from the immune cells (Mannering & Deloria, 1986). A survey of the literature reveals numerous studies on the effect of viral infections such as mouse-adapted influenza virus (Corbett & Nettesheim, 1973), Newcastle disease virus (Singh & Renton, 1981), encephalomyocarditis virus (Renton, 1981), chronic active hepatitis and cirrhosis (Schoene et al., 1972; Wilkinson, 1997) and HIV infection (Lee et al., 1993) on alteration of gene expression and activity of DMEs and oxidative pathways in animals and humans. Decreased levels of hepatic CYP1A2 were detected in children suffering from upper respiratory tract viral infections during an influenza outbreak (Chang et al., 1978; Kraemer et al., 1982). With exceptions of CYP2D6 mRNA and CYP1A2 activity, other major CYPs such as CYP2C9, 2C19, and 3A4 in HCV-infected PXB mice (chimeric mouse with human hepatocytes) were comparable to the non-infected controls (Kikuchi et al., 2010). Recombinant adenovirus injections in Sprague-Dawley rats led to significant down-regulation of renal CYP2E1 and hepatic CYP3A2 and CYP2C11 expression and activity, and induction of CYP4A protein expression (Callahan et al., 2005; Le et al., 2006).

2.2.2 Drug transporters

A recent study showed that HIV-type 1 viral envelope glycoprotein gp120 decreased P-gp and Mrp expression levels in rat astrocytes (Ronaldson & Bendayan, 2006). However, due to the fact that HIV infected patients are on highly active antiretroviral therapy (HAART) consisting of numerous drugs, both, induction and suppression of drug transporters in HIV infection are reported (Giraud et al., 2010). Polyinosinic/polycytidylic acid [poly (I:C)] is widely used as a model of in vivo viral-induced inflammation. Poly (I:C) can induce interferons (IFNs) and pro-inflammatory cytokines such as interleukin (IL)-6, IL-10, IL-12, and tumor necrosis factor (TNF)-α. A significant down-regulation of key maternal hepatic and placental drug transporters and their endogenous substrates was observed upon i.p injection of poly (I:C) in pregnant rats (Petrovic & Piquette-Miller, 2010) However, Abcb1b (ATP-binding cassette sub-family B member 1) and Abcc3 (ATP-binding cassette sub-family C) were significantly induced. A recent study in PXB mice infected with hepatitis C virus (HCV) reported significantly higher expression of MRP4 and OATP2B1 and lower expression of OCT1 compared to non-infected mice (Kikuchi et al., 2010).

2.2.3 PK/PD studies

During the 1982 influenza B outbreak in King County, Washington, 11 children whose asthma had previously been controlled with a stable theophylline dose, developed theophylline toxicity on this same dose (Kraemer et al., 1982). These children had a significant decrease in CL and increase in $T_{1/2}$ of theophylline. HIV infections could also lead to altered PK of levofloxacin and fluconazole (Goodwin *et al.*, 1994; Tett *et al.*, 1995). End-stage liver disease, which is largely the result of HCV infection, now accounts for up to 50% of deaths among persons with HIV-1 infection (Bica *et al.*, 2001). A clinical study in HIV-HCV-coinfected patients showed significantly lower nelfinavir oral clearances in HIV+ and HCV+ patients with and without cirrhosis compared to HIV+ and HCV-negative patients (Regazzi *et al.*, 2005). This presses the need for therapeutic drug monitoring in individualizing nelfinavir dosage in HIV-HCV-coinfected patients. In addition, an increase in AUC and C_{max} of several anti-retrovirals are reported in HCV-infected patients with moderate liver impairment (Veronese *et al.*, 2000; Wyles & Gerber, 2005). Other studies have also shown significantly higher AUC of docetaxel and reduced glomerular filtration rate, suggesting changes in renal CYP in rats injected with the recombinant adenovirus expressing β-galactosidase (Le *et al.*, 2006; Wonganan *et al.*, 2009). On the contrary, significantly reduced C_{max} and AUC of ceftiofur hydrochloride were observed in pigs infected with porcine reproductive and respiratory syndrome virus compared to the uninfected pigs (Tantituvanont *et al.*, 2009).

2.3 Mechanisms for altered drug metabolism in infections and inflammation

Bacterial or viral infections lead to activation of Toll-like receptor (TLR) signaling pathway, which leads to the induction of pro-inflammatory cytokines, IL-1β, IL-6 and TNF-α in the immune cells. In the liver, TLRs are present on the cell surface of various immune cells (the resident macrophages or Kupffer cells) as well as the hepatocytes (Scott *et al.*, 2009). Out of the 13 TLRs identified in mammals, TLR4 is activated by the gram-negative component, LPS, and TLR2 is activated by the gram-positive component, LTA (Aliprantis *et al.*, 1999; Takeuchi *et al.*, 1999). We and others have shown down-regulation of Cyp3a11 and P-gp in LPS sensitive TLR4 *wild type* (C3HeB/FeJ) mice could not be detected in TLR4-mutant (C3H/HeJ) mice (Ghose *et al.*, 2008; Goralski *et al.*, 2003; 2005). Recent data from our lab showed that down-regulation of gene expression of key hepatic phase I and phase II DMEs in TLR2+/+ mice by LTA was blocked in TLR2-/- mice (Ghose *et al.*, 2009). We also observed that LTA down-regulated Mrp2, had no effect on Mrp3 and induced Mdr1b expression. Although, most of the studies have cited the role of Kupffer cell-derived TLRs in hepatic drug metabolism, we and others have also shown that LPS or LTA treatment of primary mouse hepatocytes can directly affect the DMEs via TLRs present on the hepatocytes, independent of cytokines (Ferrari *et al.*, 2001; Ghose *et al.*, 2011a). TLR-mediated signaling is initiated by the down-stream adaptor protein, Toll-interleukin 1 receptor domain containing adaptor protein (TIRAP) (Kagan & Medzhitov, 2006; O'Neill & Bowie, 2007). We showed that TIRAP was involved only in TLR2-mediated regulation of DME and transporter genes (Ghose *et al.*, 2011a), and not by TLR4 (Ghose *et al.*, 2008).

Cytokines are involved in alteration of DMEs and transporters *in vitro* (Barker *et al.*, 1992; Muntane-Relat *et al.*, 1995). LPS-treatment of primary rat cocultures of hepatocytes and Kupffer cells significantly suppressed phenobarbital-mediated induction of CYP2B1 (Milosevic *et al.*, 1999). This decrease was associated with a 5-fold induction in TNF-α released from the Kupffer cells in cocultures. *In vitro* studies with cytokine-treated rat or human hepatocytes led to decreased expression and activity of several drug transporters including efflux pumps such as P-gp, MRP2, 3 and 4, and BCRP, sodium-taurocholate cotransporting polypeptide (NTCP), a major sinusoidal transporter handling bile acids, uptake transporters such as OATP-B, OATP-C, and OATP-8 (Diao *et al.*, 2010; Le Vee *et al.*, 2008; Lee & Piquette-Miller, 2003; Sukhai *et al.*, 2000; Vee *et al.*, 2009).

However, recent evidence suggests cytokines may not be playing a major role in regulation of DMEs. Earlier studies in TNF-$\alpha^{-/-}$ and IL-6$^{-/-}$ knockout mice revealed that DMEs were still down-regulated (Warren *et al.*, 1999; 2001). A recent study by *Kinloch et al* in TNFR1$^{-/-}$, IL1R1$^{-/-}$ and Kupffer cell depleted mice showed that only TNF-α, but not IL-1β and Kupffer cells, was involved in regulation of CYP3A11 and 3A25 oral *C. rodentium* infection (Kinloch *et al.*, 2011). In addition, we showed that although down-regulation of DMEs was blocked in LTA-treated TIRAP$^{-/-}$ mice, hepatic cytokine gene expression remained unchanged (Ghose *et al.*, 2011a).

Nitric oxide (NO), released from macrophages and hepatocytes during inflammation is also known to regulate DMEs (Morris & Billiar, 1994). However, contrasting results have been reported for the role of NO in regulation of DMEs in cytokine-treated primary rat hepatocytes (Carlson & Billings, 1996; Sewer & Morgan, 1997). IL-1β and TNF-α-mediated down-regulation of CYP protein was NO dependent, but not in IL-6 mediated down-regulation (Carlson & Billings, 1996). NO was also shown to regulate the suppression of UGT activities in cytokine-treated hepatocytes (Monshouwer *et al.*, 1996).

Several studies have shown that inflammation-mediated activation of NF-κB plays a significant role in down-regulation of DMEs (Abdulla *et al.*, 2005; Gilmore, 2006; Ke *et al.*, 2001). NF-κB can either indirectly regulate CYP gene expression through mutual repression between NF-κB and nuclear receptors, or can directly regulate CYP gene expression through binding to NF-κB response element in the promoter region of CYP genes (Pascussi *et al.*, 2003). Interaction of NF-κB with nuclear receptors during pathophysiological conditions can alter expression of DMEs (Gu *et al.*, 2006). Inflammation-mediated activation of mitogen activated protein kinase (MAPK), c-Jun-N-terminal kinase (JNK), also regulates nuclear receptors and DMEs (Adam-Stitah *et al.*, 1999; Yu *et al.*, 1999). Recent experiments in human gastric carcinoma and pancreatic carcinoma cell lines suggested a prominent role of JNK activation in down-regulation of P-gp protein expression (Zhou *et al.*, 2006). However, further detailed studies using *in vitro* models such as cell lines or primary hepatocytes, and specific inhibitors of these cell signaling components will significantly contribute in understanding the mechanistic regulation of DMEs and transporters during inflammation.

We speculate that down-regulation of nuclear receptors during inflammation might be involved in regulating the gene expression of DMEs and transporters in animal models (Ghose *et al.*, 2004, 2008, 2009; Synold *et al.*, 2001). We also showed that down-regulation of nuclear receptors by LPS in TLR4$^{+/+}$ or by LTA in TLR2$^{+/+}$ mice was blocked in TLR4 mutant or TLR2$^{-/-}$ mice (Ghose *et al.*, 2008, 2009, 2011a). On the contrary, mRNA and protein expression of several CYPs did not differ in PXR$^{-/-}$ or PPAR$^{-/-}$ mice treated with LPS (Richardson & Morgan, 2005). Similarly, it was shown that PXR was least important in regulating several efflux and uptake drug transporters using PXR *wild type* or PXR *null* mice treated with LPS (Teng & Piquette-Miller, 2005). However, the down-regulation of Bsep and Mrp2 mRNA in IL6-treated *wild type* mice was attenuated in the PXR *null* mice. Thus, involvement of nuclear receptors in inflammation-mediated regulation of DMEs and transporters may depend on the nature of the inflammatory stimuli.

3. Cancer

3.1 Drug metabolizing enzymes

Owing to the fact that, most anticancer drugs have a very low or narrow therapeutic index, alteration of DMEs can lead to life-threatening adverse drug reactions or increased risk of treatment failure in patients undergoing chemotherapy. Decreased hepatic microsomal DME activity was detected in tumor bearing rats with Walker carcinosarcoma 256, where impaired metabolism of hexobarbital, strychnine and meprobamate was observed (Kato *et al.*, 1963). Due to difficulties in obtaining human liver tissue from cancer patients, an Engelbreth-Holm-Swarm (EHS) sarcoma mouse model bearing transgenic CYP3A4/lacZ gene was developed (Charles *et al.*, 2006). Reduced hepatic levels of the transgene-derived β-galactosidase, as quantified by o-nitrophenyl-β-D-galactopyranoside assay, and *Cyp3a11* mRNA and protein was observed in these mice (Charles *et al.*, 2006). Tumors derived from the surface of the ovary account for the vast majority of ovarian tumors (approximately 80%). Altered gene expression ratio of CYP3A4/ABCB1 (P-gp) in cancer cells grown from epithelial ovarian tumors had significant contribution in altering docetaxel disposition (DeLoia *et al.*, 2008). On the other hand, there was no significant correlation in CYP2C8/ABCB1 ratio suggesting that paclitaxel disposition may require additional critical gene products. The expression of several phase II DMEs was also characterized in EHS tumor-bearing mice (Charles *et al.*, 2006). Out of 8 GSTs studied, six were reduced and two unchanged; SULT1A1 was increased while SULT2A1 and UGT2B5 were reduced, and no change was observed in UGT1A7. Tamoxifen remains the first-line targeted treatment for the estrogen receptor α-positive breast cancer patients and undergoes metabolism in the breast tissue which also consists of several DMEs (Williams & Phillips, 2000). In a study examining the role of methylation patterns of genes responsible for tamoxifen metabolism, higher methylation rate of N-acetyl transferase-1 (NAT1), a phase II DME gene, was observed in human breast cancer tissues compared to control breast tissues (Kim *et al.*, 2010).

3.2 Drug transporters

Changes in the genetic variability in clinical specimens as well as over expression of ABC transporter family in tumors have been shown to play a critical role in multidrug resistance to several anticancer drugs (Hoffmeyer *et al.*, 2000; Robinson *et al.*, 1997; Yoh *et al.*, 2004; Young *et al.*, 1999). A recent study showed significant reductions in the mRNA levels of Mdr2, Mrp2, Mrp3, Ntcp, Oatp 2, bile salt export pump (Bsep), Bcrp, whereas Mdr1a and Oatp1 remained unchanged (Sharma *et al.*, 2008).

3.3 PK/PD studies

Cancer-induced changes in the PK and PD profiles of several drugs have been documented since the late 1960s (Kato *et al.*, 1968; Rosso *et al.*, 1968, 1971). In a clinical study, the absorption rate constant, apparent V_d and serum CL of penbutolol (antihypertensive drug) were significantly reduced in the cancer group (Aguirre *et al.*, 1996). PD effect (reduction in heart rate) of penbutolol did not vary statistically in respect to baseline values in cancer patients (Aguirre *et al.*, 1996). Reduction in the metabolism of omeprazole (CYP2C19 substrate) has also been observed in patients with advanced cancer (Williams *et al.*, 2000). Reduced CYP3A expression resulted in >2 fold increase in the sleep time in tumor bearing mice receiving the widely used sedative-hypnotic, midazolam, (CYP3A specific substrate) (Charles *et al.*, 2006).

3.4 Mechanisms of cancer-mediated altered drug metabolism

Since the 1800s, it was observed that chronic inflammation is frequently associated with the onset and progression of various cancers (Balkwill & Mantovani, 2001). A strong association between cancer progression and induction of cytokines or acute phase reactive proteins in tumors is documented (Burke & Balkwill, 1996; Burke *et al.*, 1996; Naylor *et al.*, 1993). E.g. EHS tumor-bearing mice had significantly higher circulating plasma levels of IL-6 (25 pg/ml) compared to the control mice (below detection limit). IL-6 mediated activation of JNK was also evident in EHS tumor-bearing mice, which again prompts the important role of JNK in regulation of DMEs. Studies have shown that TLR expression is enhanced in tumor cells lines (Yu & Chen, 2008). However, the role of TLRs in alteration of DMEs and transporters in cancer has never been investigated.

The role of NF-κB activation in acute inflammation has been suggested in carcinogenesis (Karin *et al.*, 2002; Lind *et al.*, 2001). Cancer-mediated alteration of DMEs and transporters may possibly be regulated by over-expression of NF-κB. A recent study highlighted the role of extra hepatic malignancies in down-regulation of PXR and CAR in tumor-bearing mice (Kacevska *et al.*, 2011). This study prompts to link the reduction in nuclear receptors with altered drug metabolism in cancer. However, additional studies with nuclear receptor knockout animal models with tumors will help identify their direct role in regulation of DMEs and transporters. Overall, all these studies imply that tumor-mediated inflammation may play an integral role in drug response and toxicity of various anticancer agents.

4. Diabetes and obesity

4.1 Drug metabolizing enzymes

Another prevalent pathophysiological condition affecting millions of people in the world is the occurrence of diabetes and obesity. As per the latest statistical report, 366 million people in the world will have diabetes by 2030 (Wild *et al.*, 2004). *Dixon et al* demonstrated that alloxan-induced diabetes decreased hexobarbital, chlorpromazine, and codeine metabolism in male rats (Dixon *et al.*, 1961, 1963). Although, streptozotocin-induced diabetes in rats and hamsters significantly induced hepatic and renal CYP2E1 and 4A2 protein levels (Chen *et al.*, 1996; Shimojo *et al.*, 1993), suggesting altered metabolism of ketones and fatty acids in diabetes, hepatic CYP2E1 protein levels remained unchanged in streptozotocin-induced diabetic mice livers (Chen *et al.*, 1996; Sakuma *et al.*, 2001). A recent study showed differential effects of alloxan-induced diabetes on protein expression and activity of CYP2E1 (increased) and CYP2B4 (decreased) in rabbits (Arinc *et al.*, 2005). Altered gene expression of DMEs in genetically obese zucker fatty rats (reduction in CYP2B1/2 and Mrp3) and *db/db* mice (increase in CYP2B10) are also reported (Xiong *et al.*, 2002; Yoshinari *et al.*, 2006a). Studies have reported interesting results on DME gene and protein expression for different diet-induced obese (DIO) animal models. E.g. Although Cyp3a11 gene and protein expression were significantly reduced in both long term (12 weeks) and short term treatment (1 week) of high fat diet (HFD), Cyp2c9 gene expression was significantly reduced only in the short term HFD treatment (Yoshinari *et al.*, 2006b). We recently showed that mRNA levels of the phase II DMEs (Ugt1a1, Sult1a1, Sultn) were reduced ~30-60% in mice fed high-fat diet (HFD, 60% kcal fat for 14 weeks) compared to low fat diet (LFD, 10% kcal fat) mice (Ghose et al., 2011b). RNA levels of Cyp2e1 and Cyp1a2 were unaltered in HFD mice. These findings indicate that regulation of CYPs is dependent on the model of diabetes and obesity, and is tissue, isoform and species-specific.

4.2 Drug transporters

Streptozotocin treatment in rats increased hepatic levels of Mdr2, leading to increased phospholipid secretion into bile (van Waarde et al., 2002). Another study also showed that the hepatic expression of uptake transporters (Oatp1a1, 1a4, 1b2, 1a6, 2b1, and Ntcp) in diabetic mice decreased significantly compared to the wild type controls (Cheng et al., 2008). Our recent study showed no effect of high fat in DIO mice on gene expression of hepatic transporters (Mrp2 and 3, and Mdr1b) (Ghose et al., 2011b).

4.3 PK/PD studies

Obesity-associated alterations in phase II metabolism were reported in 1980's. E.g. clearances of oxazepam and lorazepam, widely used benzodiazepines and excreted as glucuronide conjugates, were significantly increased in obese patients (Abernethy et al., 1983). Similarly, increased metabolism of chlorzoxazone (CYP2E1 substrate) to 6-hydroxychlorzoxazone was observed in obese individuals. This was attributed to increased CYP2E1 activity associated with obesity (O'Shea et al., 1994). Animal studies performed using a diabetes mellitus rat model (induced by alloxan or streptozotocin treatment) have reported altered PK of drugs such as acetaminophen, chlorzoxazone, theophylline, clarithromycin, furosemide, and methotrexate (Baek et al., 2006; Kim et al., 2005a, 2005b; Park et al., 1996, 1998; Watkins & Sherman, 1992). Although, no changes in PD of atracurium were reported in obese animals compared to lean control (Varin et al., 1990), triazolam-induced sedation in obese humans increased significantly compared to normal weight men (Derry et al., 1995). We also observed similar disparities in the PD of midazolam, CYP3A substrate, (increased sleep time) and zoxazolamine, CYP2E1 substrate (no change) in DIO mice (Ghose et al., 2011b). This can be attributed to decrease in CYP3A and no change in CYP2E1 expression. Thus, the differential effects of obesity on PD of drugs may depend on the DME, or the drug or the target organ itself.

4.4 Mechanisms of altered drug metabolism in diabetes/obesity

The major pathophysiological manifestation in diabetes/obesity is characterized by low-level chronic and local inflammation, such as release or over expression of TNF-α and C-reactive protein in adipose tissue (Hotamisligil et al., 1993; Wellen & Hotamisligil, 2005). However, the role of inflammation in regulation of DMEs and transporters in diabetes/obesity remains unclear. Hormonal regulation of DMEs in diabetes/obesity has also been addressed before (Thummel & Schenkman, 1990). Although an increase in mRNA or protein levels of CYP2E1 have been observed in obese patients (Lucas et al., 1998), db/db mice showed no such effects (Yoshinari et al., 2006a). This can possibly be due to hyperinsulinemia leading to a faster turnover (shorter CYP2E1 mRNA half-life) by insulin (De Waziers et al., 1995). Various studies have shown that phosphatidylinositol-3-kinase

(PI3K) signaling, using PI3K inhibitors, wortmannin and LY294002, ameliorated insulin-mediated decrease in CYP2E1 and phase II enzymes (α-GST) mRNA (Kim *et al.*, 2006; Kim & Novak, 2007; Woodcroft *et al.*, 2002).

Interestingly, lower expression of CAR and CYP2B in obese Zucker rats and ~2 fold induction in obese and genetically diabetic mice (*db/db*) on HFD (Xiong *et al.*, 2002; Yoshinari *et al.*, 2006b) were reported. This discrepancy in obese Zucker rats and *db/db* mice in regulating expression profiles of CYPs and nuclear receptors can be explained by the difference in the position of mutation of leptin receptor gene (Chua *et al.*, 1996; Lee *et al.*, 1996). We recently showed that expression of PXR and CAR; and protein levels of RXRα were significantly reduced in HFD mice (Ghose *et al.*, 2011b). Thus, a complex set of processes including but not limited to cytokines, nuclear receptors, insulin sensitization or downstream signaling molecules, may regulate DMEs and transporters in diabetes/obesity.

5. Non-alcoholic fatty liver disease

5.1 Drug metabolizing enzymes

Non-alcoholic fatty liver disease (NAFLD) is highly prevalent with an estimated world population between 14% and 24% being affected. NAFLD comprises of symptoms ranging from simple steatosis (fatty liver) to the more severe non-alcoholic steatohepatitis (NASH, fatty liver with infiltration of inflammatory cells) to progressive hepatic fibrosis and to cirrhosis (Reynaert *et al.*, 2005). Alteration of hepatic CYP2E1 was first noted in humans with NASH (Weltman *et al.*, 1998). Later studies have shown significant contribution of NAFLD (comprising of both, simple stage fatty liver as well as NASH) on expression and activity of DMEs in animals (Fisher *et al.*, 2008, 2009a, 2009b). Similarly, *in vitro* studies in primary human or animal hepatocyte cell cultures from steatotic or non-steatotic livers showed a profound impact of steatosis on the metabolic functionality of hepatocytes (Donato *et al.*, 2007; Fisher *et al.*, 2004; Gomez-Lechon *et al.*, 2004). Significant reductions in CYP1A2, 2C9, 2E1 and 3A4 activities in fat-overloaded hepatocytes were observed compared with control hepatocytes obtained from the same liver sample (Fisher *et al.*, 2008).

5.2 Drug transporters

Decreased mRNA and protein expression of uptake transporters such as NTCP, OATP1a1, 1a4, 1b2 and 2b1; and OAT 2 and 3 were observed in NAFLD (Fisher *et al.*, 2009a).

5.3 PK/PD studies

Studies have shown interesting results with acetaminophen (APAP) PK in rats and humans with NAFLD. Children with NAFLD had significantly higher concentrations of APAP-glucuronide (APAP-G) in serum and urine compared with controls, with no significant differences in PK of APAP among the 2 groups (Barshop *et al.*, 2011). Another study showed that biliary concentrations of APAP-sulfate (APAP-S), APAP-G, and APAP-glutathione were reduced in MCD (methionine- and choline-deficient) rats (Lickteig *et al.*, 2007a). However, plasma levels of APAP-G were also elevated in MCD rats, similar to that observed in children (Barshop *et al.*, 2011). A clinical study evaluated the effect of NAFLD on PK of silymarin (Schrieber *et al.*, 2008). The AUC_{0-24h} for the sum of total silymarin flavonolignans was ~3-4 fold higher in patients with NAFLD ($p<0.03$), compared with healthy volunteers.

5.4 Mechanisms of altered drug metabolism in NAFLD

Several mechanisms have been proposed for the effect of NAFLD on altered drug metabolism. Deposition of fat in human hepatocytes can lead to a marked impairment in CYP mRNA and activity (Donato *et al.*, 2006). *Fisher et al* observed intense staining for IL-1β in steatotic livers, indicating that experimental steatosis and NASH results in increased hepatocellular inflammation (Fisher *et al.*, 2009a). Studies have shown ambiguous results on expression of nuclear receptors and transcription factors in NAFLD (Fisher *et al.*, 2009b; Hardwick *et al.*, 2010; Lickteig *et al.*, 2007b). Except for PXR, which was significantly increased by 1.4 fold, the other nuclear receptors (AhR, CAR, PPARα and Nrf2) were not altered (Fisher *et al.*, 2008). Therefore, various factors need to be taken into account for improved pharmacotherapy in patients with NAFLD.

6. Cardiovascular disorders

6.1 Drug metabolizing enzymes

CYPs in humans are responsible for metabolizing a large number of cardiovascular medications, including β-blockers, calcium channel blockers and angiotensin receptor antagonists (Abernethy & Flockhart, 2000). Alteration in DMEs could be of particular clinical relevance in patients with heart failure because these patients take more than 10 medications on average. Although, not detected in the normal human heart, failing hearts expressed CYP11B1 and 11B2 (Young *et al.*, 2001). Surprisingly, an up-regulation in CYP2J2, 1B1, 2E1, 4A10 and 2F2 gene expression was reported in the failing heart (Tan *et al.*, 2002). Increased cardiac CYP11B2 mRNA was associated with increased myocardial fibrosis and the severity of left ventricular dysfunction in patients with heart failure (Satoh *et al.*, 2002). It was shown that the production of testosterone metabolites, including dihydrotestosterone and androstenedione, was significantly increased in hypertrophic human hearts (Thum & Borlak, 2002). Transient ischemic attacks (TIA) are risk factors for strokes. A recent study showed that cerebral infarct size was reduced in TIA-preconditioned animals and CYP2C11 mRNA and protein were coincidentally increased in the brain after experimentally induced TIA (Johnston, 2004). Genetic polymorphisms of DMEs are commonly associated with heart failure and hypertension (Kivisto *et al.*, 2005). E.g. a study in Japanese subjects reported that CYP2C9 *wild type* carriers had lower systolic blood pressure after losartan (metabolizes to the active metabolite EXP3174) therapy than poor metabolizers (Sekino *et al.*, 2003).

6.2 Drug transporters

A recent study demonstrated a selective disease-dependent regulation of the high-affinity carnitine transporter, OCTN2, in patients with dilated cardiomyopathy, whereas the other OCT(N)s were unaffected (Grube *et al.*, 2011).

6.3 PK/PD studies

It was shown that lidocaine plasma clearance was significantly decreased in patients with cardiac failure and this was associated with decreased liver blood flow (Thomson *et al.*, 1971). Another group also observed reduced plasma clearance of lignocaine in patients suffering from myocardial infarction without cardiac failure (Prescott *et al.*, 1976). Thus, the mounting evidence for the effect of CVDs on DMEs and transporters needs to be extended for further PK/PD studies.

6.4 Mechanisms of altered drug metabolism in CVDs

Failing or hypertensive hearts are susceptible to infiltration by pro-inflammatory cytokines and reactive oxygen species induced by stress (Fliser *et al.*, 2004). Studies have shown that increased circulating levels of TNF-α and IL-6 in patients with congestive heart failure were inversely proportional to CYP2C19 and CYP1A2 activity (Frye *et al.*, 2002). Similarly, down-regulation of OCTN2 expression in patients with dilated cardiomyopathy inversely correlated with cardiac CD3+ T-cell count (Grube *et al.*, 2011). In addition, cardiac cytokine release may affect OCTN2 expression during cardiomyopathy associated with inflammation.

7. Rheumatoid Arthritis (RA)

7.1 Drug metabolizing enzymes

Rheumatic diseases are estimated to affect up to 1.1% of the world's population (Harris, 1980). Various studies have shown that gene expressions of DMEs are altered in adjuvant arthritis (AA) rats (Achira *et al.*, 2002b, 2002c; Projean *et al.*, 2005). Similarly, activities of CYP3A were significantly decreased in AA rats compared to control rats (Uno *et al.*, 2007).

7.2 Drug transporters

Decreased activity of hepatic P-gp in the isolated perfused liver of AA rats was reported (Achira *et al.*, 2002c; Uno *et al.*, 2007). Decrease in P-gp activity corresponded with the decreased levels of Mdr1a mRNA and P-gp protein in AA rats.

7.3 PK/PD studies

PK/PD changes such as elevated plasma levels of acebutolol, cyclosporin A, propranolol and prolongation of sleep time with pentobarbital were observed in AA rats compared to normal rats (Dipasquale *et al.*, 1974; Piquette-Miller & Jamali, 1992, 1993; Shibata *et al.*, 1993). Based on these early observations, recent studies have also shown altered PK of methotrexate, T-5557 (novel anti-inflammatory agent) and doxorubicin in AA animals (Achira *et al.*, 2002a, 2002b; 2002d). Although, a significant increase in the plasma concentrations of verapamil in rats and humans with underlying arthritis were reported, there were no changes in the PD of verapamil (prolongation of PR interval) (Mayo *et al.*, 2000; Sattari *et al.*, 2003). This discrepancy was then attributed to a decrease in the receptor-ligand affinity in inflammation (Laporte *et al.*, 1998; Shore *et al.*, 1997).

7.4 Mechanisms of altered drug metabolism in RA

AA animal models represent a systemic inflammatory disease with bone and cartilage changes similar to those observed in RA (Williams *et al.*, 1992). Down-regulation of hepatic P-gp in AA rats was attributed to elevated levels of cytokines such as TNF-α and IL-6 but not IL-1β (Philippe *et al.*, 1997). Similarly, increased plasma concentrations of drugs in AA rats correlated with increased serum TNF-α level (Sattari *et al.*, 2003). Several *in vitro* and *in vivo* studies have shown up-regulation of NF-κB in RA and osteoarthritis (Handel *et al.*, 1995; Mor *et al.*, 2005). It was recently demonstrated that PXR and CAR expression in small intestine was decreased in arthritis (Kawase *et al.*, 2007b). In another study, bilirubin elimination was significantly decreased in collagen-induced arthritis (CIA) rats compared to normal rats (Kawase *et al.*, 2007a), which was attributed to decreased expression of CAR in CIA rats. Thus, overall these studies imply that inflammatory pathways may be involved in the regulation of DMEs and transporters in arthritis.

8. Conclusion

A common theme of this chapter is that a multiplex of mechanisms are responsible for alterations of DMEs, transporters and PK/PD of drugs in different pathophysiological conditions. It is well-established that changes in gene expression of enzymes and transporters can lead to disruption in drug disposition in altered pathophysiological conditions including infection/inflammation, cancer, obesity, CVD, rheumatoid arthritis, etc. Studies show that induction of inflammatory mediators is an underlying factor common to all these pathophysiological conditions and may contribute to altered drug disposition in disease states. In addition, the generally accepted role of cytokines in alterations of DMEs and transporters needs further evaluation. We have established the involvement of Toll-like receptor signaling pathway in the regulation of DMEs and transporters, and our studies point to the role of cytokine-independent pathways in the liver. The role of transcription factors and nuclear receptors in the regulation of DMEs and transporters in disease states need further investigation. There is an urgent need to develop models for delineating the roles of individual inflammatory mediators or nuclear receptors in altered drug disposition in disease states. Understanding alterations of drug disposition in disease states is critical in predicting and preventing undesirable effects of clinically-relevant medications.

9. References

Abdulla, D.; Goralski, K. B.; Del Busto Cano, E. G. & Renton, K. W. (2005). The signal transduction pathways involved in hepatic cytochrome P450 regulation in the rat during a lipopolysaccharide-induced model of central nervous system inflammation. *Drug Metab Dispos* 33 1521-1531.

Abernethy, D. R. & Flockhart, D. A. (2000). Molecular basis of cardiovascular drug metabolism: implications for predicting clinically important drug interactions. *Circulation* 101 1749-1753.

Abernethy, D. R.; Greenblatt, D. J.; Divoll, M. & Shader, R. I. (1983). Enhanced glucuronide conjugation of drugs in obesity: studies of lorazepam, oxazepam, and acetaminophen. *J Lab Clin Med* 101 873-880.

Achira, M.; Totsuka, R.; Fujimura, H. & Kume, T. (2002a). Decreased hepatobiliary transport of methotrexate in adjuvant arthritis rats. *Xenobiotica* 32 1151-1160.

Achira, M.; Totsuka, R.; Fujimura, H. & Kume, T. (2002b). Tissue-specific regulation of expression and activity of P-glycoprotein in adjuvant arthritis rats. *Eur J Pharm Sci* 16 29-36.

Achira, M.; Totsuka, R. & Kume, T. (2002c). Decreased activity of hepatic P-glycoprotein in the isolated perfused liver of the adjuvant arthritis rat. *Xenobiotica* 32 963-973.

Achira, M.; Totsuka, R. & Kume, T. (2002d). Differences in pharmacokinetics and hepatobiliary transport of a novel anti-inflammatory agent between normal and adjuvant arthritis rats. *Xenobiotica* 32 1139-1149.

Adam-Stitah, S.; Penna, L.; Chambon, P. & Rochette-Egly, C. (1999). Hyperphosphorylation of the retinoid X receptor alpha by activated c-Jun NH2-terminal kinases. *J Biol Chem* 274 18932-18941.

Aguirre, C.; Troconiz, I. F.; Valdivieso, A.; Jimenez, R. M.; Gonzalez, J. P.; Calvo, R. & Rodriguez-Sasiain, J. M. (1996). Pharmacokinetics and pharmacodynamics of penbutolol in healthy and cancer subjects: role of altered protein binding. *Res Commun Mol Pathol Pharmacol* 92 53-72.

Aitken, A. E.; Richardson, T. A. & Morgan, E. T. (2006). Regulation of drug-metabolizing enzymes and transporters in inflammation. *Annu Rev Pharmacol Toxicol* 46 123-149.

Aliprantis, A. O.; Yang, R. B.; Mark, M. R.; Suggett, S.; Devaux, B.; Radolf, J. D.; Klimpel, G. R.; Godowski, P. & Zychlinsky, A. (1999). Cell activation and apoptosis by bacterial lipoproteins through toll-like receptor-2. *Science* 285 736-739.

Alkayed, N. J.; Goyagi, T.; Joh, H. D.; Klaus, J.; Harder, D. R.; Traystman, R. J. & Hurn, P. D. (2002). Neuroprotection and P450 2C11 upregulation after experimental transient ischemic attack. *Stroke* 33 1677-1684.

Arinc, E.; Arslan, S. & Adali, O. (2005). Differential effects of diabetes on CYP2E1 and CYP2B4 proteins and associated drug metabolizing enzyme activities in rabbit liver. *Arch Toxicol* 79 427-433.

Baek, H. W.; Bae, S. K.; Lee, M. G. & Sohn, Y. T. (2006). Pharmacokinetics of chlorzoxazone in rats with diabetes: Induction of CYP2E1 on 6-hydroxychlorzoxazone formation. *J Pharm Sci* 95 2452-2462.

Balkwill, F. & Mantovani, A. (2001). Inflammation and cancer: back to Virchow? *Lancet* 357 539-545.

Barker, C. W.; Fagan, J. B. & Pasco, D. S. (1992). Interleukin-1 beta suppresses the induction of P4501A1 and P4501A2 mRNAs in isolated hepatocytes. *J Biol Chem* 267 8050-8055.

Barshop, N. J.; Capparelli, E. V.; Sirlin, C. B.; Schwimmer, J. B. & Lavine, J. E. (2011). Acetaminophen pharmacokinetics in children with nonalcoholic fatty liver disease. *J Pediatr Gastroenterol Nutr* 52 198-202.

Bica, I.; McGovern, B.; Dhar, R.; Stone, D.; McGowan, K.; Scheib, R. & Snydman, D. R. (2001). Increasing mortality due to end-stage liver disease in patients with human immunodeficiency virus infection. *Clin Infect Dis* 32 492-497.

Burke, F. & Balkwill, F. R. (1996). Cytokines in animal models of cancer. *Biotherapy* 8 229-241.

Burke, F.; Relf, M.; Negus, R. & Balkwill, F. (1996). A cytokine profile of normal and malignant ovary. *Cytokine* 8 578-585.

Callahan, S. M.; Ming, X.; Lu, S. K.; Brunner, L. J. & Croyle, M. A. (2005). Considerations for use of recombinant adenoviral vectors: dose effect on hepatic cytochromes P450. *J Pharmacol Exp Ther* 312 492-501.

Carlson, T. J. & Billings, R. E. (1996). Role of nitric oxide in the cytokine-mediated regulation of cytochrome P-450. *Mol Pharmacol* 49 796-801.

Chaluvadi, M. R.; Kinloch, R. D.; Nyagode, B. A.; Richardson, T. A.; Raynor, M. J.; Sherman, M.; Antonovic, L.; Strobel, H. W.; Dillehay, D. L. & Morgan, E. T. (2009). Regulation of hepatic cytochrome P450 expression in mice with intestinal or systemic infections of citrobacter rodentium. *Drug Metab Dispos* 37 366-374.

Chang, K. C.; Bell, T. D.; Lauer, B. A. & Chai, H. (1978). Altered theophylline pharmacokinetics during acute respiratory viral illness. *Lancet* 1 1132-1133.

Charles, K. A.; Rivory, L. P.; Brown, S. L.; Liddle, C.; Clarke, S. J. & Robertson, G. R. (2006). Transcriptional repression of hepatic cytochrome P450 3A4 gene in the presence of cancer. *Clin Cancer Res* 12 7492-7497.

Chen, T. L.; Chen, S. H.; Tai, T. Y.; Chao, C. C.; Park, S. S.; Guengerich, F. P. & Ueng, T. H. (1996). Induction and suppression of renal and hepatic cytochrome P450-dependent monooxygenases by acute and chronic streptozotocin diabetes in hamsters. *Arch Toxicol* 70 202-208.

Chen, Y.; Ferguson, S. S.; Negishi, M. & Goldstein, J. A. (2004). Induction of human CYP2C9 by rifampicin, hyperforin, and phenobarbital is mediated by the pregnane X receptor. *J Pharmacol Exp Ther* 308 495-501.

Cheng, Q.; Aleksunes, L. M.; Manautou, J. E.; Cherrington, N. J.; Scheffer, G. L.; Yamasaki, H. & Slitt, A. L. (2008). Drug-metabolizing enzyme and transporter expression in a mouse model of diabetes and obesity. *Mol Pharm* 5 77-91.

Chua, S. C., Jr.; White, D. W.; Wu-Peng, X. S.; Liu, S. M.; Okada, N.; Kershaw, E. E.; Chung, W. K.; Power-Kehoe, L.; Chua, M.; Tartaglia, L. A. & Leibel, R. L. (1996). Phenotype of fatty due to Gln269Pro mutation in the leptin receptor (Lepr). *Diabetes* 45 1141-1143.

Corbett, T. H. & Nettesheim, P. (1973). Effect of PR-8 viral respiratory infection of benz[a]pyrene hydroxylase activity in BALB/c mice. *J Natl Cancer Inst* 50 779-782.

De Waziers, I.; Garlatti, M.; Bouguet, J.; Beaune, P. H. & Barouki, R. (1995). Insulin down-regulates cytochrome P450 2B and 2E expression at the post-transcriptional level in the rat hepatoma cell line. *Mol Pharmacol* 47 474-479.

DeLoia, J. A.; Zamboni, W. C.; Jones, J. M.; Strychor, S.; Kelley, J. L. & Gallion, H. H. (2008). Expression and activity of taxane-metabolizing enzymes in ovarian tumors. *Gynecol Oncol* 108 355-360.

Deng, X.; Luyendyk, J. P.; Ganey, P. E. & Roth, R. A. (2009). Inflammatory stress and idiosyncratic hepatotoxicity: hints from animal models. *Pharmacol Rev* 61 262-282.

Derry, C. L.; Kroboth, P. D.; Pittenger, A. L.; Kroboth, F. J.; Corey, S. E. & Smith, R. B. (1995). Pharmacokinetics and pharmacodynamics of triazolam after two intermittent doses in obese and normal-weight men. *J Clin Psychopharmacol* 15 197-205.

Diao, L.; Li, N.; Brayman, T. G.; Hotz, K. J. & Lai, Y. (2010). Regulation of MRP2/ABCC2 and BSEP/ABCB11 expression in sandwich cultured human and rat hepatocytes exposed to inflammatory cytokines TNF-{alpha}, IL-6, and IL-1{beta}. *J Biol Chem* 285 31185-31192.

Dietrich, C. G.; de Waart, D. R.; Ottenhoff, R.; Schoots, I. G. & Elferink, R. P. (2001). Increased bioavailability of the food-derived carcinogen 2-amino-1-methyl-6-phenylimidazo[4,5-b]pyridine in MRP2-deficient rats. *Mol Pharmacol* 59 974-980.

Dipasquale, G.; Welaj, P. & Rassaert, C. L. (1974). Prolonged pentobarbital sleeping time in adjuvant-induced polyarthritic rats. *Res Commun Chem Pathol Pharmacol* 9 253-264.

Dixon, R. L.; Hart, L. G. & Fouts, J. R. (1961). The metabolism of drugs by liver microsomes from alloxan-diabetic rats. *J Pharmacol Exp Ther* 133 7-11.

Dixon, R. L.; Hart, L. G.; Rogers, L. A. & Fouts, J. R. (1963). The Metabolism of Drugs by Liver Microsomes from Alloxan-Diabetic Rats: Long Term Diabetes. *J Pharmacol Exp Ther* 142 312-317.

Donato, M. T.; Jimenez, N.; Serralta, A.; Mir, J.; Castell, J. V. & Gomez-Lechon, M. J. (2007). Effects of steatosis on drug-metabolizing capability of primary human hepatocytes. *Toxicol In Vitro* 21 271-276.

Donato, M. T.; Lahoz, A.; Jimenez, N.; Perez, G.; Serralta, A.; Mir, J.; Castell, J. V. & Gomez-Lechon, M. J. (2006). Potential impact of steatosis on cytochrome P450 enzymes of human hepatocytes isolated from fatty liver grafts. *Drug Metab Dispos* 34 1556-1562.

Ferrari, L.; Peng, N.; Halpert, J. R. & Morgan, E. T. (2001). Role of nitric oxide in down-regulation of CYP2B1 protein, but not RNA, in primary cultures of rat hepatocytes. *Mol Pharmacol* 60 209-216.

Fisher, C. D.; Jackson, J. P.; Lickteig, A. J.; Augustine, L. M. & Cherrington, N. J. (2008). Drug metabolizing enzyme induction pathways in experimental non-alcoholic steatohepatitis. *Arch Toxicol* 82 959-964.

Fisher, C. D.; Lickteig, A. J.; Augustine, L. M.; Oude Elferink, R. P.; Besselsen, D. G.; Erickson, R. P. & Cherrington, N. J. (2009a). Experimental non-alcoholic fatty liver disease results in decreased hepatic uptake transporter expression and function in rats. *Eur J Pharmacol* 613 119-127.

Fisher, C. D.; Lickteig, A. J.; Augustine, L. M.; Ranger-Moore, J.; Jackson, J. P.; Ferguson, S. S. & Cherrington, N. J. (2009b). Hepatic cytochrome P450 enzyme alterations in humans with progressive stages of nonalcoholic fatty liver disease. *Drug Metab Dispos* 37 2087-2094.

Fisher, R. A.; Bu, D.; Thompson, M.; Wolfe, L. & Ritter, J. K. (2004). Optimization of conditions for clinical human hepatocyte infusion. *Cell Transplant* 13 677-689.

Fliser, D.; Buchholz, K. & Haller, H. (2004). Antiinflammatory effects of angiotensin II subtype 1 receptor blockade in hypertensive patients with microinflammation. *Circulation* 110 1103-1107.

Frapolli, R.; Zucchetti, M.; Sessa, C.; Marsoni, S.; Vigano, L.; Locatelli, A.; Rulli, E.; Compagnoni, A.; Bello, E.; Pisano, C.; Carminati, P. & D'Incalci, M. (2010). Clinical pharmacokinetics of the new oral camptothecin gimatecan: the inter-patient variability is related to alpha1-acid glycoprotein plasma levels. *Eur J Cancer* 46 505-516.

Frye, R. F.; Schneider, V. M.; Frye, C. S. & Feldman, A. M. (2002). Plasma levels of TNF-alpha and IL-6 are inversely related to cytochrome P450-dependent drug metabolism in patients with congestive heart failure. *J Card Fail* 8 315-319.

Garcia Del Busto Cano, E. & Renton, K. W. (2003). Modulation of hepatic cytochrome P450 during Listeria monocytogenes infection of the brain. *J Pharm Sci* 92 1860-1868.

Ghose, R.; Guo, T. & Haque, N. (2009). Regulation of gene expression of hepatic drug metabolizing enzymes and transporters by the Toll-like receptor 2 ligand, lipoteichoic acid. *Arch Biochem Biophys* 481 123-130.

Ghose, R.; Guo, T.; Vallejo, J. G. & Gandhi, A. (2011a). Differential role of Toll-interleukin 1 receptor domain-containing adaptor protein in Toll-like receptor 2-mediated regulation of gene expression of hepatic cytokines and drug-metabolizing enzymes. *Drug Metab Dispos* 39 874-881.

Ghose, R.; Omoluabi, O.; Gandhi, A.; Shah, P.; Strohacker, K.; Carpenter, K. C.; McFarlin, B. & Guo, T. (2011b). Role of high-fat diet in regulation of gene expression of drug metabolizing enzymes and transporters. *Life Sci* 89 57-64.

Ghose, R.; White, D.; Guo, T.; Vallejo, J. & Karpen, S. J. (2008). Regulation of hepatic drug-metabolizing enzyme genes by Toll-like receptor 4 signaling is independent of Toll-interleukin 1 receptor domain-containing adaptor protein. *Drug Metab Dispos* 36 95-101.

Ghose, R.; Zimmerman, T. L.; Thevananther, S. & Karpen, S. J. (2004). Endotoxin leads to rapid subcellular re-localization of hepatic RXRalpha: A novel mechanism for reduced hepatic gene expression in inflammation. *Nucl Recept* 2 4.

Gilmore, T. D. (2006). Introduction to NF-kappaB: players, pathways, perspectives. *Oncogene* 25 6680-6684.

Ginsburg, I. (2002). Role of lipoteichoic acid in infection and inflammation. *Lancet Infect Dis* 2 171-179.

Giraud, C.; Manceau, S.; Decleves, X.; Goffinet, F.; Morini, J. P.; Chappuy, H.; Batteux, F.; Chouzenoux, S.; Yousif, S.; Scherrmann, J. M.; Blanche, S. & Treluyer, J. M. (2010). Influence of development, HIV infection, and antiretroviral therapies on the gene expression profiles of ABC transporters in human lymphocytes. *J Clin Pharmacol* 50 226-230.

Godellas, C. V.; Williams, J. F. & Fabri, P. J. (1995). Mixed-function oxidase activity in sepsis. *J Surg Res* 59 783-786.

Gomez-Lechon, M. J.; Donato, M. T.; Castell, J. V. & Jover, R. (2004). Human hepatocytes in primary culture: the choice to investigate drug metabolism in man. *Curr Drug Metab* 5 443-462.

Gonzalez, F. J. & Lee, Y. H. (1996). Constitutive expression of hepatic cytochrome P450 genes. *Faseb J* 10 1112-1117.

Goodwin, B.; Hodgson, E.; D'Costa, D. J.; Robertson, G. R. & Liddle, C. (2002). Transcriptional regulation of the human CYP3A4 gene by the constitutive androstane receptor. *Mol Pharmacol* 62 359-365.

Goodwin, S. D.; Gallis, H. A.; Chow, A. T.; Wong, F. A.; Flor, S. C. & Bartlett, J. A. (1994). Pharmacokinetics and safety of levofloxacin in patients with human immunodeficiency virus infection. *Antimicrob Agents Chemother* 38 799-804.

Goralski, K. B.; Abdulla, D.; Sinal, C. J.; Arsenault, A. & Renton, K. W. (2005). Toll-like receptor-4 regulation of hepatic Cyp3a11 metabolism in a mouse model of LPS-induced CNS inflammation. *Am J Physiol Gastrointest Liver Physiol* 289 G434-443.

Goralski, K. B.; Hartmann, G.; Piquette-Miller, M. & Renton, K. W. (2003). Downregulation of mdr1a expression in the brain and liver during CNS inflammation alters the in vivo disposition of digoxin. *Br J Pharmacol* 139 35-48.

Gous, A. G.; Dance, M. D.; Lipman, J.; Luyt, D. K.; Mathivha, R. & Scribante, J. (1995). Changes in vancomycin pharmacokinetics in critically ill infants. *Anaesth Intensive Care* 23 678-682.

Gray, J. D.; Renton, K. W. & Hung, O. R. (1983). Depression of theophylline elimination following BCG vaccination. *Br J Clin Pharmacol* 16 735-737.

Grube, M.; Ameling, S.; Noutsias, M.; Kock, K.; Triebel, I.; Bonitz, K.; Meissner, K.; Jedlitschky, G.; Herda, L. R.; Reinthaler, M.; Rohde, M.; Hoffmann, W.; Kuhl, U.; Schultheiss, H. P.; Volker, U.; Felix, S. B.; Klingel, K.; Kandolf, R. & Kroemer, H. K. (2011). Selective regulation of cardiac organic cation transporter novel type 2 (OCTN2) in dilated cardiomyopathy. *Am J Pathol* 178 2547-2559.

Gu, X.; Ke, S.; Liu, D.; Sheng, T.; Thomas, P. E.; Rabson, A. B.; Gallo, M. A.; Xie, W. & Tian, Y. (2006). Role of NF-kappaB in regulation of PXR-mediated gene expression: a mechanism for the suppression of cytochrome P-450 3A4 by proinflammatory agents. *J Biol Chem* 281 17882-17889.

Guengerich, F. P. (1999). Cytochrome P-450 3A4: regulation and role in drug metabolism. *Annu Rev Pharmacol Toxicol* 39 1-17.

Guirguis, M. S. & Jamali, F. (2003). Disease-drug interaction: Reduced response to propranolol despite increased concentration in the rat with inflammation. *J Pharm Sci* 92 1077-1084.

Handel, M. L.; McMorrow, L. B. & Gravallese, E. M. (1995). Nuclear factor-kappa B in rheumatoid synovium. Localization of p50 and p65. *Arthritis Rheum* 38 1762-1770.

Hardwick, R. N.; Fisher, C. D.; Canet, M. J.; Lake, A. D. & Cherrington, N. J. (2010). Diversity in antioxidant response enzymes in progressive stages of human nonalcoholic fatty liver disease. *Drug Metab Dispos* 38 2293-2301.

Harris, M. (1980). Careers in nursing: caring for children with rheumatoid arthritis. *Nursing (Lond)* 880-881.

Hartmann, G.; Kim, H. & Piquette-Miller, M. (2001). Regulation of the hepatic multidrug resistance gene expression by endotoxin and inflammatory cytokines in mice. *Int Immunopharmacol* 1 189-199.

Hartmann, G.; Vassileva, V. & Piquette-Miller, M. (2005). Impact of endotoxin-induced changes in P-glycoprotein expression on disposition of doxorubicin in mice. *Drug Metab Dispos* 33 820-828.

Hasegawa, T.; Nadai, M.; Wang, L.; Haghgoo, S.; Nabeshima, T. & Kato, N. (1994). Influence of endotoxin and lipid A on the renal handling and accumulation of gentamicin in rats. *Biol Pharm Bull* 17 1651-1655.

Higgins, L. M.; Frankel, G.; Douce, G.; Dougan, G. & MacDonald, T. T. (1999). Citrobacter rodentium infection in mice elicits a mucosal Th1 cytokine response and lesions similar to those in murine inflammatory bowel disease. *Infect Immun* 67 3031-3039.

Hoffmeyer, S.; Burk, O.; von Richter, O.; Arnold, H. P.; Brockmoller, J.; Johne, A.; Cascorbi, I.; Gerloff, T.; Roots, I.; Eichelbaum, M. & Brinkmann, U. (2000). Functional polymorphisms of the human multidrug-resistance gene: multiple sequence variations and correlation of one allele with P-glycoprotein expression and activity in vivo. *Proc Natl Acad Sci U S A* 97 3473-3478.

Hotamisligil, G. S.; Shargill, N. S. & Spiegelman, B. M. (1993). Adipose expression of tumor necrosis factor-alpha: direct role in obesity-linked insulin resistance. *Science* 259 87-91.

Ishikawa, M.; Ohzeki, R.; Takayanagi, Y. & Sasaki, K. (1990). Potentiation of cisplatin lethality by bacterial lipopolysaccharide pretreatment in mice. *Res Commun Chem Pathol Pharmacol* 70 375-378.

Jancova, P.; Anzenbacher, P. & Anzenbacherova, E. (2010). Phase II drug metabolizing enzymes. *Biomed Pap Med Fac Univ Palacky Olomouc Czech Repub* 154 103-116.

Johnston, S. C. (2004). Ischemic preconditioning from transient ischemic attacks? Data from the Northern California TIA Study. *Stroke* 35 2680-2682.

Kacevska, M.; Downes, M. R.; Sharma, R.; Evans, R. M.; Clarke, S. J.; Liddle, C. & Robertson, G. R. (2011). Extrahepatic cancer suppresses nuclear receptor-regulated drug metabolism. *Clin Cancer Res* 17 3170-3180.

Kagan, J. C. & Medzhitov, R. (2006). Phosphoinositide-mediated adaptor recruitment controls Toll-like receptor signaling. *Cell* 125 943-955.

Karin, M.; Cao, Y.; Greten, F. R. & Li, Z. W. (2002). NF-kappaB in cancer: from innocent bystander to major culprit. *Nat Rev Cancer* 2 301-310.

Kast, H. R.; Goodwin, B.; Tarr, P. T.; Jones, S. A.; Anisfeld, A. M.; Stoltz, C. M.; Tontonoz, P.; Kliewer, S.; Willson, T. M. & Edwards, P. A. (2002). Regulation of multidrug resistance-associated protein 2 (ABCC2) by the nuclear receptors pregnane X receptor, farnesoid X-activated receptor, and constitutive androstane receptor. *J Biol Chem* 277 2908-2915.

Kato, R. (1977). Drug metabolism under pathological and abnormal physiological states in animals and man. *Xenobiotica* 7 25-92.

Kato, R.; Frontino, G. & Vassanellip (1963). Decreased activities of liver microsomal drug-metabolizing enzymes in the rats bearing Walker carcinosarcoma. *Experientia* 19 31-32.

Kato, R.; Takanaka, A. & Oshima, T. (1968). Drug metabolism in tumor-bearing rats. II. In vivo metabolisms and effects of drugs in tumor-bearing rats. *Jpn J Pharmacol* 18 245-254.

Kawase, A.; Tsunokuni, Y. & Iwaki, M. (2007a). Effects of alterations in CAR on bilirubin detoxification in mouse collagen-induced arthritis. *Drug Metab Dispos* 35 256-261.

Kawase, A.; Yoshida, I.; Tsunokuni, Y. & Iwaki, M. (2007b). Decreased PXR and CAR inhibit transporter and CYP mRNA Levels in the liver and intestine of mice with collagen-induced arthritis. *Xenobiotica* 37 366-374.

Ke, S.; Rabson, A. B.; Germino, J. F.; Gallo, M. A. & Tian, Y. (2001). Mechanism of suppression of cytochrome P-450 1A1 expression by tumor necrosis factor-alpha and lipopolysaccharide. *J Biol Chem* 276 39638-39644.

Kikuchi, R.; McCown, M.; Olson, P.; Tateno, C.; Morikawa, Y.; Katoh, Y.; Bourdet, D. L.; Monshouwer, M. & Fretland, A. J. (2010). Effect of hepatitis C virus infection on the mRNA expression of drug transporters and cytochrome p450 enzymes in chimeric mice with humanized liver. *Drug Metab Dispos* 38 1954-1961.

Kim, S. J.; Kang, H. S.; Jung, S. Y.; Min, S. Y.; Lee, S.; Kim, S. W.; Kwon, Y.; Lee, K. S.; Shin, K. H. & Ro, J. (2010). Methylation patterns of genes coding for drug-metabolizing enzymes in tamoxifen-resistant breast cancer tissues. *J Mol Med (Berl)* 88 1123-1131.

Kim, S. K.; Abdelmegeed, M. A. & Novak, R. F. (2006). Identification of the insulin signaling cascade in the regulation of alpha-class glutathione S-transferase expression in primary cultured rat hepatocytes. *J Pharmacol Exp Ther* 316 1255-1261.

Kim, S. K. & Novak, R. F. (2007). The role of intracellular signaling in insulin-mediated regulation of drug metabolizing enzyme gene and protein expression. *Pharmacol Ther* 113 88-120.

Kim, Y. C.; Lee, A. K.; Lee, J. H.; Lee, I.; Lee, D. C.; Kim, S. H.; Kim, S. G. & Lee, M. G. (2005a). Pharmacokinetics of theophylline in diabetes mellitus rats: induction of CYP1A2 and CYP2E1 on 1,3-dimethyluric acid formation. *Eur J Pharm Sci* 26 114-123.

Kim, Y. C.; Lee, J. H.; Kim, S. H. & Lee, M. G. (2005b). Effect of CYP3A1(23) induction on clarithromycin pharmacokinetics in rats with diabetes mellitus. *Antimicrob Agents Chemother* 49 2528-2532.

Kinloch, R. D.; Lee, C. M.; van Rooijen, N. & Morgan, E. T. (2011). Selective role for tumor necrosis factor-alpha, but not interleukin-1 or Kupffer cells, in down-regulation of CYP3A11 and CYP3A25 in livers of mice infected with a noninvasive intestinal pathogen. *Biochem Pharmacol* 82 312-321.

Kivisto, K. T.; Niemi, M.; Schaeffeler, E.; Pitkala, K.; Tilvis, R.; Fromm, M. F.; Schwab, M.; Lang, F.; Eichelbaum, M. & Strandberg, T. (2005). CYP3A5 genotype is associated with diagnosis of hypertension in elderly patients: data from the DEBATE Study. *Am J Pharmacogenomics* 5 191-195.

Klotz, U.; McHorse, T. S.; Wilkinson, G. R. & Schenker, S. (1974). The effect of cirrhosis on the disposition and elimination of meperidine in man. *Clin Pharmacol Ther* 16 667-675.

Kraemer, M. J.; Furukawa, C. T.; Koup, J. R.; Shapiro, G. G.; Pierson, W. E. & Bierman, C. W. (1982). Altered theophylline clearance during an influenza B outbreak. *Pediatrics* 69 476-480.

Kulmatycki, K. M.; Abouchehade, K.; Sattari, S. & Jamali, F. (2001). Drug-disease interactions: reduced beta-adrenergic and potassium channel antagonist activities of sotalol in the presence of acute and chronic inflammatory conditions in the rat. *Br J Pharmacol* 133 286-294.

Laporte, J. D.; Moore, P. E.; Panettieri, R. A.; Moeller, W.; Heyder, J. & Shore, S. A. (1998). Prostanoids mediate IL-1beta-induced beta-adrenergic hyporesponsiveness in human airway smooth muscle cells. *Am J Physiol* 275 L491-501.

Lazarou, J.; Pomeranz, B. H. & Corey, P. N. (1998). Incidence of adverse drug reactions in hospitalized patients: a meta-analysis of prospective studies. *Jama* 279 1200-1205.

Le, H. T.; Boquet, M. P.; Clark, E. A.; Callahan, S. M. & Croyle, M. A. (2006). Renal pathophysiology after systemic administration of recombinant adenovirus: changes in renal cytochromes P450 based on vector dose. *Hum Gene Ther* 17 1095-1111.

Le Vee, M.; Gripon, P.; Stieger, B. & Fardel, O. (2008). Down-regulation of organic anion transporter expression in human hepatocytes exposed to the proinflammatory cytokine interleukin 1beta. *Drug Metab Dispos* 36 217-222.

Lee, B. L.; Wong, D.; Benowitz, N. L. & Sullam, P. M. (1993). Altered patterns of drug metabolism in patients with acquired immunodeficiency syndrome. *Clin Pharmacol Ther* 53 529-535.

Lee, G. & Piquette-Miller, M. (2003). Cytokines alter the expression and activity of the multidrug resistance transporters in human hepatoma cell lines; analysis using RT-PCR and cDNA microarrays. *J Pharm Sci* 92 2152-2163.

Lee, G. H.; Proenca, R.; Montez, J. M.; Carroll, K. M.; Darvishzadeh, J. G.; Lee, J. I. & Friedman, J. M. (1996). Abnormal splicing of the leptin receptor in diabetic mice. *Nature* 379 632-635.

Leemans, J. C.; Vervoordeldonk, M. J.; Florquin, S.; van Kessel, K. P. & van der Poll, T. (2002). Differential role of interleukin-6 in lung inflammation induced by lipoteichoic acid and peptidoglycan from Staphylococcus aureus. *Am J Respir Crit Care Med* 165 1445-1450.

Lickteig, A. J.; Fisher, C. D.; Augustine, L. M.; Aleksunes, L. M.; Besselsen, D. G.; Slitt, A. L.; Manautou, J. E. & Cherrington, N. J. (2007a). Efflux transporter expression and acetaminophen metabolite excretion are altered in rodent models of nonalcoholic fatty liver disease. *Drug Metab Dispos* 35 1970-1978.

Lickteig, A. J.; Fisher, C. D.; Augustine, L. M. & Cherrington, N. J. (2007b). Genes of the antioxidant response undergo upregulation in a rodent model of nonalcoholic steatohepatitis. *J Biochem Mol Toxicol* 21 216-220.

Lind, D. S.; Hochwald, S. N.; Malaty, J.; Rekkas, S.; Hebig, P.; Mishra, G.; Moldawer, L. L.; Copeland, E. M., 3rd & Mackay, S. (2001). Nuclear factor-kappa B is upregulated in colorectal cancer. *Surgery* 130 363-369.

Lucas, D.; Farez, C.; Bardou, L. G.; Vaisse, J.; Attali, J. R. & Valensi, P. (1998). Cytochrome P450 2E1 activity in diabetic and obese patients as assessed by chlorzoxazone hydroxylation. *Fundam Clin Pharmacol* 12 553-558.

Maddox, J. F.; Amuzie, C. J.; Li, M.; Newport, S. W.; Sparkenbaugh, E.; Cuff, C. F.; Pestka, J. J.; Cantor, G. H.; Roth, R. A. & Ganey, P. E. (2010). Bacterial- and viral-induced inflammation increases sensitivity to acetaminophen hepatotoxicity. *J Toxicol Environ Health A* 73 58-73.

Mannering, G. J. & Deloria, L. B. (1986). The pharmacology and toxicology of the interferons: an overview. *Annu Rev Pharmacol Toxicol* 26 455-515.

Martin, G. S.; Mannino, D. M.; Eaton, S. & Moss, M. (2003). The epidemiology of sepsis in the United States from 1979 through 2000. *N Engl J Med* 348 1546-1554.

Mayo, P. R.; Skeith, K.; Russell, A. S. & Jamali, F. (2000). Decreased dromotropic response to verapamil despite pronounced increased drug concentration in rheumatoid arthritis. *Br J Clin Pharmacol* 50 605-613.

McHorse, T. S.; Klotz, U.; Wilkinson, G. & Schenker, S. (1974). Impaired elimination of meperidine in patients with liver disease. *Trans Assoc Am Physicians* 87 281-287.

Meyer, U. A. (1996). Overview of enzymes of drug metabolism. *J Pharmacokinet Biopharm* 24 449-459.

Milosevic, N.; Schawalder, H. & Maier, P. (1999). Kupffer cell-mediated differential down-regulation of cytochrome P450 metabolism in rat hepatocytes. *Eur J Pharmacol* 368 75-87.

Mizuno, N.; Niwa, T.; Yotsumoto, Y. & Sugiyama, Y. (2003). Impact of drug transporter studies on drug discovery and development. *Pharmacol Rev* 55 425-461.

Mizuno, N. & Sugiyama, Y. (2002). Drug transporters: their role and importance in the selection and development of new drugs. *Drug Metab Pharmacokinet* 17 93-108.

Modric, S.; Webb, A. I. & Derendorf, H. (1998). Pharmacokinetics and pharmacodynamics of tilmicosin in sheep and cattle. *J Vet Pharmacol Ther* 21 444-452.

Monshouwer, M.; Witkamp, R. F.; Nijmeijer, S. M.; Pijpers, A.; Verheijden, J. H. & Van Miert, A. S. (1995). Selective effects of a bacterial infection (Actinobacillus pleuropneumoniae) on the hepatic clearances of caffeine, antipyrine, paracetamol, and indocyanine green in the pig. *Xenobiotica* 25 491-499.

Monshouwer, M.; Witkamp, R. F.; Nujmeijer, S. M.; Van Amsterdam, J. G. & Van Miert, A. S. (1996). Suppression of cytochrome P450- and UDP glucuronosyl transferase-dependent enzyme activities by proinflammatory cytokines and possible role of nitric oxide in primary cultures of pig hepatocytes. *Toxicol Appl Pharmacol* 137 237-244.

Mor, A.; Abramson, S. B. & Pillinger, M. H. (2005). The fibroblast-like synovial cell in rheumatoid arthritis: a key player in inflammation and joint destruction. *Clin Immunol* 115 118-128.

Morris, S. M., Jr. & Billiar, T. R. (1994). New insights into the regulation of inducible nitric oxide synthesis. *Am J Physiol* 266 E829-839.

Muntane-Relat, J.; Ourlin, J. C.; Domergue, J. & Maurel, P. (1995). Differential effects of cytokines on the inducible expression of CYP1A1, CYP1A2, and CYP3A4 in human hepatocytes in primary culture. *Hepatology* 22 1143-1153.

Naylor, M. S.; Stamp, G. W.; Foulkes, W. D.; Eccles, D. & Balkwill, F. R. (1993). Tumor necrosis factor and its receptors in human ovarian cancer. Potential role in disease progression. *J Clin Invest* 91 2194-2206.

Nebert, D. W. & Russell, D. W. (2002). Clinical importance of the cytochromes P450. *Lancet* 360 1155-1162.

O'Neill, L. A. & Bowie, A. G. (2007). The family of five: TIR-domain-containing adaptors in Toll-like receptor signalling. *Nat Rev Immunol* 7 353-364.

O'Shea, D.; Davis, S. N.; Kim, R. B. & Wilkinson, G. R. (1994). Effect of fasting and obesity in humans on the 6-hydroxylation of chlorzoxazone: a putative probe of CYP2E1 activity. *Clin Pharmacol Ther* 56 359-367.

Park, J. H.; Lee, W. I.; Yoon, W. H.; Park, Y. D.; Lee, J. S. & Lee, M. G. (1998). Pharmacokinetic and pharmacodynamic changes of furosemide after intravenous and oral administration to rats with alloxan-induced diabetes mellitus. *Biopharm Drug Dispos* 19 357-364.

Park, J. M.; Moon, C. H. & Lee, M. G. (1996). Pharmacokinetic changes of methotrexate after intravenous administration to streptozotocin-induced diabetes mellitus rats. *Res Commun Mol Pathol Pharmacol* 93 343-352.

Pascussi, J. M.; Dvorak, Z.; Gerbal-Chaloin, S.; Assenat, E.; Maurel, P. & Vilarem, M. J. (2003). Pathophysiological factors affecting CAR gene expression. *Drug Metab Rev* 35 255-268.

Petrovic, V.; Teng, S. & Piquette-Miller, M. (2007). Regulation of drug transporters during infection and inflammation. *Mol Interv* 7 99-111.

Petrovic, V. & Piquette-Miller, M. (2010). Impact of polyinosinic/polycytidylic acid on placental and hepatobiliary drug transporters in pregnant rats. *Drug Metab Dispos* 38 1760-1766.

Philippe, L.; Gegout-Pottie, P.; Guingamp, C.; Bordji, K.; Terlain, B.; Netter, P. & Gillet, P. (1997). Relations between functional, inflammatory, and degenerative parameters during adjuvant arthritis in rats. *Am J Physiol* 273 R1550-1556.

Pinder, M.; Bellomo, R. & Lipman, J. (2002). Pharmacological principles of antibiotic prescription in the critically ill. *Anaesth Intensive Care* 30 134-144.

Piquette-Miller, M. & Jamali, F. (1992). Effect of adjuvant arthritis on the disposition of acebutolol enantiomers in rats. *Agents Actions* 37 290-296.

Piquette-Miller, M. & Jamali, F. (1993). Selective effect of adjuvant arthritis on the disposition of propranolol enantiomers in rats detected using a stereospecific HPLC assay. *Pharm Res* 10 294-299.

Pirmohamed, M.; James, S.; Meakin, S.; Green, C.; Scott, A. K.; Walley, T. J.; Farrar, K.; Park, B. K. & Breckenridge, A. M. (2004). Adverse drug reactions as cause of admission to hospital: prospective analysis of 18 820 patients. *Bmj* 329 15-19.

Prescott, L. F.; Adjepon-Yamoah, K. K. & Talbot, R. G. (1976). Impaired Lignocaine metabolism in patients with myocardial infarction and cardiac failure. *Br Med J* 1 939-941.

Projean, D.; Dautrey, S.; Vu, H. K.; Groblewski, T.; Brazier, J. L. & Ducharme, J. (2005). Selective downregulation of hepatic cytochrome P450 expression and activity in a rat model of inflammatory pain. *Pharm Res* 22 62-70.

Regazzi, M.; Maserati, R.; Villani, P.; Cusato, M.; Zucchi, P.; Briganti, E.; Roda, R.; Sacchelli, L.; Gatti, F.; Delle Foglie, P.; Nardini, G.; Fabris, P.; Mori, F.; Castelli, P. & Testa, L. (2005). Clinical pharmacokinetics of nelfinavir and its metabolite M8 in human immunodeficiency virus (HIV)-positive and HIV-hepatitis C virus-coinfected subjects. *Antimicrob Agents Chemother* 49 643-649.

Renton, K. W. (1981). Depression of hepatic cytochrome P-450-dependent mixed function oxidases during infection with encephalomyocarditis virus. *Biochem Pharmacol* 30 2333-2336.

Reynaert, H.; Geerts, A. & Henrion, J. (2005). Review article: the treatment of non-alcoholic steatohepatitis with thiazolidinediones. *Aliment Pharmacol Ther* 22 897-905.

Richardson, T. A. & Morgan, E. T. (2005). Hepatic cytochrome P450 gene regulation during endotoxin-induced inflammation in nuclear receptor knockout mice. *J Pharmacol Exp Ther* 314 703-709.

Robinson, L. J.; Roberts, W. K.; Ling, T. T.; Lamming, D.; Sternberg, S. S. & Roepe, P. D. (1997). Human MDR 1 protein overexpression delays the apoptotic cascade in Chinese hamster ovary fibroblasts. *Biochemistry* 36 11169-11178.

Ronaldson, P. T. & Bendayan, R. (2006). HIV-1 viral envelope glycoprotein gp120 triggers an inflammatory response in cultured rat astrocytes and regulates the functional expression of P-glycoprotein. *Mol Pharmacol* 70 1087-1098.

Rosso, R.; Dolfini, E. & Donelli, M. G. (1968). Prolonged effect of pentobarbital in tumor bearing rats. *Eur J Cancer* 4 133-135.

Rosso, R.; Donelli, M. G.; Franchi, G. & Garattini, S. (1971). Impairement of drug metabolism in tumor-bearing animals. *Eur J Cancer* 7 565-577.

Sakuma, T.; Honma, R.; Maguchi, S.; Tamaki, H. & Nemoto, N. (2001). Different expression of hepatic and renal cytochrome P450s between the streptozotocin-induced diabetic mouse and rat. *Xenobiotica* 31 223-237.

Satoh, M.; Nakamura, M.; Saitoh, H.; Satoh, H.; Akatsu, T.; Iwasaka, J.; Masuda, T. & Hiramori, K. (2002). Aldosterone synthase (CYP11B2) expression and myocardial fibrosis in the failing human heart. *Clin Sci (Lond)* 102 381-386.

Sattari, S.; Dryden, W. F.; Eliot, L. A. & Jamali, F. (2003). Despite increased plasma concentration, inflammation reduces potency of calcium channel antagonists due to lower binding to the rat heart. *Br J Pharmacol* 139 945-954.

Schoene, B.; Fleischmann, R. A.; Remmer, H. & von Oldershausen, H. F. (1972). Determination of drug metabolizing enzymes in needle biopsies of human liver. *Eur J Clin Pharmacol* 4 65-73.

Schrieber, S. J., Wen, Z., Vourvahis, M., Smith, P. C., Fried, M. W., Kashuba, A. D., Hawke, R. L. (2008). The pharmacokinetics of silymarin is altered in patients with hepatitis C virus and nonalcoholic Fatty liver disease and correlates with plasma caspase-3/7 activity. *Drug Metab Dispos* 36 1909-1916.

Scott, M. J.; Liu, S.; Shapiro, R. A.; Vodovotz, Y. & Billiar, T. R. (2009). Endotoxin uptake in mouse liver is blocked by endotoxin pretreatment through a suppressor of cytokine signaling-1-dependent mechanism. *Hepatology* 49 1695-1708.

Sekino, K.; Kubota, T.; Okada, Y.; Yamada, Y.; Yamamoto, K.; Horiuchi, R.; Kimura, K. & Iga, T. (2003). Effect of the single CYP2C9*3 allele on pharmacokinetics and pharmacodynamics of losartan in healthy Japanese subjects. *Eur J Clin Pharmacol* 59 589-592.

Sewer, M. B.; Koop, D. R. & Morgan, E. T. (1996). Endotoxemia in rats is associated with induction of the P4504A subfamily and suppression of several other forms of cytochrome P450. *Drug Metab Dispos* 24 401-407.

Sewer, M. B. & Morgan, E. T. (1997). Nitric oxide-independent suppression of P450 2C11 expression by interleukin-1beta and endotoxin in primary rat hepatocytes. *Biochem Pharmacol* 54 729-737.

Sharma, R.; Kacevska, M.; London, R.; Clarke, S. J.; Liddle, C. & Robertson, G. (2008). Downregulation of drug transport and metabolism in mice bearing extra-hepatic malignancies. *Br J Cancer* 98 91-97.

Shedlofsky, S. I.; Israel, B. C.; McClain, C. J.; Hill, D. B. & Blouin, R. A. (1994). Endotoxin administration to humans inhibits hepatic cytochrome P450-mediated drug metabolism. *J Clin Invest* 94 2209-2214.

Shen, G. & Kong, A. N. (2009). Nrf2 plays an important role in coordinated regulation of Phase II drug metabolism enzymes and Phase III drug transporters. *Biopharm Drug Dispos* 30 345-355.

Shibata, N.; Shimakawa, H.; Minouchi, T. & Yamaji, A. (1993). Pharmacokinetics of cyclosporin A after intravenous administration to rats in various disease states. *Biol Pharm Bull* 16 1130-1135.

Shimamoto, Y.; Kitamura, H.; Hoshi, H.; Kazusaka, A.; Funae, Y.; Imaoka, S.; Saito, M. & Fujita, S. (1998). Differential alterations in levels of hepatic microsomal cytochrome P450 isozymes following intracerebroventricular injection of bacterial lipopolysaccharide in rats. *Arch Toxicol* 72 492-498.

Shimojo, N.; Ishizaki, T.; Imaoka, S.; Funae, Y.; Fujii, S. & Okuda, K. (1993). Changes in amounts of cytochrome P450 isozymes and levels of catalytic activities in hepatic and renal microsomes of rats with streptozocin-induced diabetes. *Biochem Pharmacol* 46 621-627.

Shore, S. A.; Laporte, J.; Hall, I. P.; Hardy, E. & Panettieri, R. A., Jr. (1997). Effect of IL-1 beta on responses of cultured human airway smooth muscle cells to bronchodilator agonists. *Am J Respir Cell Mol Biol* 16 702-712.

Singh, G. & Renton, K. W. (1981). Interferon-mediated depression of cytochrome P-450-dependent drug biotransformation. *Mol Pharmacol* 20 681-684.

Sonne, J.; Dossing, M.; Loft, S. & Andreasen, P. B. (1985). Antipyrine clearance in pneumonia. *Clin Pharmacol Ther* 37 701-704.

Sukhai, M.; Yong, A.; Kalitsky, J. & Piquette-Miller, M. (2000). Inflammation and interleukin-6 mediate reductions in the hepatic expression and transcription of the mdr1a and mdr1b Genes. *Mol Cell Biol Res Commun* 4 248-256.

Synold, T. W.; Dussault, I. & Forman, B. M. (2001). The orphan nuclear receptor SXR coordinately regulates drug metabolism and efflux. *Nat Med* 7 584-590.

Takeuchi, O.; Hoshino, K.; Kawai, T.; Sanjo, H.; Takada, H.; Ogawa, T.; Takeda, K. & Akira, S. (1999). Differential roles of TLR2 and TLR4 in recognition of gram-negative and gram-positive bacterial cell wall components. *Immunity* 11 443-451.

Tan, F. L.; Moravec, C. S.; Li, J.; Apperson-Hansen, C.; McCarthy, P. M.; Young, J. B. & Bond, M. (2002). The gene expression fingerprint of human heart failure. *Proc Natl Acad Sci U S A* 99 11387-11392.

Tantituvanont, A.; Yimprasert, W.; Werawatganone, P. & Nilubol, D. (2009). Pharmacokinetics of ceftiofur hydrochloride in pigs infected with porcine reproductive and respiratory syndrome virus. *J Antimicrob Chemother* 63 369-373.

Teng, S. & Piquette-Miller, M. (2005). The involvement of the pregnane X receptor in hepatic gene regulation during inflammation in mice. *J Pharmacol Exp Ther* 312 841-848.

Tett, S.; Moore, S. & Ray, J. (1995). Pharmacokinetics and bioavailability of fluconazole in two groups of males with human immunodeficiency virus (HIV) infection compared with those in a group of males without HIV infection. *Antimicrob Agents Chemother* 39 1835-1841.

Thomson, P. D.; Rowland, M. & Melmon, K. L. (1971). The influence of heart failure, liver disease, and renal failure on the disposition of lidocaine in man. *Am Heart J* 82 417-421.

Thum, T. & Borlak, J. (2002). Testosterone, cytochrome P450, and cardiac hypertrophy. *Faseb J* 16 1537-1549.

Thummel, K. E. & Schenkman, J. B. (1990). Effects of testosterone and growth hormone treatment on hepatic microsomal P450 expression in the diabetic rat. *Mol Pharmacol* 37 119-129.

Tirona, R. G.; Lee, W.; Leake, B. F.; Lan, L. B.; Cline, C. B.; Lamba, V.; Parviz, F.; Duncan, S. A.; Inoue, Y.; Gonzalez, F. J.; Schuetz, E. G. & Kim, R. B. (2003). The orphan nuclear receptor HNF4alpha determines PXR- and CAR-mediated xenobiotic induction of CYP3A4. *Nat Med* 9 220-224.

Uno, S.; Kawase, A.; Tsuji, A.; Tanino, T. & Iwaki, M. (2007). Decreased intestinal CYP3A and P-glycoprotein activities in rats with adjuvant arthritis. *Drug Metab Pharmacokinet* 22 313-321.

van Waarde, W. M.; Verkade, H. J.; Wolters, H.; Havinga, R.; Baller, J.; Bloks, V.; Muller, M.; Sauer, P. J. & Kuipers, F. (2002). Differential effects of streptozotocin-induced diabetes on expression of hepatic ABC-transporters in rats. *Gastroenterology* 122 1842-1852.

Varin, F.; Ducharme, J.; Theoret, Y.; Besner, J. G.; Bevan, D. R. & Donati, F. (1990). Influence of extreme obesity on the body disposition and neuromuscular blocking effect of atracurium. *Clin Pharmacol Ther* 48 18-25.

Vee, M. L.; Lecureur, V.; Stieger, B. & Fardel, O. (2009). Regulation of drug transporter expression in human hepatocytes exposed to the proinflammatory cytokines tumor necrosis factor-alpha or interleukin-6. *Drug Metab Dispos* 37 685-693.

Veronese, L.; Rautaureau, J.; Sadler, B. M.; Gillotin, C.; Petite, J. P.; Pillegand, B.; Delvaux, M.; Masliah, C.; Fosse, S.; Lou, Y. & Stein, D. S. (2000). Single-dose pharmacokinetics of amprenavir, a human immunodeficiency virus type 1 protease inhibitor, in subjects with normal or impaired hepatic function. *Antimicrob Agents Chemother* 44 821-826.

Warren, G. W.; Poloyac, S. M.; Gary, D. S.; Mattson, M. P. & Blouin, R. A. (1999). Hepatic cytochrome P-450 expression in tumor necrosis factor-alpha receptor (p55/p75) knockout mice after endotoxin administration. *J Pharmacol Exp Ther* 288 945-950.

Warren, G. W.; van Ess, P. J.; Watson, A. M.; Mattson, M. P. & Blouin, R. A. (2001). Cytochrome P450 and antioxidant activity in interleukin-6 knockout mice after induction of the acute-phase response. *J Interferon Cytokine Res* 21 821-826.

Watkins, J. B., 3rd & Sherman, S. E. (1992). Long-term diabetes alters the hepatobiliary clearance of acetaminophen, bilirubin and digoxin. *J Pharmacol Exp Ther* 260 1337-1343.

Wellen, K. E. & Hotamisligil, G. S. (2005). Inflammation, stress, and diabetes. *J Clin Invest* 115 1111-1119.

Weltman, M. D.; Farrell, G. C.; Hall, P.; Ingelman-Sundberg, M. & Liddle, C. (1998). Hepatic cytochrome P450 2E1 is increased in patients with nonalcoholic steatohepatitis. *Hepatology* 27 128-133.

Wichterman, K. A.; Baue, A. E. & Chaudry, I. H. (1980). Sepsis and septic shock--a review of laboratory models and a proposal. *J Surg Res* 29 189-201.

Wild, S.; Roglic, G.; Green, A.; Sicree, R. & King, H. (2004). Global prevalence of diabetes: estimates for the year 2000 and projections for 2030. *Diabetes Care* 27 1047-1053.

Wilkinson, G. R. (1997). The effects of diet, aging and disease-states on presystemic elimination and oral drug bioavailability in humans. *Adv Drug Deliv Rev* 27 129-159.

Williams, J. A. & Phillips, D. H. (2000). Mammary expression of xenobiotic metabolizing enzymes and their potential role in breast cancer. *Cancer Res* 60 4667-4677.

Williams, M. L.; Bhargava, P.; Cherrouk, I.; Marshall, J. L.; Flockhart, D. A. & Wainer, I. W. (2000). A discordance of the cytochrome P450 2C19 genotype and phenotype in patients with advanced cancer. *Br J Clin Pharmacol* 49 485-488.

Williams, R. O.; Feldmann, M. & Maini, R. N. (1992). Anti-tumor necrosis factor ameliorates joint disease in murine collagen-induced arthritis. *Proc Natl Acad Sci U S A* 89 9784-9788.

Wonganan, P.; Zamboni, W. C.; Strychor, S.; Dekker, J. D. & Croyle, M. A. (2009). Drug-virus interaction: effect of administration of recombinant adenoviruses on the pharmacokinetics of docetaxel in a rat model. *Cancer Gene Ther* 16 405-414.

Woodcroft, K. J.; Hafner, M. S. & Novak, R. F. (2002). Insulin signaling in the transcriptional and posttranscriptional regulation of CYP2E1 expression. *Hepatology* 35 263-273.

Wyles, D. L. & Gerber, J. G. (2005). Antiretroviral drug pharmacokinetics in hepatitis with hepatic dysfunction. *Clin Infect Dis* 40 174-181.

Xie, W. (2008). *Nuclear receptors in drug metabolism*, John Wiley & Sons, Inc. ISBN: 978-0-470-08679-7, Hoboken, New Jersey.

Xiong, H.; Yoshinari, K.; Brouwer, K. L. & Negishi, M. (2002). Role of constitutive androstane receptor in the in vivo induction of Mrp3 and CYP2B1/2 by phenobarbital. *Drug Metab Dispos* 30 918-923.

Yoh, K.; Ishii, G.; Yokose, T.; Minegishi, Y.; Tsuta, K.; Goto, K.; Nishiwaki, Y.; Kodama, T.; Suga, M. & Ochiai, A. (2004). Breast cancer resistance protein impacts clinical outcome in platinum-based chemotherapy for advanced non-small cell lung cancer. *Clin Cancer Res* 10 1691-1697.

Yoshinari, K.; Takagi, S.; Sugatani, J. & Miwa, M. (2006a). Changes in the expression of cytochromes P450 and nuclear receptors in the liver of genetically diabetic db/db mice. *Biol Pharm Bull* 29 1634-1638.

Yoshinari, K.; Takagi, S.; Yoshimasa, T.; Sugatani, J. & Miwa, M. (2006b). Hepatic CYP3A expression is attenuated in obese mice fed a high-fat diet. *Pharm Res* 23 1188-1200.

Young, L. C.; Campling, B. G.; Voskoglou-Nomikos, T.; Cole, S. P.; Deeley, R. G. & Gerlach, J. H. (1999). Expression of multidrug resistance protein-related genes in lung cancer: correlation with drug response. *Clin Cancer Res* 5 673-680.

Young, M. J.; Clyne, C. D.; Cole, T. J. & Funder, J. W. (2001). Cardiac steroidogenesis in the normal and failing heart. *J Clin Endocrinol Metab* 86 5121-5126.

Yu, L. & Chen, S. (2008). Toll-like receptors expressed in tumor cells: targets for therapy. *Cancer Immunol Immunother* 57 1271-1278.

Yu, R.; Lei, W.; Mandlekar, S.; Weber, M. J.; Der, C. J.; Wu, J. & Kong, A. N. (1999). Role of a mitogen-activated protein kinase pathway in the induction of phase II detoxifying enzymes by chemicals. *J Biol Chem* 274 27545-27552.

Zhou, J.; Liu, M.; Aneja, R.; Chandra, R.; Lage, H. & Joshi, H. C. (2006). Reversal of P-glycoprotein-mediated multidrug resistance in cancer cells by the c-Jun NH2-terminal kinase. *Cancer Res* 66 445-452.

Zordoky, B. N. & El-Kadi, A. O. (2009). Role of NF-kappaB in the regulation of cytochrome P450 enzymes. *Curr Drug Metab* 10 164-178.

5

Anticancer Drug Metabolism: Chemotherapy Resistance and New Therapeutic Approaches

Hanane Akhdar[1], Claire Legendre[1], Caroline Aninat and Fabrice Morel
Inserm, UMR991, Liver Metabolisms and Cancer, Rennes,
University of Rennes 1, Rennes,
France

1. Introduction

Over the last decades, several studies have demonstrated that cancer cells have a unique metabolism compared to normal cells (Herling et al., 2011). Metabolic changes occurring in cancer cells are considered to be fundamental for the transformation of normal cells into cancer cells and are also responsible for the resistance to different types of chemotherapeutic drugs (Cree, 2011). Therefore, resistance to chemotherapy represents a major problem in the treatment of several tumor types. Among the different metabolic and signalling pathways that are altered in cancer cells, variations in the expression and activity of several drug-metabolizing enzymes play a critical role in drug resistance (Rochat, 2009). Resistance can occur prior to drug treatment (primary or innate resistance) or may develop over time following exposure to the drug (acquired resistance). In some patients, prolonged exposure to a single chemotherapeutic agent may lead to the development of resistance to multiple other structurally unrelated compounds, known as cross resistance or multidrug resistance.

Cancer cell metabolism is also closely linked to molecular oxygen concentration. Indeed, weak blood irrigation is frequently encountered in solid tumors and is responsible for hypoxic environment which is associated with invasive/aggressive phenotype and therapeutic resistance (Shannon et al., 2003). Hypoxia also contributes to drug resistance because some chemotherapeutic drugs require oxygen to generate free radicals that contribute to toxicity. Moreover, hypoxia might modulate expression of enzymes directly involved in metabolism of chemotherapeutic drugs, thereby limiting the toxic effects of these drugs on cancer cells. On the other hand, new therapeutic strategies aim at using bioreductive drugs that are selectively toxic to hypoxic cells (McKeown et al., 2007).

The proposal of this chapter is to describe the role of anticancer drug metabolism in chemotherapy resistance but also its importance for the development of new approaches, taking advantage of the specificity of cancer cells metabolism.

2. Anticancer drugs

Anticancer or chemotherapy drugs are powerful chemicals that kill cancer cells by arresting their growth at one or more checkpoints in their cell cycle. Their main role is thus to reduce

---

[1] These authors contributed equally to this work.

and prevent the growth and spread of cancer cells. However, because anticancer agents rapidly affect dividing cells, normal cells are also affected. This is especially true in tissue with high cell turnover such as the gastrointestinal tract, bone marrow, skin, hair roots, nails... Consequently, side effects are commonly observed with various types of chemotherapies. More than 100 different drugs are used today for chemotherapy, either alone or in combination with other treatments.

For several years, the most effective drugs used in cancer chemotherapy were DNA-damaging agents (Gurova, 2009). These drugs can be divided into different categories based on their mechanism of action. Inhibitors of DNA synthesis inhibit essential biosynthetic processes or are incorporated into macromolecules (DNA and RNA). These drugs are either structural analogues for heterocyclic bases or agents interfering with folate metabolism (heterocyclic bases and folic acid are DNA building blocks) and they inhibit main steps in the formation of purine and pyrimidine bases as well as nucleotides (Parker, 2009). This class of agent includes antifolates (methotrexate, pemetrixed) (Goldman et al., 2010), antipyrimidines (5-fluorouracil, capecitabine, eniluracile, hydroxyurea) (Longley et al., 2003) and antipurines (6-mercaptopurine, 6-thioguanine). Another class of drugs directly damages DNA by adding methyl or other alkyl groups onto nucleotide bases (Izbicka and Tolcher, 2004). This in turn inhibits their correct utilization by base pairing leading to mutation, DNA fragmentation as well as inhibition of DNA replication and transcription. These anticancer drugs include alkylating agents (cyclophosphamide, ifosfamide, melphalan, chlorambucil), platinum-based drugs (cisplatin, carboplatin), antibiotics (anthracyclines, dactinomycin, bleomycin, adriamycin, etoposide) and topoisomerase II inhibitors (camptothecine, irinotecan, topotecan). Molecules belonging to the third class affect synthesis or breakdown of the mitotic spindle (Risinger et al., 2009). These drugs disrupt the cell division by either inhibiting the tubulin polymerization and therefore the formation of the mitotic spindle (vinblastine, vincristine) or by stabilizing microtubules (paclitaxel, docetaxel).

Over the past 20 years, the elucidation of different signal-transduction networks that are responsible for neoplastic transformation has led to rationally designed anticancer drugs that target specific molecular events. These targeted cancer drug candidates include protein kinase inhibitors that represent an important and still emerging class of therapeutic agents. Clinically approved kinase-targeted oncology agents include 1) small molecules such as imatinib (targeting Abl, Platelet-Derived Growth Factor Receptor (PDGFR)), gefitinib and erlotinib (targeting epidermal growth factor Receptor (EGFR)), sorafenib (targeting PDGFR, EGFR, Raf-1, c-kit) or 2) antibodies such as Cetuximab or Bevacizumab that inhibit EGFR and vascular endothelial growth factor receptor (VEGFR), respectively (Sebolt-Leopold and English, 2006). Unfortunately, these new targeted drugs also face major obstacles similar to those that challenge traditional agents.

3. Anticancer drug metabolism and resistance

3.1 Anticancer drug metabolism

In vivo, after absorption in the organism, xenobiotics (including anticancer drugs) are typically metabolized through a number of parallel and/or sequential reactions. Metabolism occurred through two distinct consecutive phases named "phase I" and "phase II", although this order is not exclusive (phase I not always followed by phase II; phase II not always preceded by phase I) (Iyanagi, 2007). Phase I reactions are most commonly described as "functionalization" reactions and include oxidations, reductions, and hydrolysis (Guengerich, 2007, 2008). These reactions introduce a new polar functional group to the parent drug (oxidation), modify an existing functional group in order to be more polar (reduction) or unmask existing polar functional group (hydrolysis). The most common functional groups exposed or introduced in the phase I reactions are hydroxyl (-OH), amino (-NH$_2$), and carboxylic acid (-COOH).

Phase II reactions are most commonly described as conjugation reactions and include glucuronidation, sulfonation, glycine/glutamine conjugation, acetylation, methylation, and glutathione (GSH) conjugation (Bock et al., 1987; Jancova et al., 2010). Conjugations allow linking a new group either to the parent drug or to phase I metabolites. Some conjugations cause a dramatic increase in the polarity and thus favor excretion of a drug by adding an ionized functional group: sulfonation, glucuronidation, and amino acid conjugation. Other conjugation reactions are just likely to cause termination of therapeutic activity: methylation and acetylation. GSH conjugation reaction protects against reactive metabolites.

In this chapter, we will be interested mainly by two distinct families of enzymes, cytochrome P450s (CYP) and glutathione transferases (GST) belonging to phase I and phase II metabolism, respectively.

3.1.1 Cytochrome P450s

CYP enzymes are key players in the phase I-dependent metabolism, mostly catalyse oxidations of drugs and other xenobiotics. More than 57 active human CYP genes and 58 pseudogenes have been described (Sim and Ingelman-Sundberg, 2010). Most of these genes are polymorphic and more than 434 different alleles of genes encoding CYP enzymes have been identified. The CYP3A (CYP belonging to family 3, subfamily A) enzymes are involved in the metabolism of about 50% of all drugs currently on the market (Bu, 2006). CYPs also participate in the metabolic activation of several carcinogens such as aflatoxin B$_1$ (Langouet et al., 1995). As a result of the CYP-dependent metabolism, intermediates that exert toxicity or carcinogenicity can be formed. In most cases, these metabolites are targets for phase II enzyme dependent reactions, rendering them inactive polar products suitable for excretion *via* the kidneys. Concerning anticancer agents, CYPs are involved not only in cytotoxic drugs detoxication but also in the activation of prodrugs making them therapeutically effective (McFadyen et al., 2004). Prodrugs are inactive agents that are converted to active cytotoxic drugs upon exposure to tumor tissues exhibiting high expression of activating enzymes. This targeting strategy minimizes toxicity towards normal tissues while it increases delivery of active agent to the tumor tissue. Cyclophosphamide, ifosfamide, dacarbazine, procarbazine, tegafur, and thiotepa are metabolized by CYPs in the liver and this activation reaction is required for therapeutic activity (Rodriguez-Antona and Ingelman-Sundberg, 2006). Another example is 1,4-bis-([2-(dimethylamino-N-oxide)ethyl]amino)5,8-dihydroxy anthracene-9,10-dione (AQ4N), a bioreductive prodrug that needs activation by CYP2S1 and CYP2W1 in tumor tissues to be converted to a topoisomerase II inhibitor (Nishida et al., 2010). Therefore, because CYPs are involved in either the bioactivation or the inactivation of both carcinogens and anticancer drugs (Huttunen et al., 2008), they play important roles in the etiology of cancer diseases and as determinants of cancer therapy (Oyama et al., 2004).

3.1.2 Glutathione transferases

GSTs are a family of ubiquitous intracellular enzymes that catalyze the conjugation of GSH to many exogenous and endogenous compounds (Hayes et al., 2005). These include chemical carcinogens, therapeutic drugs and products of oxidative stress. In addition to their major role in catalyzing the conjugation of electrophilic substrates to GSH, these enzymes have GSH-dependent peroxidase (Hurst et al., 1998) and isomerase (Johansson and Mannervik, 2001) activities. GSTs play an important role in the protection against reactive molecules such as electrophilic xenobiotics (anticancer drugs, pollutants or carcinogens) or endogenous alpha,beta-unsaturated aldehydes, quinones, epoxides, and hydroperoxides formed as secondary metabolites during oxidative stress. Over the last decade, different studies have demonstrated that GSTs also have a non-catalytic function *via* their interaction with some kinases (Adler et al., 1999; Cho et al., 2001; Gilot et al., 2002) or other proteins (Dulhunty et al., 2001; Wu et al., 2006) thus playing critical roles in stress response, apoptosis and proliferation. GSTs are members of at least three gene families: the cytosolic (or soluble) GSTs that are divided in seven families: alpha, mu, pi, theta, sigma, zeta and omega (Hayes et al., 2005); the mitochondrial GST (kappa class) (Morel and Aninat, 2011) and the membrane-associated proteins involved in eicosanoid and glutathione metabolism (MAPEG) (Jakobsson et al., 2000; Jakobsson et al., 1999). The cancer chemotherapeutic agents adriamycin, 1,3-bis(2-chloroethyl)-1-nitrosourea (BCNU), busulfan, carmustine, chlorambucil, cisplatin, crotonyloxymethyl-2-cyclohexenone, cyclophosphamide, melphalan, mitozantrone and thiotepa are potent substrates of GSTs (Hamilton et al., 2003; Hayes and Pulford, 1995; Lien et al., 2002). Metabolism of these anticancer drugs by GSTs is related to several drug resistance phenomena and adverse toxicity effects (Townsend and Tew, 2003b).

3.1.3 Drug transporters

Drug passage across biological membranes is possible through two different mechanisms. The first one involves passive *trans*-cellular transport and concerned lipophilic molecules. The second one depends on carrier-mediated transporters, among which, we distinguish those requiring ATP-dependent hydrolysis as the first step in catalysis (ABC transporters such as multidrug resistance protein (MDR), multidrug resistance-associated protein (MRP), and breast cancer resistance protein (BCRP)) from those driven by an exchange or co-transport of intracellular and/or extracellular ions with the substrate (organic anion transporter (OAT), organic anion-transporting polypeptide (OATP), sodium taurocholate co-transporting peptide (NTCP), organic cation transporter (OCT), novel organic cation transporter (OCTN) and oligopeptide transporter (PEPT)) (Keppler, 2011; Li et al., 2010; Ni et al., 2010; Svoboda et al., 2011).

Active transporters are of great interest to pharmacologists since they are responsible for both the uptake and the efflux of drugs and are key elements of the pharmacokinetic characteristics of a drug (Degorter et al., 2011). Indeed, it has now become clear that transporters are essential for the uptake, accumulation, distribution and efflux of drugs. For example, drug efflux transporters including the P-glycoprotein pump (Pgp), the multidrug-resistant protein-1 (MRP1) and the BCRP actively pump drugs such as chemotherapeutics out of the cells, thereby reducing their intracellular accumulation and making the cell insensitive to different drugs such as anthracyclines, vinca-alkaloids or taxanes. Among the major known ABC transporters,

ABCB1 gene, also known as *MDR1*, encoding Pgp is by far the best characterized and understood efflux transporter (Goda et al., 2009; Wu et al., 2011). It is predominantly expressed in several tissues including the luminal surface of intestinal epithelia, the renal proximal tubule, the bile canalicular membrane of hepatocytes and the blood brain barrier (Ho and Kim, 2005). Pgp plays an important role in limiting intestinal drug absorption and brain penetration as well as in facilitating renal or biliary excretion of drugs. The MRPs are involved in the drug efflux from the liver or kidney into the peripheral blood (e.g. MRP1, MRP3, and MRP6), or from the liver, kidney and small intestines into the bile, urine and intestinal lumen respectively (MRP2) (Keppler, 2011). Since GSH-, glucuronide-, sulfate-conjugates and organic anions such as methotrexate, indinavir, cisplatin, vincristine and etoposide are all MRP substrates, MRPs are also crucial in human drug disposition and toxicity.

3.2 Anticancer drug resistance

The development of chemotherapy resistance remains a major problem to the effective treatment of many tumor types. Resistance can occur prior to drug treatment (primary or innate resistance) or may develop over time following exposure (acquired resistance). In some patients, prolonged exposure to a single chemotherapeutic agent may lead to the development of resistance to multiple other structurally unrelated compounds. This process is known as cross resistance or multidrug resistance (MDR). In primary resistance, MDR can occur without prior exposure to chemotherapy. Several mechanisms, including alterations in drug pharmacokinetic and metabolism, modification of drug target expression or function, drug compartmentalization in cellular organelles, altered repair of drug-induced DNA damages, changes in apoptotic signaling pathways or expression of proteins directly affecting cellular drug transport are responsible of anticancer drug resistance (Figure 1).

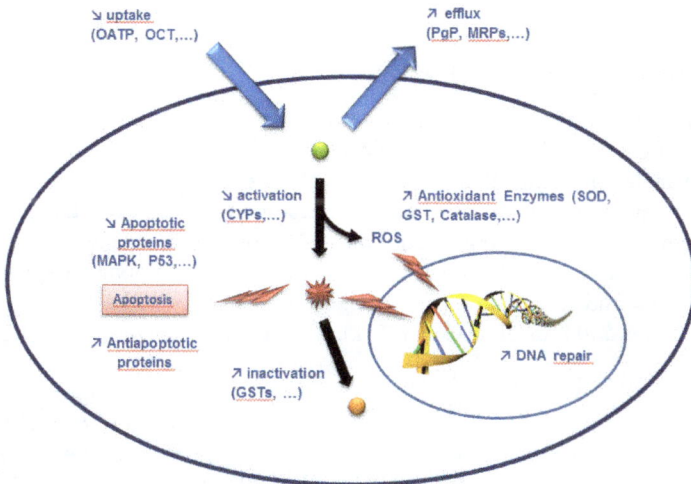

Fig. 1. Representation of different mechanisms involved in anticancer drug resistance. ↗: increase; ↘: decrease; OATP: organic anion-transporting polypeptide ; OCT : organic cation transporter ; Pgp: P-glycoprotein; MRP: multidrug resistance associated proteins; CYP: cytochrome P-450; SOD: superoxide dismutase; GST: glutathione transferase; MAPK: mitogen activated protein kinase.

3.2.1 Drug transport

Drug transporters are the key determinants for the uptake, accumulation, distribution and efflux of several chemotherapeutic drugs. Interestingly, overexpression of these drug transporters in tumors has been demonstrated by several studies. Pgp is expressed in approximately 40% of all breast carcinomas (Trock et al., 1997), although another study reported values as high as 66% (Larkin et al., 2004). MRP3 was found to be the predominant MRP isoform in gallbladder carcinomas and cholangiocellular carcinomas and the intrinsic multidrug resistance in these carcinomas seems to be dependent on the expression of MRP3 (Rau et al., 2008). The *MRP4* (also named *cMOAT* or *ABCC4*) gene is overexpressed in cisplatin resistant human cancer cell lines with decreased drug accumulation (Taniguchi et al., 1996). Platinum-resistant tumor cells are capable of eliminating platinum GSH-conjugates in an ATP-dependent manner through an active efflux mechanism mediated by a GS-X pumps (Ishikawa et al., 2000; Suzuki et al., 2001). MRP8, encoded by *ABCC11* gene, is able to confer resistance to fluoropyrimidines by mediating the MgATP-dependent transport of the cytotoxic metabolite 5'-fluoro-2'-deoxyuridine monophosphate (Guo et al., 2003). MRP2 expression has been suggested to affect the efficacy of cisplatin treatment in patients with hepatocellular carcinoma (Korita et al., 2010). Overexpression of these pumps in tumor cells gives them the ability to evade the treatment by drugs such as cisplatin, fluoropyrimidines, doxorubicin and etoposide in different types of cancer (Jedlitschky et al., 1996; Kool et al., 1997; Xu et al., 2010; Zelcer et al., 2001). Therefore, the use of chemomodulators to inhibit efflux transport has been tested in an attempt to overcome this resistance (Baumert and Hilgeroth, 2009; Zhou et al., 2008). In this way, a recent study has demonstrated that indomethacin and SC236 inhibit Pgp and MRP1 expression and thus enhance the cytotoxicity of doxorubicin in human hepatocellular carcinoma cells (Ye et al., 2011).

3.2.2 Drug inactivation/detoxification

Drug-metabolizing enzymes can also play an important role in reducing the intracellular concentration of drugs and in affecting cancer drug resistance. Interestingly, certain drugs require to be metabolized by these enzymes before exerting their cytotoxic effects. The expression of drug-metabolizing enzymes can therefore either potentiate or reduce the toxicity of chemicals and variations in both the activation and the inactivation pathways are important variables that can lead to drug resistance. In model systems, it appears that both oxidation (phase I) and conjugation (phase II) enzymes play critical roles in protecting cells against many drugs and thus play a key role in drug resistance.

3.2.2.1 Involvement of cytochrome P450s

As previously mentioned, CYPs are involved in both activation and detoxication of xenobiotics, including therapeutic drugs. CYP3A4 plays an important role in the metabolism of several anticancer agents (e.g. taxanes, vinca-alkaloids and new drugs such as imatinib, sorafenib and gefitinib). CYP3A4 metabolizes docetaxel to inactive hydroxylated derivatives. Therefore, a high CYP3A4 activity would result in a poor therapeutic outcome of the drug. Accordingly, in cancer patients treated with docetaxel in combination with the potent CYP3A4 inhibitor ketoconazole, a 49% decrease in docetaxel clearance was found (Engels et al., 2004). A low expression of CYP3A4 in breast tumors resulted in a better response to docetaxel (Miyoshi et al., 2005). Similarly, hepatic CYP3A4 activity measured by the erythromycin breath test and midazolam clearance predicted docetaxel clearance and demonstrated a higher toxicity in patients with the lowest CYP3A4 activity (Goh et al., 2002). Similarly to docetaxel, irinotecan is inactivated by CYP3A4 and induction of CYP3A4 in patients receiving irinotecan results in a significant decrease in the formation of the toxic metabolite of this drug (Mathijssen et al., 2002). Additionally, CYP3A4 phenotype, as assessed by midazolam clearance, is significantly associated with irinotecan pharmacokinetic (Mathijssen et al., 2004). More recently, a study suggested that the Pregnane X-Receptor (PXR) pathway is also involved in irinotecan resistance in colon cancer cell line *via* the upregulation of drug-metabolizing genes such as *CYP3A4* (Basseville et al., 2011).

Other CYP families also participate to anticancer drugs metabolism. For example, CYP2C19 and CYP2B6 are involved in the activation of the chemotherapeutic agent cyclophosphamide (Helsby et al., 2010) and reduced expression of these CYPs is a potential mechanism of resistance. An interesting study showed a mechanism of acquired resistance to anticancer therapy based on the induction of CYP2C8 and MDR1. In this study, Caco-2 cells were capable of increasing the expression of *CYP2C8* as a response to long-term exposure to paclitaxel (Garcia-Martin et al., 2006). Furthermore, the correlation between CYP polymorphism and anticancer drug response has been demonstrated for CYP2B6. Indeed, CYP2B6*2, CYP2B6*8, CYP2B6*9, CYP2B6*4 variant alleles are associated with response to doxorubicin- cyclophosphamide therapy in the treatment of breast cancer and with a worse outcome (Bray et al., 2010). In another study, it has been demonstrated that CYP1B1 inactivates docetaxel and showed that the overexpression of CYP1B1 in a Chinese hamster ovary fibroblast cell line (V79MZ) was correlated to a significantly decreased sensitivity towards docetaxel (McFadyen et al., 2001a; McFadyen et al., 2001b). Finally, other authors suggested that CYP1B1 does not directly inactivate docetaxel but promotes cell survival by another unknown mechanism (Martinez et al., 2008).

Altogether, these studies demonstrate that altered levels of expression or inhibition of CYPs can have profound effects on the sensitivity of target cell to toxic compounds.

3.2.2.2 Involvement of glutathione transferases

GSTs are involved in the development of resistance to anticancer drugs by different ways. Indeed, they play a role in the metabolism of a diverse array of cancer chemotherapeutic agents including adriamycin, BCNU, busulfan, carmustine, chlorambucil, cisplatin, cyclophosphamide, ethacrynic acid, melphalan or thiotepa (Chen and Waxman, 1994; Dirven et al., 1994; Paumi et al., 2001). The roles of GSTs in the metabolism of these anticancer drugs and the correlation between GST expression levels and drug sensitivity have been demonstrated in several studies. For example, the inhibition of GST Pi 1 (GSTP1) expression, through antisense cDNA, has been shown to increase the tumor sensitivity to adriamicin, cisplatin, melphalan and etoposide (Ban et al., 1996). By contrast, the overexpression of GSTP1 in human renal UOK130 tumor cells was accompanied by a decreased sensitivity to cisplatin, melphalan and chlorambucil (Wang et al., 2007). Similarly, overexpression of Alpha class GST has been correlated with the resistance to alkylating agents in Colo 320HSR cells (Xie et al., 2005) and to doxorubicin in MCF-7 human breast cancer and small cell lung cancer (H69) cell lines (Sharma et al., 2006; Wang et al., 1999).

Overexpression of Mu class GST has been associated with chlorambucil resistance in human ovarian carcinoma cell line (Horton et al., 1999) and with poor prognosis in childhood acute lymphoblastic leukaemia (Hall et al., 1994).

Interestingly, high levels of GSTs are linked either with drug resistance or cancer incidence. GSTP1 has retained much attention because many tumors and cancer cell lines are characterized by high GSTP1 expression. Moreover, increased expression of GSTP1 has been associated to acquired resistance to cancer drugs (Tew, 1994). It is noteworthy that several studies have demonstrated that altered GST catalytic activities caused by genetic polymorphisms are linked to cancer susceptibility and prognosis (McIlwain et al., 2006). For example, GST genotypes are associated with primary and post-chemotherapy tumor histology in testicular germ cell tumors (Kraggerud et al., 2009); GST polymorphisms may have a role in treatment response and osteosarcoma progression (Salinas-Souza et al., 2010) and null genotypes of GSTM1 and GSTT1 contribute to hepatocellular carcinoma risk (Wang et al., 2010).

The non-catalytic functions of GST might also play a key role in the anticancer drug sensitivity. Indeed, the direct interaction and inhibition of various MAP Kinases by GSTs have been demonstrated. These MAP kinases are involved in cell proliferation and apoptosis but also in anticancer drug responses. In the last decade, several studies have demonstrated that GSTs are involved in the control of apoptosis through the inhibition of the Jun N-terminal Kinase (JNK) signaling pathway. Indeed, JNK is inactive and sequestered into a GSTP1-JNK complex (Adler et al., 1999) whereas Apoptosis Signal Kinase 1 (ASK1) and Mitogen-activated protein kinase kinase kinase (MEKK1) interact with GSTM1 leading to their inactivation (Gilot et al., 2002; Ryoo et al., 2004). Thus, the overexpression of GSTs in many tumors or their up-regulation by drugs could represent another mechanism of drug resistance, independent of their enzymatic activity. As an example, cisplatin, chlorambucil, doxorubicin, 5-fluorouracil and carboplatin are among anticancer drugs whose toxicity require the activation of JNK and resistance to these drugs is highly associated to overexpression of GSTs in tumors (Townsend and Tew, 2003a). Therefore, development of GST inhibitors that could prevent MAPK inhibition is considered as a promising strategy to achieve new anticancer drugs in order to increase chemotherapeutic efficiency.

3.2.3 Involvement of nuclear transcription factors in drug resistance

Nuclear receptors are a superfamily of transcription factors with 48 distinct members identified within the human genome (Germain et al., 2006). In addition to the classic steroidal hormone receptors, other nuclear receptors act as metabolic sensors that respond to compounds of dietary origin, intermediates in metabolic pathways, drugs and other environmental factors, integrating homeostatic control over many metabolic processes (Sonoda et al., 2008). For example, some aspects of drug metabolism and transport are regulated by pregnane X receptor (PXR) and constitutive androstane receptor (CAR); energy and glucose metabolism are regulated in part by peroxisome proliferator-activated receptor gamma (PPARγ); fatty acid, triglyceride and lipoprotein metabolisms are controlled by PPARα, δ, and γ; reverse cholesterol transport and cholesterol absorption depends on liver X receptor (LXR) activation and bile acid metabolism is regulated by farnesoid X receptor (FXR) (Evans, 2005; Francis et al., 2003).

PXR and CAR are master xenobiotic receptors that regulate the expression of genes involved in drug metabolism and clearance, including drug-metabolizing enzymes and transporters (Evans, 2005). In this part, we will focus on nuclear factors involved in the regulation drug-metabolizing enzymes and drug transporters (PXR, CAR and Nrf2) and on their specific roles in drug resistance.

3.2.3.1 Pregnane X receptor (PXR)

In 1998, a new member of the nuclear hormone receptor family, named PXR (NR1I2), has been identified (Kliewer et al., 1998). PXR is activated primarily by pregnanes and dimerizes with retinoid X receptor (RXR) immediately after its activation by ligand binding. PXR is present in the cytoplasm where it interacts with a protein complex. After its activation, PXR translocates into the nucleus to regulate gene transcription (Squires et al., 2004). PXR recognizes a wide variety of ligands including dexamethasone, rifampicin, spironolactone and pregnenolone 16α-carbonitrile being among the best characterized (Timsit and Negishi, 2007) as well as many anticancer drugs such as microtubule-binding drugs (Raynal et al., 2010). Targets genes of PXR are *CYP3A4*, *MDR1*, *CYP2B6*, members of UGTs superfamily and *MRP3* and *OATP2* transporters (Klaassen and Slitt, 2005; Tolson and Wang, 2010).¶

Due to its capacity to recognize such compounds and to induce transcription of genes involved in the detoxification process, PXR is considered as one of the master regulator of xenobiotic clearance. Moreover, because PXR controls the expression of key genes involved in anticancer drugs disposition, recent works have focused on its potential role in drug resistance (Chen, 2010). The mechanisms of resistance induced by PXR activation probably involve up-regulation of drug-detoxifying enzymes and transporters. Supporting this hypothesis, it has been shown that PXR activation by different ligands induces PXR target genes (*CYP2B6*, *CYP3A4* and *UGT1A1*) and consequently drug resistance in ovarian cancer cells (Gupta et al., 2008). Moreover, PXR induces expression of *CYP3A4* and *MDR1* genes in multiple cell types and the products of these genes are known to detoxify microtubule-binding and topoisomerase-binding drugs. Previous studies have shown that PXR activation regulates Pgp in the blood-brain barrier (Bauer et al., 2004). Interestingly, anticancer drugs such as vincristine, tamoxifen, vinblastine, docetaxel, cyclophosphamide, flutamide, ifosfamide and paclitaxel activate PXR-mediated Pgp induction and thus affect the cytotoxic activity and accumulation of the Pgp substrate rhodamine 123 (Harmsen et al., 2010).

Increased expression of PXR leads to higher resistance of HEC-1 cells to paclitaxel and cisplatin (Chen, 2010) and of human colon adenocarcinoma to doxorubicin (Harmsen et al., 2010). In osteocarcinoma, the effectiveness of etoposide was reduced due to activation of PXR and the co-administration of PXR agonists enhanced the clearance of all-trans-retinoic acid (ATRA). This mechanism could potentially contribute to ATRA resistance in the treatment of acute promyelocytic leukemia (APL) and several solid tumors (Wang, T. et al., 2008). However, other mechanisms of resistance (e.g., down-regulation of apoptotic genes) may also play a dominant role (Zhou et al., 2008).

3.2.3.2 Constitutive androstane receptor (CAR)

The constitutive androstane receptor (CAR) is a sister xenobiotic receptor of PXR. CAR was first purified from hepatocytes as a protein bound to the phenobarbital responsive element in the *CYP2B* gene promoter. CAR was subsequently shown to bind to the *CYP2B* gene promoter as a heterodimer with retinoid X receptor (RXR). Transfected CAR exhibited a high basal activity and was once termed a "constitutively active receptor." The name of constitutive androstane receptor was conceived due to the binding and inhibition of CAR activity by androstanes (Forman et al., 1998). CAR is retained in the cytoplasm by forming a complex with phosphatase 2A, HSP90 and cytosolic CAR retention protein (Kobayashi et al., 2003). Phenobarbital, 5β-pregnane-3,20-dione, and 5-androstan-3-ol are known CAR ligands (Moore et al., 2000). The hepatomitogen 1,4-Bis[2-(3,5-dichloropyridyloxy)] benzene (TCPOBOP) is a synthetic agonist for murine CAR (Tzameli et al., 2000) and 6-(4-chlorophenyl)imidazo[2,1-b] [1,3]thiazole-5-carbaldehydeO-(3,4-dichlorobenzyl)oxime (CITCO) is an imidazothiazole derivative that functions as a selective agonist for human CAR (Ikeda et al., 2005). Upon activation with specific agonist, CAR translocates into the nucleus and binds to the response elements as monomer or CAR/RXR heterodimer. CAR functions as a xenobiotic receptor that participates in the regulation of transcription of drug transporter genes such as MRPs (*MRP2*, *MRP3* and *MRP4*), *OATP2* and *MDR1* ((Urquhart et al., 2007). CAR promotes the detoxification and elimination of potentially toxic compounds by modulating the phase I and phase II drug-metabolizing enzymes. Therefore, CAR-mediated expression of xenobiotic-metabolizing enzymes is generally protective, but can be deleterious if toxic metabolites are produced. CAR agonists are able to induce hepatocyte proliferation that depends on c-Myc-FoxM1 function (Blanco-Bose et al., 2008) but also to inhibit Fas-induced hepatocyte apoptosis by depleting the proapoptotic proteins Bak (Bcl-2 antagonistic killer) and Bax (Bcl-2-associated X protein) and increasing the expression of the antiapoptotic effector myeloid cell leukaemia factor-1 (Baskin-Bey et al., 2006).

3.2.3.3 Nuclear factor-erythroid 2p45 (NF-E2)-related factor 2 (NRF2)

The transcription factor Nrf2 (nuclear factor-erythroid 2p45 (NF-E2)-related factor 2) is a major regulator in the basal and inducible expression of various phase II detoxifying and antioxidant enzymes. In the resting state, kelch-like ECH-associated protein 1 (Keap1) functions as an intracellular redox receptor, which binds Nrf2 and targets it for proteosomal degradation. When cells are exposed to oxidative damage, Nrf2 is liberated from Keap1 and translocated into the nucleus where it specifically recognizes an enhancer sequence known as Antioxidant Response Element (ARE). This binding of Nrf2 on ARE sequence results in the activation of redox balancing genes (e.g. heme-oxygenase–1), phase II detoxifying genes (e.g. GSTs and NAD(P)H quinine oxidoreductase-1) and drug transporters (e.g. MRP) (Baird and Dinkova-Kostova, 2011; Taguchi et al., 2011). Several studies have suggested that the activation of Nrf2 protects against chronic diseases such as cardiovascular diseases, neurodegenerative disorders, lung inflammation, fibrosis, diabetes and nephropathy. However, in recent years, the dark side of Nrf2 has emerged and growing evidences suggest that Nrf2 constitutive up-regulation is associated with cancer development, progression and resistance to chemotherapy (Hayes and McMahon, 2006, 2009; Konstantinopoulos et al., 2011; Wang X.J. et al., 2008). Many anticancer drugs are responsible for the production of ROS in cancer cells, a phenomenon which contributes to drug-induced apoptosis. Such species are scavenged by the catalytic activities of superoxide dismutase, catalase, GSH peroxidase, γ-glutamylcysteine synthetase and heme oxygenase-1. These enzymes are members of the ARE-gene battery and are often overexpressed during carcinogenesis and it seems likely that Nrf2 may be responsible for this phenotype.

The down-regulation of Nrf2-dependent response by overexpression of its negative regulator, Keap1, or transient-transfection of Nrf2-siRNA in lung carcinoma, breast adenocarcinoma, neuroblastoma, ovarian cancer and colon cancer rendered cancer cells more susceptible to cisplatin, etoposide, doxorubicin and 5-fluorouracil (Akhdar et al., 2009; Cho et al., 2008; Homma et al., 2009; Wang, X.J. et al., 2008). Induction of nuclear translocation and activation of Nrf2 by 5-fluorouracil, which in turn leads to antioxidant enzymes up-regulation and increases resistance toward cytotoxic effects of this anticancer drug has been recently demonstrated (Akhdar et al., 2009). The inhibition of Nrf2 by a specific flavone, lutolein, leads to negative regulation of the Nrf2/ARE pathway and to the sensitization of human lung carcinoma cells to therapeutic drugs (Tang et al., 2011). *KEAP1* gene deletion provoked an aberrant Nrf2 activation and is one of the molecular mechanisms explaining chemotherapeutic resistance against 5-FU in gallbladder cells (Shibata et al., 2008a; Shibata et al., 2008b). Several studies have reported mutations of the interacting domain between Keap1 and Nrf2 leading to a permanent Nrf2 activation in non-small cell lung cancer (Ohta et al., 2008; Padmanabhan et al., 2006). Somatic mutations of the *KEAP1* gene were also reported in patients affected by gall bladder tumors and in breast cancer cell line (Nioi and Nguyen, 2007; Shibata et al., 2008a). Although recent studies demonstrated low or no expression of *KEAP1* in more than half of non-small cell lung cancers, only two papers investigated the epigenetic alterations of *KEAP1* in this type of tumor. An aberrant hypermethylation at the *KEAP1* gene promoter in lung cancer cell lines and in five lung cancer tissues has been demonstrated (Wang, R. et al., 2008). More recently, two alterations in *KEAP1* gene were detected in one third of the non-small cell lung cancers suggesting that both copies of the gene might be inactivated (Muscarella et al., 2011). In these cases, Keap1 function is impaired, leading to constitutive stabilization of Nrf2 and increased activation of its cytoprotective target genes (Okawa et al., 2006).

All of these findings support the idea that increased Nrf2 expression could facilitate cell growth, survival, resistance to chemotherapy through the activation of cytoprotective factors. Thus, investigating the deregulation of Keap1/Nrf2 pathway may shed light into the understanding of molecular mechanism of chemoresistance.

3.2.3.4 Hypoxia and Hypoxia Inducible Factor-1 (HIF-1)

Hypoxia and HIF-1α are found in solid tumors

Around fifty percent of locally advanced solid tumors exhibit hypoxic and/or anoxic tissue areas, heterogeneously distributed within the mass tumors (Vaupel and Mayer, 2007). Consequently, partial pressure of oxygen (PO$_2$) in tumors is variable and can reach values between 10 to 30 mmHg (equivalent to 1 to 3% O$_2$), in contrast to a PO$_2$ of 50–80 mmHg in most normal tissues (Grigoryan et al., 2005). Three converging mechanisms lead to this limited oxygenation in cancer cells. The first one is due to cell proliferation which is responsible for an increase of the tumor mass. The second one is characterized by a loss of structural organization of blood vessels already present or newly formed (angiogenesis) in the solid tumor. This process leads to a decreased irrigation of the tumor. In addition, hematologic status of patients with cancer is frequently modified by the disease itself or by chemotherapy and numbers of them suffer from anemia triggering a reduced oxygen-carrying capacity of the blood (Vaupel and Harrison, 2004; Vaupel and Mayer, 2007). HIF-1 transcription factor is a master regulator of the hypoxic response and HIF-1α subunit is stabilized during hypoxia. Therefore, overexpression of HIF-1α has been found in many human cancers such as bladder, brain, breast, colon, ovarian, pancreatic, prostate and renal carcinomas (Talks et al., 2000).

Metabolic adaptation to hypoxia and angiogenesis in solid tumor: HIF-1 and HIF-target genes

In order to fight against hypoxia, a metabolic adaptation of solid tumors is observed compared to the surrounding normal tissue. This phenomena has been first described by Otto Warburg (Warburg, 1956) fifty years ago. He found that, in contrast to normal tissue where glycolysis is used to produce approximately 10% of ATP (the remaining 90% being obtained by oxidative phosphorylation via the tricarboxylic acid (TCA) cycle); solid tumors produced over 50% of ATP by anaerobic glycolysis, i.e. without oxidative phosphorylation and with lactate production. Interestingly, this phenomenon occurs even if oxygen is available for the mitochondrial function. This altered energy dependency is known as the "Warburg effect" and is a hallmark of cancer cells. Several explanations have been given to understand the use of anaerobic glycolysis rather than oxidative phosphorylation for production of ATP, while this is less efficient for energy production. The first one is linked to the accumulation of mutations in the mitochondrial genome that prevent the proper functioning of mitochondria (Carew and Huang, 2002). As a consequence, oxidative phosphorylation is not enough efficient, forcing the cancer cells to use anaerobic glycolysis for ATP production. The second one involves the activation of a transcription factor specifically activated in cell response to hypoxia: the transcription factor hypoxia-inducible factor-1 (HIF-1).

HIF-1 transcription factor is composed of two protein subunits, HIF-1α and HIF-1β (Wang and Semenza, 1995). Its transcriptional activity depends on the stabilization of HIF-1α. While HIF-1β subunit is constitutively expressed into the cells, expression of HIF-1α protein is thinly regulated at a post-translational level. Hydroxylation of HIF-1α by prolyl hydroxylase domain (PHD) proteins, which target its subsequent proteasomal degradation, is one of the major mechanisms of regulation of HIF-1α cellular levels (Jaakkola et al., 2001). Since the activity of PHD enzymes is inhibited by low oxygen tension, HIF-1α protein is stabilized during hypoxia. As a result, upon hypoxic signal, HIF-1α subunit is stabilized translocated into the nucleus where it binds to HIF-1β to form the active HIF-1 complex. HIF-1 binds to hypoxia-responsive elements (HRE), consensus sequences in the promoter region of more than one hundred genes involved in cell proliferation, differentiation and survival, angiogenesis and energy metabolism that allow the cell, tissue, and organism to adapt to reduced oxygen conditions (Semenza, 2003).

Regarding glycolysis metabolism, several HIF-1 gene targets are directly involved in the switch between aerobic to anaerobic glycolysis. Glucose cell uptake and its metabolism are very active in cancer cells. This high activity is correlated with the induction of expression of both the glucose transporter GLUT1 and the glycolysis enzymes aldolase C and phosphoglycerate kinase 1 (PGK1) (Seagroves et al., 2001; Semenza, 2003). Furthermore, HIF-1 facilitates the conversion of pyruvate into lactic acid by the induction of lactate dehydrogenase A (LDHA) (Firth et al., 1995) and pyruvate dehydrogenase kinase 1 (PDK1) expressions (Kim et al., 2006; Papandreou et al., 2006). PDK1, by inhibiting the activity of the pyruvate dehydrogenase (PDH) (Patel and Korotchkina, 2001), prevents conversion of pyruvate into acetyl-CoA, promotes the conversion of pyruvate into lactate and reduces the metabolic activities of the TCA cycle and the mitochondrial oxidative phosphorylation. Finally, in order to prevent acidosis due to lactate accumulation, intracellular pH homeostasis is maintained by induction of the expression of the carbonic anhydrase 9 and 12 (CA9 and CA12) (Potter and Harris, 2004), the lactate transporter MCT-4 (Ullah et al., 2006) and the Na+/H+ exchanger NHE1 (Shimoda et al., 2006), all direct gene targets of HIF-1. Thus, those metabolic adaptations confer a selective growth advantage and, combined with angiogenesis, are a prerequisite for metastasis.

HIF-1 also plays a key role in angiogenesis, which is a process describing the growth of new blood vessels (neovascularization) from preexisting vessels. Angiogenesis is critical for tumor development since supply of oxygen and nutriments becomes limited to cancer cells located around 70-100 microns of a blood vessel (Carmeliet and Jain, 2000). Ability of tumor cells to induce angiogenesis occurs by a multi-step process, regulated by many pro-angiogenic factors. One of the strongest stimuli of angiogenesis is hypoxia and its transcription factor HIF-1 (Pugh and Ratcliffe, 2003). Indeed, HIF-1 can directly induce the expression of a number of proangiogenic factors such as the vascular endothelial growth factor (VEGF) and its receptors VEGFR1 and VEGFR2, the angiopoietins (ANG-1 and -2) and their receptors (Tie-1 and Tie-2) and the platelet-derived growth factor PDGF-β (Hickey and Simon, 2006). Of all the pro-angiogenic factors induced by HIF-1, VEGF is the factor that is most expressed in tumors (Dvorak, 2002). In several *in vitro* and *in vivo* models, HIF-1 signaling is required for VEGF production and the ability of tumor cells to promote angiogenesis. As such, stem cells HIF-1α-/- injected into nude mice form teratocarcinomas substantially smaller and less vascularized than WT embryonic cells (Ryan et al., 1998).

HIF-1 and HIF-target genes: Actors for drug resistance

Hypoxia and HIF-1 contribute to the poor response to anticancer therapy by several mechanisms (Cosse and Michiels, 2008; Tredan et al., 2007; Wouters et al., 2007). Indeed, HIF-1 activation allows expression of a battery of genes involved in survival and cell resistance to chemotherapy. For examples, studies have shown that hypoxia is directly involved in the induction of genes coding for the ABC transporters (*MDR1*, *MRP1* and *LRP*), responsible for HepG2 cells resistance toward 5-Fluorouracil (Comerford et al., 2002; Zhu et al., 2005). Moreover, a recent study has demonstrated that, by down-regulating the expression of the MAPK-specific phosphatase dual-specificity phosphatase-2 (DUSP2), HIF-1 is involved in the resistance of HeLa and HCT116 cells to cisplatin, oxaliplatin, and paclitaxel (Lin et al., 2011). Hypoxia, by modulating expression of enzymes directly involved in metabolism of chemotherapeutic drugs, such as CYPs, could also limit the toxic effects of these drugs on cancer cells. As such, paclitaxel metabolism into 6α-hydroxypaclitaxel is reduced upon hypoxic conditions compared to normoxic conditions in HepaRG cells (Legendre et al., 2009). Furthermore, cytotoxic anticancer drugs require the presence of oxygen to exert their effects via the production of ROS, damaging DNA and inducing cell cycle arrest and death by apoptosis. Therefore, lack of oxygen could interfere for the efficiency of those molecules such as doxorubicin, which exerts its cytotoxic effect by the production of superoxide anion (Grigoryan et al., 2005). Another important point is that solid tumors are often poorly irrigated, leading to a decreased accessibility of anticancer agents to the tumor. Decreased drug concentrations, because of limited drug penetration into tumor masses, participates actively to resistance of the tumor to chemotherapy (Tredan et al., 2007). Finally, hypoxic environment of solid tumors is often correlated with a decrease of extracellular pH (acidosis) that also modulates the accumulation and/or cell toxicity of anticancer agents (Gerweck, 1998; Reichert et al., 2002). For example, resistance to mitoxantrone in MCF-7 cells is related to the acidification of extracellular pH (Greijer et al., 2005). Taken together, hypoxia and HIF-1 play a key role in anticancer drug resistance.

3.2.4 Other mechanisms

Modification of drug target

Cells survival depends on a balanced assembly and disassembly of the highly conserved cytoskeletal filaments formed from actin and tubulin. Microtubules are assembled from α-tubulin and β-tubulin heterodimers, along with other proteins such as microtubule-associated proteins. Some anticancer drugs (such as vinca-alkaloids) bind to and stabilize free tubulin, causing microtubule depolymerization and others (such as taxanes) bind to and stabilize microtubules, causing a net increase in tubulin polymerization (Zhou and Giannakakou, 2005). These two mechanisms of action inhibit cell division and thereby trigger apoptosis of cells. Altered expression of β-tubulin isotypes (overexpression or mutation) and microtubule-associated proteins is found in many cancer cell lines and xenografts resistant to microtubule inhibitors. These alterations may be associated with the primary or acquired resistance to tubulin-binding agents observed clinically in many tumors (Kamath et al., 2005; Wang and Cabral, 2005). Recently, a novel skeleton microtubule inhibitor, chamaecypanone C, with anticancer activity triggering caspase 8-Fas/FasL dependent apoptotic pathway in human cancer cells has been identified and its cytotoxicity in a variety human tumor cell lines has been studied (Hsieh et al., 2010). The authors considered that chamaecypanone C is a promising anticancer compound that has potential for management of various malignancies, particularly for patients with drug resistance.

DNA repair and cellular damages

Many anticancer drugs exert their effects by inducing DNA damages. Thus, alterations in enzymes involved in DNA repair can affect drug resistance. Topoisomerase II is a critical enzyme that is involved in DNA replication and repair and reduced topoisomerase II expression or function can contribute to resistance to agents such as anthracyclines (Nitiss, 2009). DNA mismatch repair mediates damage repair from many drugs including alkylating agents, platinum compounds and anthracyclines and this mechanism has been implicated in drug resistance in cancer cells (Bignami et al., 2003).

Apoptosis

Resistance can also arise from a failure of the cells to undergo apoptosis following DNA damages or other cellular injuries. Alterations in genes regulating the apoptotic pathway such as BCL2, BCLX (anti-apoptotic proteins) or TP53 promote resistance to anticancer drugs (O'Connor et al., 1997). P53 can trigger elimination of the damaged cells by promoting apoptosis through the induction of pro-apoptotic genes, such as FAS and BAX, and the down-regulation of anti-apoptotic BCL2. Studies have reported that loss of p53 function reduces cellular sensitivity to anticancer drugs. Mutations in the TP53 gene are found in most human breast cancer cell lines, and certain mutations have been linked to de novo resistance to doxorubicin (Aas et al., 1996). On the other hand, the use of adenovirus-mediated TP53 gene therapy reverses resistance of breast cancer cells to adriamycin (Qi et al., 2011).

4. Taking advantage of cancer cell metabolism for drug targeting

4.1 Nuclear factors: Targets for new therapeutic strategies

4.1.1 PXR and CAR

During the last years, several groups have studied the role of PXR antagonists as potential pharmaceuticals for the reversal of drug resistance and enhancement of drug delivery (Biswas et al., 2009; Harmsen et al., 2010). Ketoconazole was originally described as a PXR antagonist (Takeshita et al., 2002). However, significant side effects of ketoconazole were reported mainly because of its off-target effects (e.g., cortisol synthesis, hepatic toxicity), some of which are related to its capacity to inhibit CYP activities. Recently, the development and characterization of a first-in-class novel azole analog [1-(4-(4-(((2R,4S)-2-(2,4-difluorophenyl)-2-methyl-1,3-dioxolan-4-yl)methoxy)phenyl)piperazin-1-yl)ethanone (FLB-12)] that antagonizes the activated state of PXR has been published (Venkatesh et al., 2011). This analog has limited effects on other related nuclear receptors LXR, FXR, estrogen receptor α, PPARγ, and mouse CAR. FLB-12 was demonstrated to abrogate endogenous PXR activation *in vitro* and *in vivo* and was less toxic to liver cells *in vivo* compared to ketoconazole. Interestingly, FLB-12 significantly abrogates PXR-mediated resistance to 7-ethyl-10-hydroxycamptothecin (SN-38) in colon cancer cells *in vitro*. These drugs will not only serve as valuable chemical tools for probing PXR action but will also be important adjuncts for novel targeted approaches against cancer drug resistance.

Thus, the concept that down-regulating PXR can sensitize cancer cells to chemotherapeutic agents has been proposed and investigated in several studies. In the prostate cancer cell line PC-3, treatment with the PXR agonist SR12813 activates PXR and increases both the expression of *MDR1* and the resistance of PC-3 cells to the anticancer drugs paclitaxel and vinblastine. Inversely, the targeted knock-down of PXR by using short hairpin RNA (shRNA) enhanced the sensitivity of PC-3 to paclitaxel and vinblastine, suggesting that the effectiveness of anticancer drugs can be enhanced in PXR-positive cancers by decreasing the expression of PXR. Down-regulation of PXR by small interfering RNA (siRNA) in the endometrial cancer cell line HEC-1 also decreased the expression of *MDR1* and sensitized cells to anticancer agent and PXR agonist paclitaxel and cisplatin (Masuyama et al., 2003; Masuyama et al., 2007). Other reports suggest that down-regulation of PXR may contribute to apoptotic and drug sensitivity in cancer cells (Gong et al., 2006; Masuyama et al., 2007). Finally, expression of PXR in human colorectal cancer cells led to irinotecan chemoresistance through enhancement of its glucuronidation catalyzed by UGT1A1. The opposite effect was obtained with pharmacological inactivation of PXR or shRNA-mediated PXR down-regulation, confirming the direct involvement of PXR in irinotecan chemoresistance (Raynal et al., 2010). Altogether, these studies demonstrate that PXR represents a potential therapeutic target for clinical applications relevant drug resistance.

Although the properties of CAR and its agonists in xenobiotic metabolism have been extensively studied, its anticancer property was not known until very recently. Indeed, a recent study showed that CAR is a positive regulator of *MDR1* (Pgp), *MRP2* and *BCRP* expression in rat and mouse brain capillaries (Wang, B. et al., 2010). Moreover, another study demonstrated that CITCO inhibits the growth and expansion of brain tumor cancer stem cells by inducing cell cycle arrest and apoptosis *in vitro* (Chakraborty et al., 2011). Although the CAR-mediated antineoplastic effect is not known, these results support the use of CAR agonists as a new therapy to target brain tumor cancer stem cells for the treatment of glioma.

4.1.2 HIF-1 and its target genes

The adaptive cellular response of cancer cells to hypoxia offers new pharmacological targets, including the central regulator of molecular and cellular response to hypoxia HIF-1 as well as some of its target genes, particularly the VEGF and the carbonic CA9 (see Table 1). Validation of HIF-1 as a therapeutic target has been based on studies using genetic manipulation. When HIF-1α expression is increased in human cancer cells, angiogenesis capacity and metastasis spread are observed. Conversely, inhibition of the HIF-1α expression reverses those effects (Semenza, 2007). Accordingly, injection of tumor cells overexpressing HIF-1α into immunodeficient mice has demonstrated the capacity of HIF-1 to promote tumorigenesis (Maxwell et al., 1997). A growing number of novel anticancer agents have been shown to inhibit HIF-1 through a variety of molecular mechanisms. One of these promising molecules, the YC-1 ((3-(5'-Hydroxymethyl-2'-furyl)-1-benzylindazole), decreases the levels of HIF-1α protein through inhibition of the PI3K/AKT/mTor pathway (Sun et al., 2007). It has been shown that inhibition of HIF-1α activity in tumors from YC-1-treated mice is associated with blocked angiogenesis and an inhibition of tumor growth (Yeo et al., 2003).

Target	Agent	Mechanism of action
Hypoxia	Mitomycin C	DNA damages
	Banoxantrone (AQ4N)	DNA damages and topoisomerase II inhibitor
	Tirapazamine (TPZ)	DNA damages
HIF-1 pathway	YC-1[a]	PI3K/AKT/mTor inhibitor
	Tanespimycin (17-AAG)	HSP90 inhibitor
	PX-12[b]	Thioredoxin inhibitor
	Topotecan	Topoisomerase I inhibitor
HIF-1 target genes		
CA9	CAI17	CA9-specific small molecule inhibitor
VEGF	Sorafenib	Tyrosine kinase inhibitor
	Bevacizumab	Anti-VEGF antibody
GLUT1	Fasentin	Interacts with GLUT1 transporter and block glucose uptake

Table 1. Examples of pharmacological approaches to target hypoxic cancer cells. [a] 3-(5'-Hydroxymethyl-2'-furyl)-1-benzylindazole; [b] 1-methylpropyl 2-imidazolyl disulfide.

Angiogenesis has been described as one of the hallmarks of cancer, playing an essential role in tumor growth, invasion, and metastasis. For this reason, inhibition of angiogenesis has become a major challenge in the development of new anticancer agents, particularly in targeting the VEGF pathway. Sorafenib, a multitargeted inhibitor of tyrosine kinase, inhibits the receptor tyrosine kinase VEGFR2 and PDGFR and the Ras/Raf pathway

(Keating and Santoro, 2009). Currently, this anticancer molecule demonstrated encouraging result for palliative therapy and can prolong the overall survival for patients with advanced hepatocellular carcinoma (Cheng et al., 2009). Moreover, anti-angiogenic therapy seems efficient to improve survival from patients with hepatocellular carcinoma and the anti-VEGF monoclonal antibody bevacizumab has shown promising results (Llovet and Bruix, 2008).

Increased expression of CA9 has been found in many cancers and has been associated to an unfavorable prognosis (Kaluz et al., 2009; Pastorekova et al., 2008; Potter and Harris, 2004). Silencing both CA9 and CA12 resulted in marked inhibition of the growth of LS174 human colon carcinoma cell xenograft tumors (Chiche et al., 2010). Therefore, CA9 seems to be a new candidate for the development of new anticancer strategy. Interestingly, novel CA9-specific small molecule inhibitors such as the sulfonamide-based CAIX inhibitor CAI17 resulted in significant inhibition of tumor growth and metastasis formation in both spontaneous and experimental models of metastasis.

4.2 Bioreductive agents

It has been suggested that hypoxic environment in tumor tissues could be used as an advantage to target cancer cells with prodrugs that are metabolized into toxic metabolites only in hypoxic areas (McKeown et al., 2007). These drugs, also named bioreductive agents, are divided into 4 groups: quinones, nitroaromatics or nitro-heterocyclic, aliphatic N-oxides and heteroaromatic N-oxides.

Mitomycin C that belongs to the quinone family is an alkylating antineoplastic agent and is frequently used for chemoembolization therapy. Bioreduction and activation of mitomycin C are facilitated upon a hypoxic environment. Indeed, electrons gain (reduction) of mitomycin products a semiquinone radical anion, which forms a covalent interaction with DNA. In the presence of oxygen, this radical anion is quickly degraded, thus giving the selectivity of hypoxia for generation of cytotoxic species (Kennedy et al., 1980).

AQ4N or banoxantrone, is part of the aliphatic N-oxides. AQ4N is reduced into AQ4 under hypoxic condition. AQ4 exerts its cytotoxic activity by binding DNA and acting as an inhibitor of topoisomerase II. Used in combination with other anticancer agents, it has anti-proliferative effects on tumor cells (Patterson and McKeown, 2000).

4.3 Activation of prodrugs by glutathione transferases

As previously mentioned, a feature of cancer cell is to overexpress certain drug-metabolizing enzymes and transporters. Pathways involving such proteins that are aberrantly expressed in cancer cells are preferentially targeted for drug intervention. For example, the enhanced expression of GSTP1 in several tumors makes this protein a promising target for prodrug therapy. In order to take advantage of GSTP1 overexpression in cancer cells, two strategies have been performed. The first one consists in designing and developing inhibitors of GSTP1. Initially, this strategy was developed in order to decrease the metabolism of several active anticancer drugs known to be inactivated by GST. Furthermore, in 1999, evidence for a direct interaction of mouse GST pi with JNK was demonstrated (Adler et al., 1999). Their work showed that, under a monomeric state, GST pi acts as a direct JNK inhibitor in non-stressed cells by forming a complex with JNK and c-Jun. Oxidative stress (UV, H_2O_2...) induces the dimerization of GST pi and activation of c-jun through its phosphorylation on Ser-63 and Ser-73 residues. Subsequently, several other studies have corroborated this model in other cell lines (Bernardini et al., 2000; Castro-Caldas et al., 2009) and have shown that overexpression of GSTP1 in several tumor tissues lead to an inhibition of apoptosis pathways. Thus, inhibitor of GSTP1 triggering the disruption of this interaction could induce apoptosis in the cancer cell. TLK199 is one of them (Raza et al., 2009). The second strategy consists in designing prodrug activated by this enzyme in order to target specifically the tumor cells overexpressing GSTP1. Thus, novel alkylating agents have been synthetized (Lyttle et al., 1994; Satyam et al., 1996). Cleavage of these molecules by GSTP1 lead to the release of two metabolites: an inactive GSH conjugate and a phosphorodiamide compound. The phosphorodiamide spontaneously gives an alkylating moiety (a nitrogen mustard alkylating agent) which is responsible for the cytotoxicity. Among all the products synthetized, one has been actively studied and is tested in phase 2 and 3 studies (Kavanagh et al., 2010; Vergote et al., 2009). Initially named TER286, then TLK286, it is now designate with the International Nonproprietary Name (INN) canfosfamide (Telcita®). Several *in vitro* and *in vivo* studies, either on cell lines or on xenograft models, have linked the cytotoxicity of this molecule with the high level expression of GSTP1 and the formation of the alkylating moiety (Izbicka et al., 1997; Morgan et al., 1998; Rosario et al., 2000). Furthermore, Townsend et al. (Townsend et al., 2002) have demonstrated that canfosfamide is able to inhibit an enzyme involved in double strand break DNA repair, the DNA-dependent protein-kinase (DNA-PK). Interestingly, up-regulation of this DNA-PK leads to a resistance of adriamycin and cisplatin, suggesting that canfosfamide could be used in combination with these drugs. Several phase I studies have been realized in order to determine the safety and the pharmacokinetic of canfosfamide in human. These tests have been performed in advanced refractory solid cancers and have shown that canfosfamide is well tolerated with mild or moderate adverse effects such as nausea, vomiting, fatigue and anemia (grade 1 or 2) (Rosen et al., 2003; Rosen et al., 2004). Furthermore canfosfamide seems to be active in a large range of cancer including advanced non-small cell lung tumor (Sequist et al., 2009). Phase 2 and 3 clinical studies have also been done on resistant epithelial ovarian cancer (Kavanagh et al., 2010; Vergote et al., 2009).

Another family of compounds is under development. These compounds own an O^2-aryl diazeniumdiolate structure and are also metabolized by GSTP1 in a non-stable metabolite owning a Meisenheimer complex intermediate, which gives a GSH metabolite (PABA-GSH) and nitrogen monoxide (NO). Several of them have been designed (Andrei et al., 2008; Chakrapani et al., 2008; Saavedra et al., 2006) but the most specific and the most studied is the PABA/NO (O2-[2,4-dinitro-5-(p-methylaminobenzoato)] 1-(N, N-dimethylamino)diazen-1-ium-1,2-diolate) (Ji et al., 2008). Antiproliferative proprieties have been observed in several cell lines, including the mouse skin fibroblast NIH3T3 (Findlay et al., 2004), the human promyelocytic leukemia HL60 (Hutchens et al., 2010), the human leukemia U-937, the non-small-cell lung cancer H441, the colon cancer (HCT-116, HCT-15 and HT-29), the ovarian cancer OVCAR-3 (Andrei et al., 2008) and the U87 gliomas cell lines (Kogias et al., 2011). Antitumor activity was also demonstrated in an A2780 human ovarian cancer xenograft model in female SCID mice (Findlay et al., 2004). Mechanisms of cytotoxicity of PABA/NO involve several pathways which are due to the NO production and the nitrosylation and S-glutathionylation of some proteins. Townsend et al. (2005) have shown that PABA/NO is able to induce S-glutathionylation of several proteins, including the protein disulfide isomerase (PDI) (Townsend et al., 2005). Glutathionylation of PDI triggers a decrease of the folding protein capacity response, leading to cytotoxic effects. Activation of the apoptosis pathway through activation of JNK and p38 has also been observed (Townsend et al., 2005). Furthermore, GSH metabolite of PABA/NO is also able to inhibit sarco/endoplasmic reticulum calcium ATPases iso-enzymes, leading to an intracellular Ca^{2+} increase, triggering activation of the calmodulin pathway and thus increasing production of NO by endothelial Nitric Oxide Synthase (Manevich et al., 2010).

5. Conclusion

During the last years, several mechanisms involved in resistance phenomena have been elucidated and showed that, in many cases, drug-metabolizing enzymes and drug transporters are key factors in the failure of cancer therapies. In some cases, these discoveries led to useful strategies to identify "sensitive" tumors and direct clinical decisions for the choice of therapy. Furthermore, the molecular classification of several tumor types based on genome-wide investigations and identification of patient subclasses according to drug responsiveness should help to propose a more personalized medicine and to overcome anticancer drug resistance. Another promising field of investigation is to take advantage of cancer cell specificity in order to develop new tumor-targeted approaches that afford tumor specificity and limited toxicity.

6. References

Aas, T., Borresen, A.L., Geisler, S., Smith-Sorensen, B., Johnsen, H., Varhaug, J.E., Akslen, L.A., and Lonning, P.E. (1996). Specific P53 mutations are associated with de novo resistance to doxorubicin in breast cancer patients. *Nat Med*, Vol.2, No.7, 811-814.

Adler, V., Yin, Z., Fuchs, S.Y., Benezra, M., Rosario, L., Tew, K.D., Pincus, M.R., Sardana, M., Henderson, C.J., Wolf, C.R., Davis, R.J., and Ronai, Z. (1999). Regulation of JNK signaling by GSTp. *EMBO J*, Vol.18, No.5, 1321-1334.

Akhdar, H., Loyer, P., Rauch, C., Corlu, A., Guillouzo, A., and Morel, F. (2009). Involvement of Nrf2 activation in resistance to 5-fluorouracil in human colon cancer HT-29 cells. *Eur J Cancer*, Vol.45, No.12, 2219-2227.

Andrei, D., Maciag, A.E., Chakrapani, H., Citro, M.L., Keefer, L.K., and Saavedra, J.E. (2008). Aryl bis(diazeniumdiolates): potent inducers of S-glutathionylation of cellular proteins and their in vitro antiproliferative activities. *J Med Chem*, Vol.51, No.24, 7944-7952.

Baird, L., and Dinkova-Kostova, A.T. (2011). The cytoprotective role of the Keap1-Nrf2 pathway. *Arch Toxicol*, Vol.85, No.4, 241-272.

Ban, N., Takahashi, Y., Takayama, T., Kura, T., Katahira, T., Sakamaki, S., and Niitsu, Y. (1996). Transfection of glutathione S-transferase (GST)-pi antisense complementary DNA increases the sensitivity of a colon cancer cell line to adriamycin, cisplatin, melphalan, and etoposide. *Cancer Res*, Vol.56, No.15, 3577-3582.

Baskin-Bey, E.S., Huang, W., Ishimura, N., Isomoto, H., Bronk, S.F., Braley, K., Craig, R.W., Moore, D.D., and Gores, G.J. (2006). Constitutive androstane receptor (CAR) ligand,

TCPOBOP, attenuates Fas-induced murine liver injury by altering Bcl-2 proteins. *Hepatology*, Vol.44, No.1, 252-262.

Basseville, A., Preisser, L., de Carne Trecesson, S., Boisdron-Celle, M., Gamelin, E., Coqueret, O., and Morel, A. (2011). Irinotecan induces steroid and xenobiotic receptor (SXR) signaling to detoxification pathway in colon cancer cells. *Mol Cancer*, Vol.10, No.1, 80.

Bauer, B., Hartz, A.M., Fricker, G., and Miller, D.S. (2004). Pregnane X receptor up-regulation of P-glycoprotein expression and transport function at the blood-brain barrier. *Mol Pharmacol*, Vol.66, No.3, 413-419.

Baumert, C., and Hilgeroth, A. (2009). Recent advances in the development of P-gp inhibitors. *Anticancer Agents Med Chem*, Vol.9, No.4, 415-436.

Bernardini, S., Bernassola, F., Cortese, C., Ballerini, S., Melino, G., Motti, C., Bellincampi, L., Iori, R., and Federici, G. (2000). Modulation of GST P1-1 activity by polymerization during apoptosis. *J Cell Biochem*, Vol.77, No.4, 645-653.

Bignami, M., Casorelli, I., and Karran, P. (2003). Mismatch repair and response to DNA-damaging antitumour therapies. *Eur J Cancer*, Vol.39, No.15, 2142-2149.

Biswas, A., Mani, S., Redinbo, M.R., Krasowski, M.D., Li, H., and Ekins, S. (2009). Elucidating the 'Jekyll and Hyde' nature of PXR: the case for discovering antagonists or allosteric antagonists. *Pharm Res*, Vol.26, No.8, 1807-1815.

Blanco-Bose, W.E., Murphy, M.J., Ehninger, A., Offner, S., Dubey, C., Huang, W., Moore, D.D., and Trumpp, A. (2008). C-Myc and its target FoxM1 are critical downstream effectors of constitutive androstane receptor (CAR) mediated direct liver hyperplasia. *Hepatology*, Vol.48, No.4, 1302-1311.

Bock, K.W., Lilienblum, W., Fischer, G., Schirmer, G., and Bock-Henning, B.S. (1987). The role of conjugation reactions in detoxication. *Arch Toxicol*, Vol.60, No.1-3, 22-29.

Bray, J., Sludden, J., Griffin, M.J., Cole, M., Verrill, M., Jamieson, D., and Boddy, A.V. (2010). Influence of pharmacogenetics on response and toxicity in breast cancer patients treated with doxorubicin and cyclophosphamide. *Br J Cancer*, Vol.102, No.6, 1003-1009.

Bu, H.Z. (2006). A literature review of enzyme kinetic parameters for CYP3A4-mediated metabolic reactions of 113 drugs in human liver microsomes: structure-kinetics relationship assessment. *Curr Drug Metab*, Vol.7, No.3, 231-249.

Carew, J.S., and Huang, P. (2002). Mitochondrial defects in cancer. *Mol Cancer*, Vol.1, 9.

Carmeliet, P., and Jain, R.K. (2000). Angiogenesis in cancer and other diseases. *Nature*, Vol.407, No.6801, 249-257.

Castro-Caldas, M., Milagre, I., Rodrigues, E., and Gama, M.J. (2009). Glutathione S-transferase pi regulates UV-induced JNK signaling in SH-SY5Y neuroblastoma cells. *Neurosci Lett*, Vol.451, No.3, 241-245.

Chakraborty, S., Kanakasabai, S., and Bright, J.J. (2011). Constitutive androstane receptor agonist CITCO inhibits growth and expansion of brain tumour stem cells. *Br J Cancer*, Vol.104, No.3, 448-459.

Chakrapani, H., Wilde, T.C., Citro, M.L., Goodblatt, M.M., Keefer, L.K., and Saavedra, J.E. (2008). Synthesis, nitric oxide release, and anti-leukemic activity of glutathione-activated nitric oxide prodrugs: Structural analogues of PABA/NO, an anti-cancer lead compound. *Bioorg Med Chem*, Vol.16, No.5, 2657-2664.

Chen, G., and Waxman, D.J. (1994). Role of cellular glutathione and glutathione S-transferase in the expression of alkylating agent cytotoxicity in human breast cancer cells. *Biochem Pharmacol*, Vol.47, No.6, 1079-1087.

Chen, T. (2010). Overcoming drug resistance by regulating nuclear receptors. *Adv Drug Deliv Rev*, Vol.62, No.13, 1257-1264.

Cheng, A.L., Kang, Y.K., Chen, Z., Tsao, C.J., Qin, S., Kim, J.S., Luo, R., Feng, J., Ye, S., Yang, T.S., *et al.* (2009). Efficacy and safety of sorafenib in patients in the Asia-Pacific region with advanced hepatocellular carcinoma: a phase III randomised, double-blind, placebo-controlled trial. *Lancet Oncol*, Vol.10, No.1, 25-34.

Chiche, J., Brahimi-Horn, M.C., and Pouyssegur, J. (2010). Tumour hypoxia induces a metabolic shift causing acidosis: a common feature in cancer. *J Cell Mol Med*, Vol.14, No.4, 771-794.

Cho, J.M., Manandhar, S., Lee, H.R., Park, H.M., and Kwak, M.K. (2008). Role of the Nrf2-antioxidant system in cytotoxicity mediated by anticancer cisplatin: implication to cancer cell resistance. *Cancer Lett*, Vol.260, No.1-2, 96-108.

Cho, S.G., Lee, Y.H., Park, H.S., Ryoo, K., Kang, K.W., Park, J., Eom, S.J., Kim, M.J., Chang, T.S., Choi, S.Y., Shim, J., Kim, Y., Dong, M.S., Lee, M.J., Kim, S.G., Ichijo, H., and Choi, E.J. (2001). Glutathione S-transferase mu modulates the stress-activated signals by suppressing apoptosis signal-regulating kinase 1. *J Biol Chem*, Vol.276, No.16, 12749-12755.

Comerford, K.M., Wallace, T.J., Karhausen, J., Louis, N.A., Montalto, M.C., and Colgan, S.P. (2002). Hypoxia-inducible factor-1-dependent regulation of the multidrug resistance (MDR1) gene. *Cancer Res*, Vol.62, No.12, 3387-3394.

Cosse, J.P., and Michiels, C. (2008). Tumour hypoxia affects the responsiveness of cancer cells to chemotherapy and promotes cancer progression. *Anticancer Agents Med Chem*, Vol.8, No.7, 790-797.

Cree, I.A. (2011). Cancer biology. *Methods Mol Biol*, Vol.731, 1-11.

Degorter, M.K., Xia, C.Q., Yang, J.J., and Kim, R.B. (2011). Drug Transporters in Drug Efficacy and Toxicity. *Annu Rev Pharmacol Toxicol*.

Dirven, H.A., van Ommen, B., and van Bladeren, P.J. (1994). Involvement of human glutathione S-transferase isoenzymes in the conjugation of cyclophosphamide metabolites with glutathione. *Cancer Res*, Vol.54, No.23, 6215-6220.

Dulhunty, A., Gage, P., Curtis, S., Chelvanayagam, G., and Board, P. (2001). The glutathione transferase structural family includes a nuclear chloride channel and a ryanodine receptor calcium release channel modulator. *J Biol Chem*, Vol.276, No.5, 3319-3323.

Dvorak, H.F. (2002). Vascular permeability factor/vascular endothelial growth factor: a critical cytokine in tumor angiogenesis and a potential target for diagnosis and therapy. *J Clin Oncol*, Vol.20, No.21, 4368-4380.

Engels, F.K., Ten Tije, A.J., Baker, S.D., Lee, C.K., Loos, W.J., Vulto, A.G., Verweij, J., and Sparreboom, A. (2004). Effect of cytochrome P450 3A4 inhibition on the pharmacokinetics of docetaxel. *Clin Pharmacol Ther*, Vol.75, No.5, 448-454.

Evans, R.M. (2005). The nuclear receptor superfamily: a rosetta stone for physiology. *Mol Endocrinol*, Vol.19, No.6, 1429-1438.

Findlay, V.J., Townsend, D.M., Saavedra, J.E., Buzard, G.S., Citro, M.L., Keefer, L.K., Ji, X., and Tew, K.D. (2004). Tumor cell responses to a novel glutathione S-transferase-activated nitric oxide-releasing prodrug. *Mol Pharmacol*, Vol.65, No.5, 1070-1079.

Firth, J.D., Ebert, B.L., and Ratcliffe, P.J. (1995). Hypoxic regulation of lactate dehydrogenase A. Interaction between hypoxia-inducible factor 1 and cAMP response elements. *J Biol Chem*, Vol.270, No.36, 21021-21027.

Forman, B.M., Tzameli, I., Choi, H.S., Chen, J., Simha, D., Seol, W., Evans, R.M., and Moore, D.D. (1998). Androstane metabolites bind to and deactivate the nuclear receptor CAR-beta. *Nature*, Vol.395, No.6702, 612-615.

Francis, G.A., Fayard, E., Picard, F., and Auwerx, J. (2003). Nuclear receptors and the control of metabolism. *Annu Rev Physiol*, Vol.65, 261-311.

Garcia-Martin, E., Pizarro, R.M., Martinez, C., Gutierrez-Martin, Y., Perez, G., Jover, R., and Agundez, J.A. (2006). Acquired resistance to the anticancer drug paclitaxel is associated with induction of cytochrome P450 2C8. *Pharmacogenomics*, Vol.7, No.4, 575-585.

Germain, P., Staels, B., Dacquet, C., Spedding, M., and Laudet, V. (2006). Overview of nomenclature of nuclear receptors. *Pharmacol Rev*, Vol.58, No.4, 685-704.

Gerweck, L.E. (1998). Tumor pH: implications for treatment and novel drug design. *Seminars in radiation oncology*, Vol.8, No.3, 176-182.

Gilot, D., Loyer, P., Corlu, A., Glaise, D., Lagadic-Gossmann, D., Atfi, A., Morel, F., Ichijo, H., and Guguen-Guillouzo, C. (2002). Liver protection from apoptosis requires both blockage of initiator caspase activities and inhibition of ASK1/JNK pathway via glutathione S-transferase regulation. *J Biol Chem*, Vol.277, No.51, 49220-49229.

Goda, K., Bacso, Z., and Szabo, G. (2009). Multidrug resistance through the spectacle of P-glycoprotein. *Curr Cancer Drug Targets*, Vol.9, No.3, 281-297.

Goh, B.C., Lee, S.C., Wang, L.Z., Fan, L., Guo, J.Y., Lamba, J., Schuetz, E., Lim, R., Lim, H.L., Ong, A.B., and Lee, H.S. (2002). Explaining interindividual variability of docetaxel pharmacokinetics and pharmacodynamics in Asians through phenotyping and genotyping strategies. *J Clin Oncol*, Vol.20, No.17, 3683-3690.

Goldman, I.D., Chattopadhyay, S., Zhao, R., and Moran, R. (2010). The antifolates: evolution, new agents in the clinic, and how targeting delivery via specific membrane transporters is driving the development of a next generation of folate analogs. *Curr Opin Investig Drugs*, Vol.11, No.12, 1409-1423.

Gong, H., Singh, S.V., Singh, S.P., Mu, Y., Lee, J.H., Saini, S.P., Toma, D., Ren, S., Kagan, V.E., Day, B.W., Zimniak, P., and Xie, W. (2006). Orphan nuclear receptor pregnane X receptor sensitizes oxidative stress responses in transgenic mice and cancerous cells. *Mol Endocrinol*, Vol.20, No.2, 279-290.

Greijer, A.E., de Jong, M.C., Scheffer, G.L., Shvarts, A., van Diest, P.J., and van der Wall, E. (2005). Hypoxia-induced acidification causes mitoxantrone resistance not mediated by drug transporters in human breast cancer cells. *Cellular oncology : the official journal of the International Society for Cellular Oncology*, Vol.27, No.1, 43-49.

Grigoryan, R., Keshelava, N., Anderson, C., and Reynolds, C.P. (2005). In vitro testing of chemosensitivity in physiological hypoxia. *Methods Mol Med*, Vol.110, 87-100.

Guengerich, F.P. (2007). Mechanisms of cytochrome P450 substrate oxidation: MiniReview. *J Biochem Mol Toxicol*, Vol.21, No.4, 163-168.

Guengerich, F.P. (2008). Cytochrome p450 and chemical toxicology. *Chem Res Toxicol*, Vol.21, No.1, 70-83.

Guo, Y., Kotova, E., Chen, Z.S., Lee, K., Hopper-Borge, E., Belinsky, M.G., and Kruh, G.D. (2003). MRP8, ATP-binding cassette C11 (ABCC11), is a cyclic nucleotide efflux pump and a resistance factor for fluoropyrimidines 2',3'-dideoxycytidine and 9'-(2'-phosphonylmethoxyethyl)adenine. *J Biol Chem*, Vol.278, No.32, 29509-29514.

Gupta, D., Venkatesh, M., Wang, H., Kim, S., Sinz, M., Goldberg, G.L., Whitney, K., Longley, C., and Mani, S. (2008). Expanding the roles for pregnane X receptor in cancer: proliferation and drug resistance in ovarian cancer. *Clin Cancer Res*, Vol.14, No.17, 5332-5340.

Gurova, K. (2009). New hopes from old drugs: revisiting DNA-binding small molecules as anticancer agents. *Future Oncol*, Vol.5, No.10, 1685-1704.

Hall, A.G., Autzen, P., Cattan, A.R., Malcolm, A.J., Cole, M., Kernahan, J., and Reid, M.M. (1994). Expression of mu class glutathione S-transferase correlates with event-free survival in childhood acute lymphoblastic leukemia. *Cancer Res*, Vol.54, No.20, 5251-5254.

Hamilton, D.S., Zhang, X., Ding, Z., Hubatsch, I., Mannervik, B., Houk, K.N., Ganem, B., and Creighton, D.J. (2003). Mechanism of the glutathione transferase-catalyzed conversion of antitumor 2-crotonyloxymethyl-2-cycloalkenones to GSH adducts. *J Am Chem Soc*, Vol.125, No.49, 15049-15058.

Harmsen, S., Meijerman, I., Febus, C.L., Maas-Bakker, R.F., Beijnen, J.H., and Schellens, J.H. (2010). PXR-mediated induction of P-glycoprotein by anticancer drugs in a human colon adenocarcinoma-derived cell line. *Cancer Chemother Pharmacol*, Vol.66, No.4, 765-771.

Hayes, J.D., and Pulford, D.J. (1995). The glutathione S-transferase supergene family: regulation of GST and the contribution of the isoenzymes to cancer chemoprotection and drug resistance. *Crit Rev Biochem Mol Biol*, Vol.30, No.6, 445-600.

Hayes, J.D., Flanagan, J.U., and Jowsey, I.R. (2005). Glutathione transferases. *Annu Rev Pharmacol Toxicol*, Vol.45, 51-88.

Hayes, J.D., and McMahon, M. (2006). The double-edged sword of Nrf2: subversion of redox homeostasis during the evolution of cancer. *Mol Cell*, Vol.21, No.6, 732-734.

Hayes, J.D., and McMahon, M. (2009). NRF2 and KEAP1 mutations: permanent activation of an adaptive response in cancer. *Trends Biochem Sci*, Vol.34, No.4, 176-188.

Helsby, N.A., Hui, C.Y., Goldthorpe, M.A., Coller, J.K., Soh, M.C., Gow, P.J., De Zoysa, J.Z., and Tingle, M.D. (2010). The combined impact of CYP2C19 and CYP2B6 pharmacogenetics on cyclophosphamide bioactivation. *Br J Clin Pharmacol*, Vol.70, No.6, 844-853.

Herling, A., Konig, M., Bulik, S., and Holzhutter, H.G. (2011). Enzymatic features of the glucose metabolism in tumor cells. *FEBS J*, Vol.278, No.14, 2436-2459.

Hickey, M.M., and Simon, M.C. (2006). Regulation of angiogenesis by hypoxia and hypoxia-inducible factors. *Current topics in developmental biology*, Vol.76, 217-257.

Ho, R.H., and Kim, R.B. (2005). Transporters and drug therapy: implications for drug disposition and disease. *Clin Pharmacol Ther*, Vol.78, No.3, 260-277.

Homma, S., Ishii, Y., Morishima, Y., Yamadori, T., Matsuno, Y., Haraguchi, N., Kikuchi, N., Satoh, H., Sakamoto, T., Hizawa, N., Itoh, K., and Yamamoto, M. (2009). Nrf2 enhances cell proliferation and resistance to anticancer drugs in human lung cancer. *Clin Cancer Res*, Vol.15, No.10, 3423-3432.

Horton, J.K., Roy, G., Piper, J.T., Van Houten, B., Awasthi, Y.C., Mitra, S., Alaoui-Jamali, M.A., Boldogh, I., and Singhal, S.S. (1999). Characterization of a chlorambucil-resistant human ovarian carcinoma cell line overexpressing glutathione S-transferase mu. *Biochem Pharmacol*, Vol.58, No.4, 693-702.

Hsieh, C.C., Kuo, Y.H., Kuo, C.C., Chen, L.T., Cheung, C.H., Chao, T.Y., Lin, C.H., Pan, W.Y., Chang, C.Y., Chien, S.C., Chen, T.W., Lung, C.C., and Chang, J.Y. (2010). Chamaecypanone C, a novel skeleton microtubule inhibitor, with anticancer activity by trigger caspase 8-Fas/FasL dependent apoptotic pathway in human cancer cells. *Biochem Pharmacol*, Vol.79, No.9, 1261-1271.

Hurst, R., Bao, Y., Jemth, P., Mannervik, B., and Williamson, G. (1998). Phospholipid hydroperoxide glutathione peroxidase activity of human glutathione transferases. *Biochem J*, Vol.332 (Pt 1), 97-100.

Hutchens, S., Manevich, Y., He, L., Tew, K.D., and Townsend, D.M. (2010). Cellular resistance to a nitric oxide releasing glutathione S-transferase P-activated prodrug, PABA/NO. *Invest New Drugs*, Vol.29, No5, 719-729.

Huttunen, K.M., Mahonen, N., Raunio, H., and Rautio, J. (2008). Cytochrome P450-activated prodrugs: targeted drug delivery. *Curr Med Chem*, Vol.15, No.23, 2346-2365.

Ikeda, S., Kurose, K., Jinno, H., Sai, K., Ozawa, S., Hasegawa, R., Komamura, K., Kotake, T., Morishita, H., Kamakura, S., *et al.* (2005). Functional analysis of four naturally occurring variants of human constitutive androstane receptor. *Mol Genet Metab*, Vol.86, No.1-2, 314-319.

Ishikawa, T., Kuo, M.T., Furuta, K., and Suzuki, M. (2000). The human multidrug resistance-associated protein (MRP) gene family: from biological function to drug molecular design. *Clin Chem Lab Med*, Vol.38, No.9, 893-897.

Iyanagi, T. (2007). Molecular mechanism of phase I and phase II drug-metabolizing enzymes: implications for detoxification. *Int Rev Cytol*, Vol.260, 35-112.

Izbicka, E., Lawrence, R., Cerna, C., Von Hoff, D.D., and Sanderson, P.E. (1997). Activity of TER286 against human tumor colony-forming units. *Anticancer Drugs*, Vol.8, No.4, 345-348.

Izbicka, E., and Tolcher, A.W. (2004). Development of novel alkylating drugs as anticancer agents. *Curr Opin Investig Drugs*, Vol.5, No.6, 587-591.

Jaakkola, P., Mole, D.R., Tian, Y.M., Wilson, M.I., Gielbert, J., Gaskell, S.J., Kriegsheim, A., Hebestreit, H.F., Mukherji, M., Schofield, C.J., Maxwell, P.H., Pugh, C.W., and Ratcliffe, P.J. (2001). Targeting of HIF-alpha to the von Hippel-Lindau ubiquitylation complex by O2-regulated prolyl hydroxylation. *Science*, Vol.292, No.5516, 468-472.

Jakobsson, P.J., Thoren, S., Morgenstern, R., and Samuelsson, B. (1999). Identification of human prostaglandin E synthase: a microsomal, glutathione-dependent, inducible enzyme, constituting a potential novel drug target. *Proc Natl Acad Sci U S A*, Vol.96, No.13, 7220-7225.

Jakobsson, P.J., Morgenstern, R., Mancini, J., Ford-Hutchinson, A., and Persson, B. (2000). Membrane-associated proteins in eicosanoid and glutathione metabolism (MAPEG). A widespread protein superfamily. *Am J Respir Crit Care Med*, Vol.161, No.2 Pt 2, S20-24.

Jancova, P., Anzenbacher, P., and Anzenbacherova, E. (2010). Phase II drug metabolizing enzymes. *Biomed Pap Med Fac Univ Palacky Olomouc Czech Repub*, Vol.154, No.2, 103-116.

Jedlitschky, G., Leier, I., Buchholz, U., Barnouin, K., Kurz, G., and Keppler, D. (1996). Transport of glutathione, glucuronate, and sulfate conjugates by the MRP gene-encoded conjugate export pump. *Cancer Res*, Vol.56, No.5, 988-994.

Ji, X., Pal, A., Kalathur, R., Hu, X., Gu, Y., Saavedra, J.E., Buzard, G.S., Srinivasan, A., Keefer, L.K., and Singh, S.V. (2008). Structure-Based Design of Anticancer Prodrug PABA/NO. *Drug Des Devel Ther*, Vol.2, 123-130.

Johansson, A.S., and Mannervik, B. (2001). Human glutathione transferase A3-3, a highly efficient catalyst of double-bond isomerization in the biosynthetic pathway of steroid hormones. *J Biol Chem*, Vol.276, No.35, 33061-33065.

Kaluz, S., Kaluzova, M., Liao, S.Y., Lerman, M., and Stanbridge, E.J. (2009). Transcriptional control of the tumor- and hypoxia-marker carbonic anhydrase 9: A one transcription factor (HIF-1) show? *Biochim Biophys Acta*, Vol.1795, No.2, 162-172.

Kamath, K., Wilson, L., Cabral, F., and Jordan, M.A. (2005). BetaIII-tubulin induces paclitaxel resistance in association with reduced effects on microtubule dynamic instability. *J Biol Chem*, Vol.280, No.13, 12902-12907.

Kavanagh, J.J., Levenback, C.F., Ramirez, P.T., Wolf, J.L., Moore, C.L., Jones, M.R., Meng, L., Brown, G.L., and Bast, R.C., Jr. (2010). Phase 2 study of canfosfamide in combination with pegylated liposomal doxorubicin in platinum and paclitaxel refractory or resistant epithelial ovarian cancer. *J Hematol Oncol*, Vol.3, 9.

Keating, G.M., and Santoro, A. (2009). Sorafenib: a review of its use in advanced hepatocellular carcinoma. *Drugs*, Vol.69, No.2, 223-240.

Kennedy, K.A., Teicher, B.A., Rockwell, S., and Sartorelli, A.C. (1980). The hypoxic tumor cell: a target for selective cancer chemotherapy. *Biochem Pharmacol*, Vol.29, No.1, 1-8.

Keppler, D. (2011). Multidrug resistance proteins (MRPs, ABCCs): importance for pathophysiology and drug therapy. *Handb Exp Pharmacol*, No.201, 299-323.

Kim, J.W., Tchernyshyov, I., Semenza, G.L., and Dang, C.V. (2006). HIF-1-mediated expression of pyruvate dehydrogenase kinase: a metabolic switch required for cellular adaptation to hypoxia. *Cell metabolism*, Vol.3, No.3, 177-185.

Klaassen, C.D., and Slitt, A.L. (2005). Regulation of hepatic transporters by xenobiotic receptors. *Curr Drug Metab*, Vol.6, No.4, 309-328.

Kliewer, S.A., Moore, J.T., Wade, L., Staudinger, J.L., Watson, M.A., Jones, S.A., McKee, D.D., Oliver, B.B., Willson, T.M., Zetterstrom, R.H., Perlmann, T., and Lehmann, J.M. (1998). An orphan nuclear receptor activated by pregnanes defines a novel steroid signaling pathway. *Cell*, Vol.92, No.1, 73-82.

Kobayashi, K., Sueyoshi, T., Inoue, K., Moore, R., and Negishi, M. (2003). Cytoplasmic accumulation of the nuclear receptor CAR by a tetratricopeptide repeat protein in HepG2 cells. *Mol Pharmacol*, Vol.64, No.5, 1069-1075.

Kogias, E., Osterberg, N., Baumer, B., Psarras, N., Koentges, C., Papazoglou, A., Saavedra, J.E., Keefer, L.K., and Weyerbrock, A. (2011). Growth-inhibitory and chemosensitizing effects of the glutathione-S-transferase-pi-activated nitric oxide donor PABA/NO in malignant gliomas. *Int J Cancer*, in press.

Konstantinopoulos, P.A., Spentzos, D., Fountzilas, E., Francoeur, N., Sanisetty, S., Grammatikos, A.P., Hecht, J.L., and Cannistra, S.A. (2011). Keap1 mutations and Nrf2 pathway activation in epithelial ovarian cancer. *Cancer Res*, Vol.71, No15, 5081-5089

Kool, M., de Haas, M., Scheffer, G.L., Scheper, R.J., van Eijk, M.J., Juijn, J.A., Baas, F., and Borst, P. (1997). Analysis of expression of cMOAT (MRP2), MRP3, MRP4, and MRP5, homologues of the multidrug resistance-associated protein gene (MRP1), in human cancer cell lines. *Cancer Res*, Vol.57, No.16, 3537-3547.

Korita, P.V., Wakai, T., Shirai, Y., Matsuda, Y., Sakata, J., Takamura, M., Yano, M., Sanpei, A., Aoyagi, Y., Hatakeyama, K., and Ajioka, Y. (2010). Multidrug resistance-associated protein 2 determines the efficacy of cisplatin in patients with hepatocellular carcinoma. *Oncol Rep*, Vol.23, No.4, 965-972.

Kraggerud, S.M., Oldenburg, J., Alnaes, G.I., Berg, M., Kristensen, V.N., Fossa, S.D., and Lothe, R.A. (2009). Functional glutathione S-transferase genotypes among testicular germ cell tumor survivors: associations with primary and post-chemotherapy tumor histology. *Pharmacogenet Genomics*, Vol.19, No.10, 751-759.

Langouet, S., Coles, B., Morel, F., Becquemont, L., Beaune, P., Guengerich, F.P., Ketterer, B., and Guillouzo, A. (1995). Inhibition of CYP1A2 and CYP3A4 by oltipraz results in reduction of aflatoxin B1 metabolism in human hepatocytes in primary culture. *Cancer Res*, Vol.55, No.23, 5574-5579.

Larkin, A., O'Driscoll, L., Kennedy, S., Purcell, R., Moran, E., Crown, J., Parkinson, M., and Clynes, M. (2004). Investigation of MRP-1 protein and MDR-1 P-glycoprotein expression in invasive breast cancer: a prognostic study. *Int J Cancer*, Vol.112, No.2, 286-294.

Legendre, C., Hori, T., Loyer, P., Aninat, C., Ishida, S., Glaise, D., Lucas-Clerc, C., Boudjema, K., Guguen-Guillouzo, C., Corlu, A., and Morel, F. (2009). Drug-metabolising enzymes are down-regulated by hypoxia in differentiated human hepatoma HepaRG cells: HIF-1alpha involvement in CYP3A4 repression. *European journal of cancer*, Vol.45, No.16, 2882-2892.

Li, Y., Yuan, H., Yang, K., Xu, W., Tang, W., and Li, X. (2010). The structure and functions of P-glycoprotein. *Curr Med Chem*, Vol.17, No.8, 786-800.

Lien, S., Larsson, A.K., and Mannervik, B. (2002). The polymorphic human glutathione transferase T1-1, the most efficient glutathione transferase in the denitrosation and inactivation of the anticancer drug 1,3-bis(2-chloroethyl)-1-nitrosourea. *Biochem Pharmacol*, Vol.63, No.2, 191-197.

Lin, S.C., Chien, C.W., Lee, J.C., Yeh, Y.C., Hsu, K.F., Lai, Y.Y., and Tsai, S.J. (2011). Suppression of dual-specificity phosphatase-2 by hypoxia increases chemoresistance and malignancy in human cancer cells. *J Clin Invest*, Vol.121, No.5, 1905-1916.

Llovet, J.M., and Bruix, J. (2008). Molecular targeted therapies in hepatocellular carcinoma. *Hepatology*, Vol.48, No.4, 1312-1327.

Longley, D.B., Harkin, D.P., and Johnston, P.G. (2003). 5-fluorouracil: mechanisms of action and clinical strategies. *Nat Rev Cancer*, Vol.3, No.5, 330-338.

Lyttle, M.H., Satyam, A., Hocker, M.D., Bauer, K.E., Caldwell, C.G., Hui, H.C., Morgan, A.S., Mergia, A., and Kauvar, L.M. (1994). Glutathione-S-transferase activates novel alkylating agents. *J Med Chem*, Vol.37, No.10, 1501-1507.

Manevich, Y., Townsend, D.M., Hutchens, S., and Tew, K.D. (2010). Diazeniumdiolate mediated nitrosative stress alters nitric oxide homeostasis through intracellular calcium and S-glutathionylation of nitric oxide synthetase. *PLoS One*, Vol.5, No.11, e14151.

Martinez, V.G., O'Connor, R., Liang, Y., and Clynes, M. (2008). CYP1B1 expression is induced by docetaxel: effect on cell viability and drug resistance. *Br J Cancer*, Vol.98, No.3, 564-570.

Masuyama, H., Hiramatsu, Y., Kodama, J., and Kudo, T. (2003). Expression and potential roles of pregnane X receptor in endometrial cancer. *J Clin Endocrinol Metab*, Vol.88, No.9, 4446-4454.

Masuyama, H., Nakatsukasa, H., Takamoto, N., and Hiramatsu, Y. (2007). Down-regulation of pregnane X receptor contributes to cell growth inhibition and apoptosis by anticancer agents in endometrial cancer cells. *Mol Pharmacol*, Vol.72, No.4, 1045-1053.

Mathijssen, R.H., de Jong, F.A., van Schaik, R.H., Lepper, E.R., Friberg, L.E., Rietveld, T., de Bruijn, P., Graveland, W.J., Figg, W.D., Verweij, J., and Sparreboom, A. (2004). Prediction of irinotecan pharmacokinetics by use of cytochrome P450 3A4 phenotyping probes. *J Natl Cancer Inst*, Vol.96, No.21, 1585-1592.

Mathijssen, R.H., Verweij, J., de Bruijn, P., Loos, W.J., and Sparreboom, A. (2002). Effects of St. John's wort on irinotecan metabolism. *J Natl Cancer Inst*, Vol.94, No.16, 1247-1249.

Maxwell, P.H., Dachs, G.U., Gleadle, J.M., Nicholls, L.G., Harris, A.L., Stratford, I.J., Hankinson, O., Pugh, C.W., and Ratcliffe, P.J. (1997). Hypoxia-inducible factor-1 modulates gene expression in solid tumors and influences both angiogenesis and tumor growth. *Proc Natl Acad Sci U S A*, Vol.94, No.15, 8104-8109.

McFadyen, M.C., Cruickshank, M.E., Miller, I.D., McLeod, H.L., Melvin, W.T., Haites, N.E., Parkin, D., and Murray, G.I. (2001a). Cytochrome P450 CYP1B1 over-expression in primary and metastatic ovarian cancer. *Br J Cancer*, Vol.85, No.2, 242-246.

McFadyen, M.C., McLeod, H.L., Jackson, F.C., Melvin, W.T., Doehmer, J., and Murray, G.I. (2001b). Cytochrome P450 CYP1B1 protein expression: a novel mechanism of anticancer drug resistance. *Biochem Pharmacol*, Vol.62, No.2, 207-212.

McFadyen, M.C., Melvin, W.T., and Murray, G.I. (2004). Cytochrome P450 enzymes: novel options for cancer therapeutics. *Mol Cancer Ther*, Vol.3, No.3, 363-371.

McIlwain, C.C., Townsend, D.M., and Tew, K.D. (2006). Glutathione S-transferase polymorphisms: cancer incidence and therapy. *Oncogene*, Vol.25, No.11, 1639-1648.

McKeown, S.R., Cowen, R.L., and Williams, K.J. (2007). Bioreductive drugs: from concept to clinic. *Clinical oncology*, Vol.19, No.6, 427-442.

Miyoshi, Y., Taguchi, T., Kim, S.J., Tamaki, Y., and Noguchi, S. (2005). Prediction of response to docetaxel by immunohistochemical analysis of CYP3A4 expression in human breast cancers. *Breast Cancer*, Vol.12, No.1, 11-15.

Moore, L.B., Parks, D.J., Jones, S.A., Bledsoe, R.K., Consler, T.G., Stimmel, J.B., Goodwin, B., Liddle, C., Blanchard, S.G., Willson, T.M., Collins, J.L., and Kliewer, S.A. (2000). Orphan nuclear receptors constitutive androstane receptor and pregnane X receptor share xenobiotic and steroid ligands. *J Biol Chem*, Vol.275, No.20, 15122-15127.

Morel, F., and Aninat, C. (2011). The glutathione transferase kappa family. *Drug Metab Rev*, Vol.43, No.2, 281-291.

Morgan, A.S., Sanderson, P.E., Borch, R.F., Tew, K.D., Niitsu, Y., Takayama, T., Von Hoff, D.D., Izbicka, E., Mangold, G., Paul, C., Broberg, U., Mannervik, B., Henner, W.D., and Kauvar, L.M. (1998). Tumor efficacy and bone marrow-sparing properties of

TER286, a cytotoxin activated by glutathione S-transferase. *Cancer Res*, Vol.58, No.12, 2568-2575.

Muscarella, L.A., Parrella, P., D'Alessandro, V., la Torre, A., Barbano, R., Fontana, A., Tancredi, A., Guarnieri, V., Balsamo, T., Coco, M., *et al.* (2011). Frequent epigenetics inactivation of KEAP1 gene in non-small cell lung cancer. *Epigenetics*, Vol.6, No.6, 710-719.

Ni, Z., Bikadi, Z., Rosenberg, M.F., and Mao, Q. (2010). Structure and function of the human breast cancer resistance protein (BCRP/ABCG2). *Curr Drug Metab*, Vol.11, No.7, 603-617.

Nioi, P., and Nguyen, T. (2007). A mutation of Keap1 found in breast cancer impairs its ability to repress Nrf2 activity. *Biochem Biophys Res Commun*, Vol.362, No.4, 816-821.

Nishida, C.R., Lee, M., and de Montellano, P.R. (2010). Efficient hypoxic activation of the anticancer agent AQ4N by CYP2S1 and CYP2W1. *Mol Pharmacol*, Vol.78, No.3, 497-502.

Nitiss, J.L. (2009). Targeting DNA topoisomerase II in cancer chemotherapy. *Nat Rev Cancer*, Vol.9, No.5, 338-350.

O'Connor, P.M., Jackman, J., Bae, I., Myers, T.G., Fan, S., Mutoh, M., Scudiero, D.A., Monks, A., Sausville, E.A., Weinstein, J.N., Friend, S., Fornace, A.J., Jr., and Kohn, K.W. (1997). Characterization of the p53 tumor suppressor pathway in cell lines of the National Cancer Institute anticancer drug screen and correlations with the growth-inhibitory potency of 123 anticancer agents. *Cancer Res*, Vol.57, No.19, 4285-4300.

Ohta, T., Iijima, K., Miyamoto, M., Nakahara, I., Tanaka, H., Ohtsuji, M., Suzuki, T., Kobayashi, A., Yokota, J., Sakiyama, T., Shibata, T., Yamamoto, M., and Hirohashi, S. (2008). Loss of Keap1 function activates Nrf2 and provides advantages for lung cancer cell growth. *Cancer Res*, Vol.68, No.5, 1303-1309.

Okawa, H., Motohashi, H., Kobayashi, A., Aburatani, H., Kensler, T.W., and Yamamoto, M. (2006). Hepatocyte-specific deletion of the keap1 gene activates Nrf2 and confers potent resistance against acute drug toxicity. *Biochem Biophys Res Commun*, Vol.339, No.1, 79-88.

Oyama, T., Kagawa, N., Kunugita, N., Kitagawa, K., Ogawa, M., Yamaguchi, T., Suzuki, R., Kinaga, T., Yashima, Y., Ozaki, S., Isse, T., Kim, Y.D., Kim, H., and Kawamoto, T. (2004). Expression of cytochrome P450 in tumor tissues and its association with cancer development. *Front Biosci*, Vol.9, 1967-1976.

Padmanabhan, B., Tong, K.I., Ohta, T., Nakamura, Y., Scharlock, M., Ohtsuji, M., Kang, M.I., Kobayashi, A., Yokoyama, S., and Yamamoto, M. (2006). Structural basis for defects of Keap1 activity provoked by its point mutations in lung cancer. *Mol Cell*, Vol.21, No.5, 689-700.

Papandreou, I., Cairns, R.A., Fontana, L., Lim, A.L., and Denko, N.C. (2006). HIF-1 mediates adaptation to hypoxia by actively downregulating mitochondrial oxygen consumption. *Cell metabolism*, Vol.3, No.3, 187-197.

Parker, W.B. (2009). Enzymology of purine and pyrimidine antimetabolites used in the treatment of cancer. *Chem Rev*, Vol.109, No.7, 2880-2893.

Pastorekova, S., Zatovicova, M., and Pastorek, J. (2008). Cancer-associated carbonic anhydrases and their inhibition. *Curr Pharm Des*, Vol.14, No.7, 685-698.

Patel, M.S., and Korotchkina, L.G. (2001). Regulation of mammalian pyruvate dehydrogenase complex by phosphorylation: complexity of multiple phosphorylation sites and kinases. *Experimental & molecular medicine*, Vol.33, No.4, 191-197.

Patterson, L.H., and McKeown, S.R. (2000). AQ4N: a new approach to hypoxia-activated cancer chemotherapy. *Br J Cancer*, Vol.83, No.12, 1589-1593.

Paumi, C.M., Ledford, B.G., Smitherman, P.K., Townsend, A.J., and Morrow, C.S. (2001). Role of multidrug resistance protein 1 (MRP1) and glutathione S-transferase A1-1 in alkylating agent resistance. Kinetics of glutathione conjugate formation and efflux govern differential cellular sensitivity to chlorambucil versus melphalan toxicity. *J Biol Chem*, Vol.276, No.11, 7952-7956.

Potter, C., and Harris, A.L. (2004). Hypoxia inducible carbonic anhydrase IX, marker of tumour hypoxia, survival pathway and therapy target. *Cell Cycle*, Vol.3, No.2, 164-167.

Pugh, C.W., and Ratcliffe, P.J. (2003). Regulation of angiogenesis by hypoxia: role of the HIF system. *Nat Med*, Vol.9, No.6, 677-684.

Qi, X., Chang, Z., Song, J., Gao, G., and Shen, Z. (2011). Adenovirus-mediated p53 gene therapy reverses resistance of breast cancer cells to adriamycin. *Anticancer Drugs*, Vol.22, No.6, 556-562.

Rau, S., Autschbach, F., Riedel, H.D., Konig, J., Kulaksiz, H., Stiehl, A., Riemann, J.F., and Rost, D. (2008). Expression of the multidrug resistance proteins MRP2 and MRP3 in human cholangiocellular carcinomas. *Eur J Clin Invest*, Vol.38, No.2, 134-142.

Raynal, C., Pascussi, J.M., Leguelinel, G., Breuker, C., Kantar, J., Lallemant, B., Poujol, S., Bonnans, C., Joubert, D., Hollande, F., Lumbroso, S., Brouillet, J.P., and Evrard, A. (2010). Pregnane X Receptor (PXR) expression in colorectal cancer cells restricts irinotecan chemosensitivity through enhanced SN-38 glucuronidation. *Mol Cancer*, Vol.9, 46.

Raza, A., Galili, N., Smith, S., Godwin, J., Lancet, J., Melchert, M., Jones, M., Keck, J.G., Meng, L., Brown, G.L., and List, A. (2009). Phase 1 multicenter dose-escalation study of ezatiostat hydrochloride (TLK199 tablets), a novel glutathione analog prodrug, in patients with myelodysplastic syndrome. *Blood*, Vol.113, No.26, 6533-6540.

Reichert, M., Steinbach, J.P., Supra, P., and Weller, M. (2002). Modulation of growth and radiochemosensitivity of human malignant glioma cells by acidosis. *Cancer*, Vol.95, No.5, 1113-1119.

Risinger, A.L., Giles, F.J., and Mooberry, S.L. (2009). Microtubule dynamics as a target in oncology. *Cancer Treat Rev*, Vol.35, No.3, 255-261.

Rochat, B. (2009). Importance of influx and efflux systems and xenobiotic metabolizing enzymes in intratumoral disposition of anticancer agents. *Curr Cancer Drug Targets*, Vol.9, No.5, 652-674.

Rodriguez-Antona, C., and Ingelman-Sundberg, M. (2006). Cytochrome P450 pharmacogenetics and cancer. *Oncogene*, Vol.25, No.11, 1679-1691.

Rosario, L.A., O'Brien, M.L., Henderson, C.J., Wolf, C.R., and Tew, K.D. (2000). Cellular response to a glutathione S-transferase P1-1 activated prodrug. *Mol Pharmacol*, Vol.58, No.1, 167-174.

Rosen, L.S., Brown, J., Laxa, B., Boulos, L., Reiswig, L., Henner, W.D., Lum, R.T., Schow, S.R., Maack, C.A., Keck, J.G., Mascavage, J.C., Dombroski, J.A., Gomez, R.F., and Brown, G.L. (2003). Phase I study of TLK286 (glutathione S-transferase P1-1 activated glutathione analogue) in advanced refractory solid malignancies. *Clin Cancer Res*, Vol.9, No.5, 1628-1638.

Rosen, L.S., Laxa, B., Boulos, L., Wiggins, L., Keck, J.G., Jameson, A.J., Parra, R., Patel, K., and Brown, G.L. (2004). Phase 1 study of TLK286 (Telcyta) administered weekly in advanced malignancies. *Clin Cancer Res*, Vol.10, No.11, 3689-3698.

Ryan, H.E., Lo, J., and Johnson, R.S. (1998). HIF-1 alpha is required for solid tumor formation and embryonic vascularization. *EMBO J*, Vol.17, No.11, 3005-3015.

Ryoo, K., Huh, S.H., Lee, Y.H., Yoon, K.W., Cho, S.G., and Choi, E.J. (2004). Negative regulation of MEKK1-induced signaling by glutathione S-transferase Mu. *J Biol Chem*, Vol.279, No.42, 43589-43594.

Saavedra, J.E., Srinivasan, A., Buzard, G.S., Davies, K.M., Waterhouse, D.J., Inami, K., Wilde, T.C., Citro, M.L., Cuellar, M., Deschamps, J.R., Parrish, D., Shami, P.J., Findlay, V.J., Townsend, D.M., Tew, K.D., Singh, S., Jia, L., Ji, X., and Keefer, L.K. (2006). PABA/NO as an anticancer lead: analogue synthesis, structure revision, solution chemistry, reactivity toward glutathione, and in vitro activity. *J Med Chem*, Vol.49, No.3, 1157-1164.

Salinas-Souza, C., Petrilli, A.S., and de Toledo, S.R. (2010). Glutathione S-transferase polymorphisms in osteosarcoma patients. *Pharmacogenet Genomics*, Vol.20, No.8, 507-515.

Satyam, A., Hocker, M.D., Kane-Maguire, K.A., Morgan, A.S., Villar, H.O., and Lyttle, M.H. (1996). Design, synthesis, and evaluation of latent alkylating agents activated by glutathione S-transferase. *J Med Chem*, Vol.39, No.8, 1736-1747.

Seagroves, T.N., Ryan, H.E., Lu, H., Wouters, B.G., Knapp, M., Thibault, P., Laderoute, K., and Johnson, R.S. (2001). Transcription factor HIF-1 is a necessary mediator of the pasteur effect in mammalian cells. *Mol Cell Biol*, Vol.21, No.10, 3436-3444.

Sebolt-Leopold, J.S., and English, J.M. (2006). Mechanisms of drug inhibition of signalling molecules. *Nature*, Vol.441, No.7092, 457-462.

Semenza, G.L. (2003). Targeting HIF-1 for cancer therapy. *Nat Rev Cancer*, Vol.3, No.10, 721-732.

Semenza, G.L. (2007). Evaluation of HIF-1 inhibitors as anticancer agents. *Drug discovery today*, Vol.12, No.19-20, 853-859.

Sequist, L.V., Fidias, P.M., Temel, J.S., Kolevska, T., Rabin, M.S., Boccia, R.V., Burris, H.A., Belt, R.J., Huberman, M.S., Melnyk, O., Mills, G.M., Englund, C.W., Caldwell, D.C., Keck, J.G., Meng, L., Jones, M., Brown, G.L., Edelman, M.J., and Lynch, T.J. (2009). Phase 1-2a multicenter dose-ranging study of canfosfamide in combination with carboplatin and paclitaxel as first-line therapy for patients with advanced non-small cell lung cancer. *J Thorac Oncol*, Vol.4, No.11, 1389-1396.

Shannon, A.M., Bouchier-Hayes, D.J., Condron, C.M., and Toomey, D. (2003). Tumour hypoxia, chemotherapeutic resistance and hypoxia-related therapies. *Cancer Treat Rev*, Vol.29, No.4, 297-307.

Sharma, A., Patrick, B., Li, J., Sharma, R., Jeyabal, P.V., Reddy, P.M., Awasthi, S., and Awasthi, Y.C. (2006). Glutathione S-transferases as antioxidant enzymes: small cell lung cancer (H69) cells transfected with hGSTA1 resist doxorubicin-induced apoptosis. *Arch Biochem Biophys*, Vol.452, No.2, 165-173.

Shibata, T., Kokubu, A., Gotoh, M., Ojima, H., Ohta, T., Yamamoto, M., and Hirohashi, S. (2008a). Genetic alteration of Keap1 confers constitutive Nrf2 activation and resistance to chemotherapy in gallbladder cancer. *Gastroenterology*, Vol.135, No.4, 1358-1368, 1368 e1351-1354.

Shibata, T., Ohta, T., Tong, K.I., Kokubu, A., Odogawa, R., Tsuta, K., Asamura, H., Yamamoto, M., and Hirohashi, S. (2008b). Cancer related mutations in NRF2 impair its recognition by Keap1-Cul3 E3 ligase and promote malignancy. *Proc Natl Acad Sci U S A*, Vol.105, No.36, 13568-13573.

Shimoda, L.A., Fallon, M., Pisarcik, S., Wang, J., and Semenza, G.L. (2006). HIF-1 regulates hypoxic induction of NHE1 expression and alkalinization of intracellular pH in pulmonary arterial myocytes. *American journal of physiology Lung cellular and molecular physiology*, Vol.291, No.5, L941-949.

Sim, S.C., and Ingelman-Sundberg, M. (2010). The Human Cytochrome P450 (CYP) Allele Nomenclature website: a peer-reviewed database of CYP variants and their associated effects. *Hum Genomics*, Vol.4, No.4, 278-281.

Sonoda, J., Pei, L., and Evans, R.M. (2008). Nuclear receptors: decoding metabolic disease. *FEBS Lett*, Vol.582, No.1, 2-9.

Squires, E.J., Sueyoshi, T., and Negishi, M. (2004). Cytoplasmic localization of pregnane X receptor and ligand-dependent nuclear translocation in mouse liver. *J Biol Chem*, Vol.279, No.47, 49307-49314.

Sun, H.L., Liu, Y.N., Huang, Y.T., Pan, S.L., Huang, D.Y., Guh, J.H., Lee, F.Y., Kuo, S.C., and Teng, C.M. (2007). YC-1 inhibits HIF-1 expression in prostate cancer cells: contribution of Akt/NF-kappaB signaling to HIF-1alpha accumulation during hypoxia. *Oncogene*, Vol.26, No.27, 3941-3951.

Suzuki, T., Nishio, K., and Tanabe, S. (2001). The MRP family and anticancer drug metabolism. *Curr Drug Metab*, Vol.2, No.4, 367-377.

Svoboda, M., Riha, J., Wlcek, K., Jaeger, W., and Thalhammer, T. (2011). Organic anion transporting polypeptides (OATPs): regulation of expression and function. *Curr Drug Metab*, Vol.12, No.2, 139-153.

Taguchi, K., Motohashi, H., and Yamamoto, M. (2011). Molecular mechanisms of the Keap1-Nrf2 pathway in stress response and cancer evolution. *Genes Cells*, Vol.16, No.2, 123-140.

Takeshita, A., Taguchi, M., Koibuchi, N., and Ozawa, Y. (2002). Putative role of the orphan nuclear receptor SXR (steroid and xenobiotic receptor) in the mechanism of CYP3A4 inhibition by xenobiotics. *J Biol Chem*, Vol.277, No.36, 32453-32458.

Talks, K.L., Turley, H., Gatter, K.C., Maxwell, P.H., Pugh, C.W., Ratcliffe, P.J., and Harris, A.L. (2000). The expression and distribution of the hypoxia-inducible factors HIF-1alpha and HIF-2alpha in normal human tissues, cancers, and tumor-associated macrophages. *Am J Pathol*, Vol.157, No.2, 411-421.

Tang, X., Wang, H., Fan, L., Wu, X., Xin, A., Ren, H., and Wang, X.J. (2011). Luteolin inhibits Nrf2 leading to negative regulation of the Nrf2/ARE pathway and sensitization of human lung carcinoma A549 cells to therapeutic drugs. *Free Radic Biol Med*, Vol.50, No.11, 1599-1609.

Taniguchi, K., Wada, M., Kohno, K., Nakamura, T., Kawabe, T., Kawakami, M., Kagotani, K., Okumura, K., Akiyama, S., and Kuwano, M. (1996). A human canalicular multispecific organic anion transporter (cMOAT) gene is overexpressed in cisplatin-resistant human cancer cell lines with decreased drug accumulation. *Cancer Res*, Vol.56, No.18, 4124-4129.

Tew, K.D. (1994). Glutathione-associated enzymes in anticancer drug resistance. *Cancer Res*, Vol.54, No.16, 4313-4320.

Timsit, Y.E., and Negishi, M. (2007). CAR and PXR: the xenobiotic-sensing receptors. *Steroids*, Vol.72, No.3, 231-246.

Tolson, A.H., and Wang, H. (2010). Regulation of drug-metabolizing enzymes by xenobiotic receptors: PXR and CAR. *Adv Drug Deliv Rev*, Vol.62, No.13, 1238-1249.

Townsend, D., and Tew, K. (2003a). Cancer drugs, genetic variation and the glutathione-S-transferase gene family. *Am J Pharmacogenomics*, Vol.3, No.3, 157-172.

Townsend, D.M., Findlay, V.L., and Tew, K.D. (2005). Glutathione S-transferases as regulators of kinase pathways and anticancer drug targets. *Methods Enzymol*, Vol.401, 287-307.

Townsend, D.M., Shen, H., Staros, A.L., Gate, L., and Tew, K.D. (2002). Efficacy of a glutathione S-transferase pi-activated prodrug in platinum-resistant ovarian cancer cells. *Mol Cancer Ther*, Vol.1, No.12, 1089-1095.

Townsend, D.M., and Tew, K.D. (2003b). The role of glutathione-S-transferase in anti-cancer drug resistance. *Oncogene*, Vol.22, No.47, 7369-7375.

Tredan, O., Galmarini, C.M., Patel, K., and Tannock, I.F. (2007). Drug resistance and the solid tumor microenvironment. *J Natl Cancer Inst*, Vol.99, No.19, 1441-1454.

Trock, B.J., Leonessa, F., and Clarke, R. (1997). Multidrug resistance in breast cancer: a meta-analysis of MDR1/gp170 expression and its possible functional significance. *J Natl Cancer Inst*, Vol.89, No.13, 917-931.

Tzameli, I., Pissios, P., Schuetz, E.G., and Moore, D.D. (2000). The xenobiotic compound 1,4-bis[2-(3,5-dichloropyridyloxy)]benzene is an agonist ligand for the nuclear receptor CAR. *Mol Cell Biol*, Vol.20, No.9, 2951-2958.

Ullah, M.S., Davies, A.J., and Halestrap, A.P. (2006). The plasma membrane lactate transporter MCT4, but not MCT1, is up-regulated by hypoxia through a HIF-1alpha-dependent mechanism. *J Biol Chem*, Vol.281, No.14, 9030-9037.

Urquhart, B.L., Tirona, R.G., and Kim, R.B. (2007). Nuclear receptors and the regulation of drug-metabolizing enzymes and drug transporters: implications for interindividual variability in response to drugs. *J Clin Pharmacol*, Vol.47, No.5, 566-578.

Vaupel, P., and Harrison, L. (2004). Tumor hypoxia: causative factors, compensatory mechanisms, and cellular response. *Oncologist*, Vol.9 Suppl 5, 4-9.

Vaupel, P., and Mayer, A. (2007). Hypoxia in cancer: significance and impact on clinical outcome. *Cancer Metastasis Rev*, Vol.26, No.2, 225-239.

Venkatesh, M., Wang, H., Cayer, J., Leroux, M., Salvail, D., Das, B., Wrobel, J.E., and Mani, S. (2011). In Vivo and In Vitro Characterization of a First-in-Class Novel Azole Analog That Targets Pregnane X Receptor Activation. *Mol Pharmacol*, Vol.80, No.1, 124-135.

Vergote, I., Finkler, N., del Campo, J., Lohr, A., Hunter, J., Matei, D., Kavanagh, J., Vermorken, J.B., Meng, L., Jones, M., Brown, G., and Kaye, S. (2009). Phase 3 randomised study of canfosfamide (Telcyta, TLK286) versus pegylated liposomal doxorubicin or topotecan as third-line therapy in patients with platinum-refractory or -resistant ovarian cancer. *Eur J Cancer*, Vol.45, No.13, 2324-2332.

Wang, B., Huang, G., Wang, D., Li, A., Xu, Z., Dong, R., Zhang, D., and Zhou, W. (2010). Null genotypes of GSTM1 and GSTT1 contribute to hepatocellular carcinoma risk: evidence from an updated meta-analysis. *J Hepatol*, Vol.53, No.3, 508-518.

Wang, G.L., and Semenza, G.L. (1995). Purification and characterization of hypoxia-inducible factor 1. *J Biol Chem*, Vol.270, No.3, 1230-1237.

Wang, K., Ramji, S., Bhathena, A., Lee, C., and Riddick, D.S. (1999). Glutathione S-transferases in wild-type and doxorubicin-resistant MCF-7 human breast cancer cell lines. *Xenobiotica*, Vol.29, No.2, 155-170.

Wang, R., An, J., Ji, F., Jiao, H., Sun, H., and Zhou, D. (2008). Hypermethylation of the Keap1 gene in human lung cancer cell lines and lung cancer tissues. *Biochem Biophys Res Commun*, Vol.373, No.1, 151-154.

Wang, T., Ma, X., Krausz, K.W., Idle, J.R., and Gonzalez, F.J. (2008). Role of pregnane X receptor in control of all-trans retinoic acid (ATRA) metabolism and its potential contribution to ATRA resistance. *J Pharmacol Exp Ther*, Vol.324, No.2, 674-684.

Wang, W., Liu, G., and Zheng, J. (2007). Human renal UOK130 tumor cells: a drug resistant cell line with highly selective over-expression of glutathione S-transferase-pi isozyme. *Eur J Pharmacol*, Vol.568, No.1-3, 61-67.

Wang, X., Sykes, D.B., and Miller, D.S. (2010). Constitutive androstane receptor-mediated up-regulation of ATP-driven xenobiotic efflux transporters at the blood-brain barrier. *Mol Pharmacol*, Vol.78, No.3, 376-383.

Wang, X.J., Sun, Z., Villeneuve, N.F., Zhang, S., Zhao, F., Li, Y., Chen, W., Yi, X., Zheng, W., Wondrak, G.T., Wong, P.K., and Zhang, D.D. (2008). Nrf2 enhances resistance of cancer cells to chemotherapeutic drugs, the dark side of Nrf2. *Carcinogenesis*, Vol.29, No.6, 1235-1243.

Wang, Y., and Cabral, F. (2005). Paclitaxel resistance in cells with reduced beta-tubulin. *Biochim Biophys Acta*, Vol.1744, No.2, 245-255.

Warburg, O. (1956). On respiratory impairment in cancer cells. *Science*, Vol.124, No.3215, 269-270.

Wouters, A., Pauwels, B., Lardon, F., and Vermorken, J.B. (2007). Review: implications of in vitro research on the effect of radiotherapy and chemotherapy under hypoxic conditions. *Oncologist*, Vol.12, No.6, 690-712.

Wu, C.P., Hsieh, C.H., and Wu, Y.S. (2011). The Emergence of Drug Transporter-Mediated Multidrug Resistance to Cancer Chemotherapy. *Mol Pharm*, in press.

Wu, Y., Fan, Y., Xue, B., Luo, L., Shen, J., Zhang, S., Jiang, Y., and Yin, Z. (2006). Human glutathione S-transferase P1-1 interacts with TRAF2 and regulates TRAF2-ASK1 signals. *Oncogene*, Vol.25, No.42, 5787-5800.

Xie, J., Shults, K., Flye, L., Jiang, F., Head, D.R., and Briggs, R.C. (2005). Overexpression of GSTA2 protects against cell cycle arrest and apoptosis induced by the DNA inter-strand crosslinking nitrogen mustard, mechlorethamine. *J Cell Biochem*, Vol.95, No.2, 339-351.

Xu, H.W., Xu, L., Hao, J.H., Qin, C.Y., and Liu, H. (2010). Expression of P-glycoprotein and multidrug resistance-associated protein is associated with multidrug resistance in gastric cancer. *J Int Med Res*, Vol.38, No.1, 34-42.

Ye, C.G., Wu, W.K., Yeung, J.H., Li, H.T., Li, Z.J., Wong, C.C., Ren, S.X., Zhang, L., Fung, K.P., and Cho, C.H. (2011). Indomethacin and SC236 enhance the cytotoxicity of doxorubicin in human hepatocellular carcinoma cells via inhibiting P-glycoprotein and MRP1 expression. *Cancer Lett*, Vol.304, No.2, 90-96.

Yeo, E.J., Chun, Y.S., Cho, Y.S., Kim, J., Lee, J.C., Kim, M.S., and Park, J.W. (2003). YC-1: a potential anticancer drug targeting hypoxia-inducible factor 1. *J Natl Cancer Inst*, Vol.95, No.7, 516-525.

Zelcer, N., Saeki, T., Reid, G., Beijnen, J.H., and Borst, P. (2001). Characterization of drug transport by the human multidrug resistance protein 3 (ABCC3). *J Biol Chem*, Vol.276, No.49, 46400-46407.

Zhou, J., and Giannakakou, P. (2005). Targeting microtubules for cancer chemotherapy. *Curr Med Chem Anticancer Agents*, Vol.5, No.1, 65-71.

Zhou, J., Liu, M., Zhai, Y., and Xie, W. (2008). The antiapoptotic role of pregnane X receptor in human colon cancer cells. *Mol Endocrinol*, Vol.22, No.4, 868-880.

Zhou, S.F., Wang, L.L., Di, Y.M., Xue, C.C., Duan, W., Li, C.G., and Li, Y. (2008). Substrates and inhibitors of human multidrug resistance associated proteins and the implications in drug development. *Curr Med Chem*, Vol.15, No.20, 1981-2039.

Zhu, H., Chen, X.P., Luo, S.F., Guan, J., Zhang, W.G., and Zhang, B.X. (2005). Involvement of hypoxia-inducible factor-1-alpha in multidrug resistance induced by hypoxia in HepG2 cells. *J Exp Clin Cancer Res*, Vol.24, No.4, 565-574.

6

Genetic and Epigenetic Factors Affecting Cytochrome P450 Phenotype and Their Clinical Relevance

Viola Tamási and András Falus
Semmelweis University,
Hungary

1. Introduction

Pharmacogenetics (or pharmacogenomics) studies the role of inherited and acquired genetic variation in drug response. Clinically relevant pharmacogenetic examples, mainly involving drug metabolism are known for decades, but the field was not evolved until the 1970s, when the discovery of the CYP2D6 polymorphism and its resultant effect on drug toxicity and response led to many observations of pharmacogenetic-based variations in pharmacokinetics. These and other discoveries and the subsequent ability to genotype led to the term pharmacogenetics. Today, as a consequence of sequencing and mapping of the human genome, pharmacogenetics is becoming the first drug discovery pipeline technology to affect the structure and economics of the pharmaceutical industry (Daly, 2010). During drug development, it is important to consider pharmacogenetic variation which could explain or even prevent discarding a drug candidate if appropriate genetic reasons are identified or when lack of response/occurrence of ADRs (adverse drug reactions) in drug therapy is experienced. Genetic variation is taken strongly into consideration also in clinic during individualized therapies. It helps to improve the number of responders and decrease the number of patients suffering from ADRs.

Beside genetic polymorphism there are other heritable phenotypic changes which play role in drug response that do not involve any alteration in nuclear DNA sequence, but affect gene transcription through DNA methylation, histone modification, miRNA regulation (called pharmacoepigenetic changes) (Berger et al., 2009). There are also non-heritable changes, which affect response to drugs, such as reactions to the environment, to drug-drug interactions through regulatory mechanisms (Tamási et al., 2003). Although fast, non-heritable responses, which alter signal transduction pathways affect the therapeutic outcome of a drug tremendously, pharmacogenetic and pharmacoepigenetic difference has to be taken also strictly into consideration in clinical practice.

In general one can envision important pharmacogenetic and pharmacoepigenetic variation

1. in genes responsible for pharmacokinetic properties of the drug (genes influencing absorption, distribution metabolism, elimination) or
2. in genes responsible for pharmacodinamic properties of the drug (genes affecting the pharmacologic effect of a drug) (Daly, 2010).

So far, it is apparent that heritable changes in genes encoding drug metabolizing enzymes often affects outcome in drug treatment to a high degree and the variability of the phase I enzymes plays major role in this respect, as evidenced by many studies (Spear et al., 2001; Ingelman-Sundberg, 2004a; Weinshilboum, 2003). In general it can be estimated that 20-25% of all drug therapies are influenced by such polymorphism to an extent that therapy outcome is changed. There are much fewer examples where the pharmacodinamic properties are influenced and it has clinical relevance (Ingelman-Sundberg, 2004b; Eichelbaum et al., 2006).

In this book chapter the polymorphic and epigenetic nature of phase I enzymes will be discussed and their role in therapy and clinic will be highlighted.

2. Pharmacogenetics

All genes encoding cytochrome P450 enzymes (CYPs) in families 1–3 are polymorphic. However, the functional importance of the variant alleles is not the same and the frequency of their distribution in different ethnic groups also differs. Polymorphisms of CYPs consist of single nucleotide polymorphisms (SNP), gene deletions, missense mutations, insertions, gene duplications and deleterious mutations creating inactive gene products. Furthermore amino acid changes might be introduced, which changes the substrate specificity of the enzyme. Mutations in intronic regions could also have relevance. An important aspect of drug metabolizing gene polymorphism would be copy number variation (CNV) where multiple functional gene copies of one allele can result in increased drug metabolism and absence of drug response at ordinary dosage. To order and standardize allelic variants, the CYP-allele nomenclature committee manages the naming and definition of CYP alleles, which are presented on an associated web site (http://www.cypalleles.ki.se). The homepage contains updated information regarding the nomenclature and properties of the variant alleles with links to the dbSNP database (http://www.ncbi.nlm.nih.gov/projects/SNP/) and relevant literature references. Based on the phenotype variability among drug metabolizers, the populations could be classified into four major groups:

1. the ultrarapid metabolizers (UM); with very high drug metabolizing capacity; usually caring more than two active gene copies
2. the extensive metabolizers (EM); with high drug metabolizing capacity; usually caring two active gene copies
3. the intermediate metabolizers (IM); with intermediate drug metabolizing capacity; usually carrying one functional and one defective allel, but may also carry two partially defective alleles
4. the poor metabolizers (PM); with slow, poor drug metabolizing capacity; usually lacking functional enzyme due to defective or deleted genes (Ingelman-Sundberg et al., 2007).

Taking CYP2D6-dependent metabolism as an example, the rate of metabolism for a certain drug can differ 1000-fold between phenotypes. Thus, the dosing required to achieve the same plasma levels of a drug metabolized mainly by CYP2D6, such as nortriptyline, differs 10–20-fold among individuals. Despite this extensive variation in metabolic capacity among patients, dosing is, at present, principally population based (i.e. doses are based on the plasma levels of the drug obtained on average in the population at a certain dosage), but not individual based.

• Lack or extended pharmacological effect	• Exacerbated drug-drug interactions
• Drug toxicity	• Drug resistance
• Lack of prodrug activation	• Adverse drug reactions
• Increased effective dose	• Idiosyncrasy
• Metabolism by alternative pathways	• Precarcinogen activation

Box 1. Potential consequences of polymorphic drug metabolism.

CYP polymorphisms affect the response of individuals to drugs in many ways (see Box 1.) and it alters the therapial regimen of many diseases such as depression, psychosis, cancer, cardiovascular disorders, ulcer and gastrointestinal disorders, pain and epilepsy and many others. The problem is that the use of genotyping or genomic methods to inform clinical decisions about drug response are not widely practiced (Varmus, 2010) but it would be necessary, expecially when drugs have narrow therapeutic indexes, when severe side effects occur or when the rate of non-responders is high. In resent years, the FDA has aggressively pursued drug-label modification when excess risk can be convincingly linked to a genetic marker. The FDA-mandated incorporation of pharmacogenomic information in drug labeling will remain an important step in the acceptance of pharmacogenomics in clinical practice (Wolf & Smith, 2000).

In the next section, relevant therapeutic areas where CYP polymorphism significantly influences the response of drugs or the incidence of adverse drug reactions will be presented.

2.1 Role of pharmacogenetics in therapies

At the present time, decisions about which medications to prescribe are made on a trial and error basis for many disorders. Under the pharmacogenomic paradigm, genetically based screening methods would allow the tailoring of drug therapy, drug selection and dosing according to an individual's ability to metabolize a drug. There are many disorders where it is already taken into consideration and applying information about the patient's genetic makeup has high impact on therapeutic outcome.

2.1.1 Cancer

Oncology is a field that is already being revolutionized by pharmacogenomics. Cancer pharmacogenomics is complicated by the fact that two genomes ar involved: the germline genome of the patient and the somatic genome of the tumor. Chemotherapeutic drugs are very sensitive to genetic background, since in general they are unspecific drugs with narrow therapeutic indexes that result frequent severe or even fatal toxicities.

Germline genetic variations in cancer cells

Tamoxifen. Tamoxifen is an estrogen receptor modulator used in hormone receptor positive breast cancers. It has been suggested that CYP2D6 activity is required for the formation of endoxifen the active metabolite of tamoxifen (Jin et al., 2005). There are several studies proving that CYP2D6 PMs have worsened relapse–free time and disease-free survival rate, but they do not experience hot flashes at the same magnitude as compared with patients carrying the wild type allele. A similar loss of effectiveness is obtained as a result of enzyme inhibition (by serotonin reuptake inhibitors, antidepressants and other CYP2D6 inhibitors).

Another CYP enzyme, CYP2C19 has been shown to metabolize tamoxifen to its active form. Carriers of CYP2C19*17 allele variants have been shown to exhibit a more favourable clinical outcome, since these patients activate tamoxifen in greater extent. This allele may be especially relevant for patients with low levels of CYP2D6 (Rodriguez-Antona et al., 2010).

Cyclophosphamide. Cyclophosphamide (CPA), a prodrug used in cancer therapy and for treatment of some autoimmune disorders is activated to 4-hydroxycyclophosphamide by CYP2C19, CYP2C9, CYP3A4 and CYP2B6. It has been shown that carriers of CYP2C19*2 or CYP2B6*5 had a significant lower CPA elimination and worse therapeutical outcome. CYP2B6 enzyme expresses also in the liver and it metabolizes ifosfamide, tamoxifen, procarbazine and thiotepa in the same manner as it activate CPA (Takada et al., 2004; Rodriguez-Antona et al., 2010).

Tegafur. Tegafur is also a prodrug which is activated to 5-fluorouracil by CYP2A6. Patients with CYP2A6*4 or CYP2A6*11 were poor metabolizer of this drug. Because other CYP enzymes influence the metabolism of tegafur (CYP3A4, CYP3A5, glutathione S-transferases) calculation of effective dose is difficult (Daigo et al., 2002).

Thalidomide. Bioactivation of thalidomide is dependent on metabolism by CYP2C19 (5-hydroxythalidomide). Another pathway producing arene oxid from thalidomide also egsists and it is mediated by CYP1A1 and CYP2E1. It was reported that in multiple myeloma, response to thalidomide and dexamethasone parallel treatment was higher in CYP2C19 EMs than in PMs. The lower response rate observed in PMs is possibly due to the reduced activity to inhibit angiogenesis. Despite these facts there is no big influence of CYP2C19 polymorphism to treatment outcome (Vangsted et al., 2010).

Somatic genetic variations in cancer cells

CYP3A4 tumor expression could be somatically altered in specific tumors and it could be useful predictor for the effectiveness of drugs that are subject to CYP3A4 metabolism (for e.g. drug resistance in cancer tissue). Vincristine, CPA, etoposide treatments in lymphoma or docetaxel in breast cancer are all substrates of tumor CYP3A4 and their local metabolism could have therapeutical consequences due to their narrow therapeutical window. CYP2B1 is also overexpressed in breast cancer and there are several therapeutic approaches focusing on higher CYP2B1 metabolism in tumor cells than in other body cells (Rodriguez Antona et al., 2010).

2.1.2 Depression

CYP2D6 and CYP2C19 metabolize virtually all of the antidepressants, many of which are also strong inhibitors of the enzyme.

Antidepressants

Tricyclic antidepressants (TCAs) are medications used to alleviate mood disorders, such as major depression dysthymia or anxiety disorders. CYP2D6 mediated metabolism of antidepressants leads to equally potent metabolites but the risk for side effects in poor metabolizers for CYP2D6 has been shown to be higher than in extensive metabolizers even if the sum of parent drug and metabolite was the same. Because of these adverse effects, in case of TCAs, there should be a dose adjustment depending on the patients genotype (for e.g. single dose paroxetine is changing 10-fold in EMs compared to PMs) (Table 1.). Genotyping for *CYP2D6* in psychiatric patients is widely accepted and is more or less the only pharmacogenetic test used in clinical practice (Kirchheiner et al., 2004).

Drug	Dosing	Usual dose (mg)	EM (%)	IM (%)	PM (%)
CYP2D6-dependent					
Amitriptyline	M	150	120	90	50
	S	50	120	80	70
Nortriptyline	M	150	120	90	50
	S	50	140	70	50
Imipramine	M	150	130	80	30
	S	50	110	100	60
Paroxetine	M	20	110	90	70
	S	20	130	70	20
Venlafaxine	M	150	130	80	20
CYP2C19-dependent					
Amitryptiline	M	150	110	80	60
Imipramine	M	150	100	80	60
	S	50	100	90	70
Clomipramine	S	50	100	90	70

Table 1. M/S dosage recommendations of antidepressants for multiple-dosing or for beginning of treatment in relation to CYP2D6 and CYP2C19 polymorphism (M-maintenance treatment, S-single dose) (Kirchheiner et al., 2001).

CYP2C19 polymorphism also influences the blood level of citalopram, amitriptyline and other antidepressants (Table 1.). Amitriptyline is demethylated to nortriptyline by CYP2C19 which is further metabolised to nonactive metabolites. CYP2C19 polymorphism alone does not affect the therapeutic outcome, since nortriptyline the metabolite is an active antidepressant, but side effects are different if the amitriptyline/nortriptilline balance is changing. The highest risk for ADRs occur when a patient is EM for CYP2C19, but PM for CYP2D6, since CYP2C19 produces a high amount of nortriptyline, but there is no CYP2D6 to metabolize it to inactive metabolites (Jornil et al., 2010).

Serotonin reuptake inhibitors

The pharmacokinetics of serotonin reuptake inhibitors (SSRIs) is complex, they are very lipid solible, high clearence drugs subjected to multiple metabolic pathways.

Fluoxetine. Fluoxetine is metabolised to norfluoxetine, which is 20 times less potent SSRI than the original molecule. CYP2D6 is responsible for R-norfluoxitene production and CYP2C9 and CYP2D6 produces S-norfluoxetine (Fuller et al., 1992). CYP3A4 can also metabolise this drug, when CYP2D6 becomes saturated (Margolis et al., 2000). Although genetic polymorphism influence greatly the level of fluoxetine, it is hard to predict the gene-concentration relationship because of several metabolic pathways.

Paroxetine. This drug is inactivated by CYP2D6 (Bloomer et al., 1992). PMs for this enzyme tolerate much smaller dose than EMs (Table 1.). Single dose or multiple dosing makes difference in paroxetine addministration, because with chronic dosing metabolism is saturable and autophenocopy could occur (Laine et al., 2001).

2.1.3 Psychosis

Antipsychotic drugs are widely prescribed for a multitude of psychiatric conditions. CYP2D6 metabolizes many psychotropic drugs, including antipsychotics like haloperidol, thioridazine, perphenazine, chlorpromazine, risperidone, and aripiprazole.

Numerous authors suggested that genotyping for families of CYP enzymes (CYP2D6, CYP1A2) could potentially aid in prescribing antipsychotic drugs, since there are significant risks associated with their polymorphism, such as movement disorders (CYP1A2, CYP2D6), and cardiovascular adverse effects (CYP2D6) (Foster et al., 2007). CYP2D6 PMs had four time higher Parkinsonism like side-effects than EMs. Also, occurence of other ADRs in response to treatment increased from CYP2D6 EMs to PMs. Furtermore, the duration of treatment was higher in PM patients, which increased the costs about 4000-6000$ (Ingelman Sundberg, 2004b).

2.1.4 Epilepsy

Effective dosing of phenytoin is highly linked to CYP2C9 genotype. Patient cariing defective alleles show more frequently side effects for e.g. ataxia, diploidia and other neurological symptoms (Lee et al., 2002). Clobazam is also used in the treatment of epilepsy. This drug is metabolized to N-demethylclobazam, which is further processed by CYP2C19 to 4-hydroxydesmethylclobazam. In CYP2C19 PM patients there is an accumulation of N-demethylclobazam, which causes side effects such as drowsiness (Kosaki et al., 2004). Diazepam, another antiepileptic and anxiolitic is metabolized by CYP2C19 and CYP3A4. Both enzymes convert it to desmethyldiazepam. CYP2C19 produces two other metabolites also, oxazepam and temazepam (Andersson et al., 1994; Jung et al., 1997). PMs for CYP2C19 enzyme metabolize slower this drug and took longer to emerge from anesthesia than for EMs (Inomata et al., 2005). Although diazepam has a clear gene-concentration effect, it is not predictable for the dose because of the many other active metabolites produced and involvement of other CYP enzymes.

2.1.5 Pain

Codeine. Codeine and tramadol needs to be metabolized to its active forms (morphine or o-desmethyltramadol), before pain relieving effects are observed. Codeine is metabolised by CYP2D6 to its active metabolite, morphine, with CYP3A4 to norcodeine and with glucuronide transferase to codeine-6-glucuronide. CYP2D6 polymorphism affects greatly the precent ratio of these metabolites, which means that PMs do not bioactivate enough codeine to morphine and EMs are at risk of CNS depression and other side effects due to elevated morphine production (Table 2.) (Leppert, 2011).

Gasche et al reported a patient who received oral codeine at daily dose of 75 mg and who experienced symptoms of morphine overdose (lack of consciusness, respiratory depression) after 4 days of treatment. The patient recovered after intravenous administration of naloxon. The cause of these sympthomes was his CYP2D6 EM phenotype as genotyping showed 3 or more functional alleles. The patient was concomitatantly treated with claritromycin and voriconazole, both known inhibitors of CYP3A4 as confirmed by low CYP3A4 activity (Gasche et al., 2004)

Effects of metabolised codeine	EM	PM
Morphine conc. (% of codeine)	3.9%	0.17%
Analgesia	Yes	No
Pricking pain threshold	Increased	No effect
Tolerance thresholds to heat and pressure	Not altered	Not altered
Peak pain and disconfort during cold pressor test	Reduced	Not changed
Adverse effects	Yes	Yes

Table 2. Effects of codeine's active metabolite, morphine in relation to different CYP2D6 polymorphisms.

Dihydrocodeine. Dihydrocodeine (DHC) is a semi-synthetic analogue of codeine and it is used as analgetic, antitussive drug or for treatment of opioid addiction. DHC is metabolised to dihydromorphine (DHM) mostly by CYP2D6 (DHM percentage of a single oral DHC dose; 9%EM, 1% PM). Although DHM display greater affinity for opioid receptors than DHC, its pharmacological role in analgesic effect is not proven. Studies performed to date indicate that DHC analgesia is independent of CYP2D6 activity (Leppert, 2011).

Tramadol. Tramadol is a very usfull pain relief medication in neonates and infants. It is primary metabolized into its more active metabolite, O-demethyl tramadol by CYP2D6. EMs for CYP2D6 enzyme react better to tramadol treatment, pain treshold tests showed better tolerance of pain, than in PMs. PMs need approximately 30% higher tramadol doses than those with extensive CYP2D6 activity (EMs) (Ingelman-Sundberg et al., 2007).

2.1.6 Cardiovascular diseases

Genetic variation influences the dose of many cardiovascular drugs, because most of them has narrow therapeutic indexes. Cardiovascular diseases are treated with many different classes of drugs, such as antianginals, antihypertensives, antiarrhythmics, anticoagulants, antiaggregating agents, lipid lowering drugs, etc. Many of these drugs are metabolized through the polymorphic CYP2D6, CYP2C9 and CYP2C19 enzymes.

For example, the antianginal perhexiline metabolism is controlled by the polymorphic CYP2D6 enzyme. After perhexiline treatment a gene-dose effect has been observed; in poor metabolizers, perhexiline plasma concentrations can be very high (6-fold higher than in EMs after a single dose of perhexiline) which explains its hepatotoxic and neuropathic side effects. Determination of the ratio between perhexiline and its metabolite early in treatment may facilitate appropriate dose adjustment which may range from 10 mg in PMs to 500 mg in EMs (Cooper et al., 1984).

Oral anticoagulants

CYP2C9 and the C1 subunit of the vitamin K epoxide reductase (VKORC1) genotypes are associated with the variability in the overall pharmacodynamic responses to oral anticoagulants, such as warfarin, acenocoumarol and phenprocoumon. All three molecules have low therapeutic indexes and the dose required to produce a normal prothrombin time is largely unpredictable. The consequences of under or over treating can be dire (thromboembolism or hemorrhage) (Gardiner & Begg, 2006).

Warfarin. S-Warfarin is 3- to 5-fold more potent than R-warfarin and its responsible for 70% of the overall anticoagulant effect. S-warfarin is mostly metabolized by CYP2C9 and in 1-1.5% by CYP4F2, whereas R-warfarin is metabolised by CYP3A4 and CYP1A2. Variations in genes central to warfarin activity (VKORC1, vitamin K reductase regulator (CALU) and gamma glutaryl carboxilase (GGCX)) are also polymorphic and they have to be taken into consideration during dose calculation (Table 3.).

Gene	Allele	Outcome
VKORC1	3673;G-1639A	GG (insensitive), GA (sensitive), AA (most sensitive)
GGCX	C>G	CC (less sensitve), CG (more sensitive), GG (most sensitive)
CALU	11G>A;R4Q	GG (less sensitive), GA (more sensitive), AA (most sensitive)
CYP4F2	C>T; V433M	CC (most sensitive), CT (more sensitive),TT (less sensitive)
CYP2C9	CYP2C9*2 ;R144C CYP2C9*3 ;I359L CYP2C9*5 CYP2C9*6	CC (*1/*1, wild type), CT (*1/*2, IM), TT (*2/*2, PM) AA (wild type), AC (-/*3, PM), CC(*3/*3, PM) CC (wild type), CG (-/*5, PM), GG (*5/*5, PM) AA (wild type), A-(-/*6, PM), --(*6/*6, PM)

Table 3. Genes and their alleles that affect warfarin therapy. Various CYP alleles are just examples. The complete list could be found on the following homepage: http://www.cypalleles.ki.se.

Two common CYP2C9 allozymes have only a fraction of the level of enzyme activity of the wild type allozyme CYP2C9*1: 12% for CYP2C9*2 and 5% for CYP2C9*3. Since VKORC1, CALU and GGCX genotype together with CYP2C9 and CYP4F2 genotype and factors such as age, body size may account just for 50-60% of the variability in warfarin dosing requirements, prothrombin time monitoring is still necessary during dose adjustment. But still, genotypization is recommended because of risk of side effects caused by the pharmacodinamic properties of warfarin (strong gene-dose relationship, strong dose-effect relationship and low therapeutic index). In 2010 the FDA revised the label on warfarin providing genotype-specific ranges of doses and suggesting that genotypes should be taken into consideration when the drug is prescribed (Wang et al., 2011; Takahashi et al., 1998).

Acenocoumarol. This drug is used in preference to warfarin in some countries, expecially in Europe. R-Acenocoumarol is metabolized by several enzymes and produces most of the effect. S-Acenocoumarol is metabolized almost exclusively by CYP2C9 and although active, it contributes comperativly little because of its fast metabolism. The presence of one CYP2C9*3 allele (PM) is associated with 20-30% lower acenocoumarol doses compared with wild type, whereas two alleles lead to very low dose requirements (1 mg/day instead of 2.5 mg/day) (Spreafico et al., 2002; Gardiner et al., 2006).

Phenprocoumaron. Phenprocoumaron exist as R and S-enantiomer and CYP2C9 is responsible for the elimination of the S form. This anticoagulant undergoes a large proportion of elimination via alternative pathways (e.g. renal and CYP3A4), so any relationship with the

CYP2C9 genotype may be less important than for warfarin or acenocoumarol (Toon et al., 1985).

Antiplatelet agents

Clopidogrel. Clopidogrel is an antiplatelet and it inhibits adenosine diphosphate (ADP)-stimulated platelet activation by binding irreversibily to a specific platelet receptor of ADP, P2Y 12, thus inhibiting platelet aggregation.

Absorption of clopidogrel in the gut is opposed by the efflux pump P-glycoprotein, encoded by the *ABCB1* gene. Once absorbed, approximately 85% of the drug is converted to an inactive metabolite by the action of esterases. The remaining 15% must undergo a two-step transformation process to become active. The first step produces 2-oxo-clopidogrel and is catalyzed in varying proportions by the cytochromes CYP2C19, CYP1A2 and CYP2B6. The second step, which produces the reactive metabolite, can be catalyzed by CYP3A4/5, CYP2B6, CYP2C19 or CYP2C9. Among so many enzymes only genetic variation in CYP2C19 and ABCB1 are associated with clopidogrel efficacy. As compared with subjects with no *CYP2C19* variant allele, subjects carrying one or two *CYP2C19* loss-of-function alleles have been shown to have lower plasma concentrations of the active metabolite of clopidogrel and a decrease in the antiplatelet effect of clopidogrel and an increased likelihood of cardiovascular event. In 2010, the FDA added a boxed warning to prescribing information for clopidogrel, stating that persons with a *CYP2C19* variant encoding a form of the enzyme associated with a low rate of metabolism might require dose adjustment or the use of a different drug (Simon et al., 2009; Ingelman-Sundberg et al., 2007).

Antiarrhythmics

Antiarrhythmia drugs are used to treat abnormal heart rhythms resulting from irregular electrical activity of the heart. Most antiarrhythmics are metabolized via CYP3A or CYP2D6 (Gardner et al., 2006).

Propafenone. Its ennatiomers have equal sodium channel blocking activity, but S-propafenone is 100-fold more potent as a β-blocker (Kroemer et al., 1989a). Propafenone is metabolised via CYP2D6 to 5-hydroxipropafenone, which has sodium channel blocking activity similar to that of the racemic parent drug but less ß-blockade and also by CYP1A2 and CYP3A4 to N-desalkylpropafenone (Kroemer at al., 1989b). Propafenone inhibits CYP2D6 strongly, with 70% phenocopying and R-propafenone inhibits the metabolism of the S-enantiomer. CYP2D6 status is generally thought to matter little for antiarrhythmic effect, but more for β-blockade and for side effects in central nervous system. Because of non linear pharmacokinetic and problems with active metabolites, enantiomers and phenocopying, it is hard to translate the proven gene-concentration ratio to clinically effective dose (Siddoway et al., 1987).

Flecainide. Flecainide is inactivated by renal elimination and in the liver by CYP2D6. Since the gene-effect relationships between CYP2D6 and flecainide seem minor, there is no need for clinical monitoring of this drug (Mikus et al., 1989).

Mexiletine. Mexiletine is a chiral, with the R-enantiomer having greater activity. It is metabolized to various metabolites by CYP2D6 and other enzymes. Due to CYP2D6, a minor gene-concentration effect seems to be present, but because of other elimination pathways it is not predictable for the dose (Labbe & Turgeon, 1999).

β-blockers

Beta-blockers reduce the effects of the sympathetic nervous system on the cardiovascular system. These drugs are effective against high blood pressure, congestive heart failure, abnormal heart rhythms or chest pain. Their pharmacokinetic is very diverse; those which are metabolised by polymorph CYP enzymes are carvedilol, metoprolol, propranolol and timolol.

Carvedilol. Beside other metabolic pathways, CYP2D6 metabolizes carvediol to its more potent ß-blocker metabolite 4-hydroxyphenylcarvedilol. Polymorphism of CYP2D6 does not affect significantly the overall effect of this drug (Oldham & Clark, 1997).

Metoprolol. Metoprolol is a ß1-selective blocker and is given as a racemate. Beside other pathways, metoprolol is under the control of CYP2D6. Metoprolol seems to have both consistent gene-concentration and gene-effect relationships in healthy volunteers, suggesting that dose reduction to 25% should occur in PMs or those phenocopied by other drugs (McGourty et al., 1985a).

Propranolol. Propranolol is metabolsed by CYP2D6, but CYP2D6 polymorphism contributes little to variation in plasma concentration of this drug (Lennard et al., 1984).

Timolol. Timolol is a non selective ß-blocker and is metabolised mainly by CYP2D6. Although the ß-blocking effect can occur with very low level of the drug, it is not necessary to genotype before determinating the dose of the drug (McGourty et al., 1985b).

Angiotensin II Blockers

CYP2C9 metabolizes several antihypertensive angiotensin II receptor antagonists, such as losartan, irbesartan, candesartan or valsartan. Although losartan and candesartan are activated, irbesartan is metabolised by CYP2C9, there is no need for genotyping of the enzyme variants during the treatment (Gardiner et al., 2006).

2.1.7 Metabolic disorders

Oral antidiabetics

CYP2C9 is the main enzyme catalyzing the biotransformation of sulphanylureas such as tolbutamide, glyburine, glimeprimide and glipizide. The total oral clearance of sulphanylureas has been shown to be 20% in PM persons of that in wild type, whereas the clearance in heterozygous carriers was between 50% and 80% of that of wild type genotype. Therefore, adverse effects of many oral antidiabetics may be reduced by CYP2C9 genotype-based dose adjustments (Gardiner et al., 2006).

2.1.8 Gastrointestinal disorders

Protone pump inhibitors

The PPIs undergo extensive hepatic biotransformation by the CYP system. The principal isoenzymes involved in the metabolism of the PPIs are CYP2C19 and CYP3A4 (Andersson et al., 1998; Pierce et al., 1996). CYP2C19 is the main enzyme involved in the metabolism of PPIs omeprazole, pantoprazole and lansoprazole and the CYP2C19 genotype is a strong determinant of the acid inhibitory effect of these drugs. Higher doses of the PPIs should be used in homozygous EMs (e.g. 40 mg), and lower doses could be used in heterozygous EMs and PMs (e.g. 10 mg).

Eradication therapy		Eradication rate (%)			Av. cure rate (%)
		EM	IM	PM	
Dual therapy	Omeprazole/Amoxicillin 20 mg 1x/500mg/two weeks 4x daily	30	60	100	63
	Omeprazole/Amoxicillin 40 mg 1x/2000mg/one week 4x daily	33	30	100	54
	Rabeprazole/Amoxicillin 10 mg 2x/500mg/two weeks 3x daily	60	92,2	92	80
Triple therapy	Omeprazole/Amoxicillin/Clarithromycin 40 mg 1x/1500mg/600 mg/one week 4x daily	81	94,5	100	92

Table 4. Dual and triple eradication therapy for H. pylori infection in relation to different CYP2C19 polymorphisms (Aoyama et al., 1999; Furuta et al., 2005).

Genotyping is also important in Helicobacter pylori eradication (Table 4.). If patients are confirmed as being PMs, dual therapy with PPI plus amoxicillin may be appropriate, as the eradication rate is likely to be high (>90%). This regimen has the advantage of being cheaper and less complex than triple therapy regimens. Individuals identified as homozygous EMs might be better to commence a triple drug regimen (PPI, amoxicillin and clarithromycin).

2.1.9 Infection

Antiretrovirals

Efavirenz. Efavirenz, a nonnucleoside reverse transcriptase inhibitor is an initial therapy during HIV infections. This drug is metabolised by CYP2B6 enzyme. In PMs for CYP2B6, efavirenz has been shown to be responsible for central nervous system side effects (sleep or mood disorders) and they also have increased risk for drug resistance (Rotger et al., 2005).

Nelfinavir. The protease inhibitor nelfinavir is metabolized mainly to nelfinavir hydroxy-t-butylamide by CYP2C9, which exhibits potent antiviral activity, and to other minor products by other CYPs that are inactive (Hirani et al., 2004). CYP2C9 polymorphism appears to have a clinical effect on nelfinovir, but the exact extent of the impact awaits additional clinical studies and confirmation. Nelfinavir is an inhibitor of CYP3A. Coadministration of nelfinavir and drugs primarily metabolized by CYP3A may result in increased plasma concentrations of the other drug that could increase or prolong both their therapeutic and adverse effects (Niemi et al., 2003; Fulco et al., 2008).

2.1.10 Rheumatoid arthritis

Nonsteroid antiinflamatory drugs (NSAID) are commonly used for rheumatoid arthritis treatment and many of them are metabolised by the CYP2C9 enzyme. The low activity alleles of CYP2C9 (CYP2C9*2, CYP2C9*3) has been shown to influence the pharmacokinetics of ibuprofen, naproxen, diclofenac and celecoxib (Kircheiner & Brockmoller, 2005). From these drugs, celexocib and ibuprofen have extensive CYP2C9 metabolism (Kircheiner et al., 2002; Lundblad et al., 2006). In PM patients for CYP2C9 these two drugs have 2-7 fold longer effects and stronger gastrointestinal side effects (Martin et al., 2001).

3. Pharmacoepigenetics

Much of the interindividual variation in drug response has been addressed by pharmacogenetics and it is imperative for clinicians to consider during determination drug efficacy and reducing side effects. But it is important to note that many inherited and acquired discrepancies cannot be resolved only by sequencing the whole genome and identifying genetic variations, there are other heritable factors affecting the activity of a gene such as covalent modification of DNA and histones, DNA packaging around nucleosomes, chromatin folding and attachment to the nuclear matrix or miRNA regulation. These changes together are called epigenetic changes and with true genetics they show how genes might interact with their surroundings to produce a phenotype. It means that beside genetic information, epigenetic factors have to be also taken into consideration during determinating variation in drug response. Beside individual variations, there could be a pharmacoepigenetic basis for other drug related effects, such as drug resistance (for e.g. doxorubicin resistance due to epigenetic regulation of ABCG2 transporter in cancer cells) (Calgano et al., 2008).

In the following section, an overview has been provided of new results in the field related to regulation by DNA methylation, histone modulation and miRNA, since they are topics of considerable current interest which may describe the large variation in expression seen for several important CYPs (Okino et al., 2006; Antilla et al., 2003; Dannenberg et al., 2006; Tamási et al., 2011).

3.1 Epigenetic regulation

DNA methylation. DNA methylation occurs predominantly at CpG sites in the mammalian genome by the DNA methyltransferase (DNMT) enzymes. The majority of CpG pairs are chemically modified by the covalent attachment of a methyl group to the C_5 position of the cytosine ring (Tate & Bird, 1993; Calcagno et al., 2008). Methylation of DNA is regarded as a means of regulating gene expression through two general mechanisms. First, DNA methylation of gene promoters may prevent the physical binding of some transcription factors to their DNA binding sites (Rountree et al., 2001). Second, the transcriptional silencing capability of DNA methylation may occur via indirect mechanisms involving changes in chromatin conformation. There is extensive evidence to support a functional role for promoter-CGI methylation in transcriptional repression (Weber et al., 2007; De Smet et al., 1999; Stein et al., 1982). DNA methylation of CpG-rich promoters of some genes correlates with tissue specific gene silencing (Futcher et al., 2002; Song et al., 2005). To date, several studies show altered DNA methylation of CYPs what could have importance in drug and endogen compound metabolism.

Histone modification. Posttranslational modifications such as phosphorylation, acetylation, methylation and ubiquitination on the N-termini of histones have been shown to play critical roles in gene regulation (Kouzarides, 2007). It is believed that the combination of modifications of the chromatin-associated histone and non-histone proteins, and the interplay between these modifications create a marking system ("histone code"), which is responsible for compact DNA (heterochromatin) or more opened, transcriptionally active (euchromatin) configuration, that allows transcription (Jenuwein & Allis, 2001).

miRNA regulation. miRNAs, another part of the epigenetic machinery, are single-stranded RNA molecules of 21-24 nucleotides in lenght that arise from miRNA genes, which when transcribed, can promote posttranscriptional regulation by binding to 3'-untranslated regions (3'UTRs) of target mRNAs promoting their degradation and cleavage as miRNA/RISC complex (RISC-RNA Induced Silencing Complex) or interfering with their translation. Besides their direct influence on mRNA transcription, some miRNAs, defined as epi-miRNAs, have an indirect impact on gene transcription by affecting the epigenetic machinery, including DNA methyltransferases, histone deacetylases and other mechanisms (Fabbri et al., 2010). Post-transcriptional regulation by miRNA could be responsible for a portion of the significant amount of unexplained interindividual variability in CYP enzyme expression and activity.

The modified histones, methylated DNA sequences and miRNAs may interact in a synergistic manner, including methyl-CpG binding protein, nuclear receptor corepressor (NCoR), associated histone deacetylases, histone methyl transferases and epi-miRNAs to regulate gene expression (Yoon et al., 2003). The mentioned epigenetic changes affect the expression of drug metabolizing enzymes and with that ultimately affect the pharmacokinetic or pharmacodinamic properties of a drug.

3.2 Epigenetic regulation of P450s

CYP1A1: CYP1A1 is mainly involved in the metabolic activation of polycyclic aromatic hydrocarbons, which are common enviromental pollutants. Important functional polymorphisms have been not described with this gene, but still there are several epigenetic processes which regulate CYP1A1.

Both hypermethylation (less active CYP1A1, slower metabolism of drugs) and hypomethylation (more active enzyme, higher metabolic rate) of CYP1A1 is described, mostly in cancer tissue. In prostate cells, CpG islands in CYP1A1 show segmented/selective methylation patterns: CpG sites from 1 to 36 are not methylated; this DNA region contains the *CYP1A1* promoter and is responsible for correct initiation of gene transcription; CpG sites 37 to 90, which corresponds to the *CYP1A1* enhancer region that mediates TCDD (2,3,7,8-Tetrachlorodibenzodioxin) inducibility, exhibits cancer cell-dependent hypermethylation and CpG sites 91 to 125 are commonly methylated, but known regulatory function has been not associated with this DNA region (Okino et al., 2006). Environmental factors, such as tobacco smoke have been shown to influence the DNA methylation of CYP1A1; smokers DNA were hypomethylated compared to non-smokers on the upstream regions, containing functional XREs. In addition, there was an inverse correlation between methylation and the number of cigarettes smoked daily. Cessation of smoking results in the methylation of CYP1A1 promoter being increased at 1–7 days after the last cigarette (Antilla et al., 2003). Although there was no correlation between ethoxyresorufin-O-deethylase (EROD) activity and the percentage of methylated DNA in a sample either in smokers or in nonsmokers, decrease in methylation caused significant higher CYP1A1 activity. A high inducibility of CYP1A1 has been connected with increased susceptibility to smoking-associated lung cancer (Kellermann et al., 1973; Stücker et al., 2000).

Chromatin structure has been suggested to play an essential role in *CYP1A1* transcription (Table 5). In the basal state, histone deacetylase 1 (HDAC1) is bound to the CYP1A1 promoter and is released in concert with the recruitment of p300 upon benz[a]pirene (B[a]P) ligand activation of the AHR. HDAC1 removal allows for several histone modification steps associated with the AHR-mediated induction of CYP1A1 expression. Removal of HDAC1 is necessary, but not sufficient to activate CYP1A1 expression (Schnekenburger et al., 2007).

miRNA regulation of CYP1A1 is also known. miRNA regulation by miRNA-18b and miRNA-20b of CYP1A1 was described by Wang and coworkers and a significant correlation was found between the mentioned miRNAs and CYP1A1 expression (Wang et al., 2009).

	Methylation		Histon modification		miRNA	
	CpG region	Compound/ disease	Modification	Compound/ disease	miRNA	Tissue/ cell
CYP1A1	Enchancer/ promoter	Cancer, tobacco smoke	Acetylation	B[a]P	Hsa-miR-18b, Hsa-miR-20b	Transformed lymphocytes
CYP1B1	Enchancer/ promoter	Cancer	-	-	Hsa-miR-27b	Cancer
					Hsa-miR-124	Brain
CYP2E1	Region not described	Ethanol	-	-	Hsa-miR-378	HEK293
CYP2W1	I.exon/ I.intron	Cancer	-	-	-	-
CYP3A	Enchancer/ promoter	Cancer	Methylation	Rifampicin	Hsa-miR-27b	HEK293
					Hsa-miR-148a	Liver

Table 5. Epigenetic regulation of drug metabolism related P450s ("-" no data).

CYP1B1: CYP1B1 activates various procarcinogens, metabolizes the antiestrogen tammoxifen, some flavonoids or benzpyrene derivatives. This enzyme is overexpressed in a variety of human tumor cells such as lung, breast, liver, gastrointestinal tract, and ovarian cancer (Murray et al., 1997). CYP1B1 may be an important tumor marker, because it hydroxylates estrogenes and activates many procarcinogenes. CYP1B1 enzyme could be methylated both on the promoter and on the enchancer of the gene. Promoter region contains the CpG sites of the core promoter region including SP1 binding sites and the enhancer region including AHR/ARNT (ARNT-Aromatic Hydrocarbone Receptor Nuclear Translocator) binding sites DRE2 and DRE3. Aberrant methylation in the CYP1B1 gene affects binding of transcription factors and enchancer molecules. Because expression of CYP1B1 is regulated by the methylation of its promoter/enhancer, this region may be a useful target for anticancer drugs and in preventive medicine (Tokizone et al., 2005).

Human CYP1B1, which is highly expressed in estrogen target tissues, catalyzes the 4-hydroxylation of 17-beta-estradiol. Tsuchiya and coworkers found an abundant amount of CYP1B1 protein in breast cancerous tissue and they identified a near-perfect matching sequence with miR-27b in the 3'-untranslated region of human CYP1B1. Human CYP1B1 is post-transcriptionally regulated by miR-27b (Tsuchya et al., 2006). Another brain-specific miRNA, miR-124, also downregulates CYP1B1 directly and modulate all AHR target genes indirectly by binding to AHR receptor (Lim et al., 2005).

CYP2E1: CYP2E1 is involved in the metabolism of various drugs, such as halothane, enflurane, theophylline or isoniazid. Methylation of the CYP2E1 gene inhibits the expression of this enzyme in prenatal period (Vieira et al., 1998). In adult tissues the methylation pattern of CYP2E1 gene differs among various tissue types such as lung, kidney, placenta, liver and skin indicating that DNA methylation results in tissue-specific regulation (Vieira et al., 1996). CYP2E1 is metabolizing ethanol to its carcinogenic metabolite acetaldehyde. Even small doses of ethanol are able to change the methylation pattern of CYP2E1 and with that, increase its transcription. Higher CYP2E1 activity could have importance in cancerogenesis, since CYP2E1 is involved in bioactivation of other small-molecule precarcinogens (Ghanayem et al., 2007).

Mohri and coworkers recently found that miR-378 is involved in the post-transcriptional regulation of CYP2E1. The overexpression of miR-378 significantly decreased CYP2E1 protein levels and enzyme activity in the cells expressing CYP2E1, including 3'-UTR, but not in the cells expressing CYP2E1 without 3'-UTR, indicating that the 3'-UTR plays a role in the miR-378-dependent repression (Mohri et al., 2010). Chronically induced CYP2E1 with ethanol or other CYP2E1 inducers is a high-risk factor for esophageal and gastrointestinal cancers, which gives importance to investigate transcriptional and post-transcriptional CYP2E1 regulatory mechanisms, as basic targets in anticancer therapy.

CYP2W1: This enzyme has been shown to metabolise arachidonic acid and benzfetamine, as well as being able to metabolically activate several procarcinogens, including polycyclic aromatic hydrocarbon dihydrodiols, aflatoxin B1 or sterigmatocystin. CYP2W1 is expressed at relatively low levels (mRNA) in the human adult non-transformed tissues whereas the expression in colorectal cancer tissues was significantly higher (both at mRNA and protein levels) (Li et al., 2009; Edler et al., 2009). CYP2W1 gene expression appears to be governed by gene methylation. The CYP2W1 gene was shown to contain one functional CpG island in the exon 1-intron 1 region which was methylated in cell lines lacking CYP2W1 expression, but unmethylated in cells expressing CYP2W1 (Karlgren et al., 2007; Gomez et al., 2007).

CYP3A: These enzymes metabolise almost 50% of currently used drugs as well as endogenous and exogenous corticosteroids. Although CYP3A enzymes are not polymorph enzymes interindividual variability is high due to epigenetic regulatory mechanisms.

Different DNA methylation pattern was found between primary hepatocytes and hepatocyte cell lines. HepG2 cells exhibit many cellular features of normal human hepatocytes, but also display characteristics resembling those of a cancerous or fetal hepatocyte. CYP3A expression in untreated HepG2 cells is fairly low, suggesting that their expression is reduced in these partially dedifferentiated cells. Dannenberg and coworkers were interested in determining whether CYP3A genes are regulated by DNA methylation in HepG2 cells. Their microarray experiments showed that after 5-aza-dC treatment (5-aza-2'-deoxycytidine, methylation inhibitor), expression of CYP3A4, CYP3A5 and CYP3A7 was 2-4-fold higher, suggesting the regulatory role of methylation with these CYPs (Dannenberg & Edenberg, 2006). Since CYP3A enzymes catalyse the transformation of many drugs, understanding their regulation would explain interindividual differences in drug response and would help to develop better personalized medicine.

CYP3A4 transcription is also regulated by a histone methyltransferase enzyme called protein arginine methyltransferase 1 (PRMT1). PRMT1 is required for the transcriptional activity of CYP3A4 by pregnane X receptor (PXR). It is recruited to 5'-region of the CYP3A4 gene to methylate histone H4 as a response to the PXR agonist rifampicin (Xie et al., 2009). CYP3A4 is also regulated by constitutive androstane receptor (CAR) albeit it at a lower rate of expression. Assenat and coworkers reported that the synthetic glucocorticoid, dexamethasone, induces histone H4 acetylation at the proximal CAR promoter region, and indirectly affects CYP3A4 induction by regulating CAR expression (Assenat et al., 2004).

Until now, one miRNA, miR-27b, has been described to regulate CYP3A4 expression by binding to the miRNA response element (MRE) within the 3'UTR region of CYP3A4 mRNA (Pan et al., 2009). Some miRNAs, such as miR-148a, which is selectively and abundantly expressed in the liver, regulates other liver specific genes, for e.g., the human PXR. miR-148a binds to the 3'-UTR region of PXR mRNA, thereby decreasing synthesis of PXR protein. Since CYP3A4 is a target for PXR, miR-148a indirectly modulates the inducible and/or constitutive levels of CYP3A4 expression (Takagi et al., 2008). Another example of indirect modulation would be the vitamine D receptor (VDR). VDR also regulates CYP3A4 and VDR could be down-regulated with miR-27b (Mohri et al., 2010).

4. Conclusion

Pharmacogenetics and pharmacoepigenetics is a scientific field which understands the role of an individual's genetic background in how well a medicine works, and also what side effects occur during drug administration. The development of pharmacogenetics/ pharmacoepigenetics (for benefits and limitations see Box 2.) provides at least one mechanism for taking prescription away from its current empiricism and progressing towards more "individualised" drug treatment.

Benefits:
- Development of drugs based on a patient's genetic/epigenetic profile will maximise therapeutic effects, but decrease ADRs and other toxic effects
- More precise dose is calculated, if beside other factors, genetic background also counts
- Revival of older drugs with retrospective studies

Limitations:
- Identification of genes that may influence drug metabolism is very difficult, since more genes are involved in how someone reacts to a drug and these changes are small
- The interactions with other drugs or environmental factors need to be determined before any conclusions are made about the genetic influence on how the drug is working

---

Box 2. Potential benefits and limitations of pharmacogenetics/pharmacoepigenetics.

The clinical applicability of pharmacogenetic testing depends on the relative importance of each polymorphism in determining therapeutic outcome. Doctors need to be aware of whether a drug they are prescribing is subject to pharmacogenetic variability and they have to know how to use this knowledge. Routine genotyping or phenotyping before drug administration can be made for very few drugs today and we are still a long way from having a pharmacogenetic DNA chip that general practitioners can use to identify all the drugs to which any particular patient is sensitive. There are many issues against testing, including specific factors that contaminate the signal, such as active metabolites/enantiomers, access and availability of the tests, complication for patients etc.

What have been changed as a result of pharmacogenetic knowledge until today is the drug-label modifications. There are more and more drug-labels where the pharmacogenetic consequence is highlighted (Table 6.). Drug labels may contain information on genomic biomarkers and can describe: drug exposure and clinical response variability, risk for adverse events, genotype-specific dosing, mechanisms of drug action, polymorphic drug target, disposition genes etc.

CYP enzymes	FDA-approved drugs with pharmacogenomic information in their labels
CYP2C9	Clopidogrel, Diazepam, Dextansoprazole, Drospirenone and Ethenyl Estradiol, Esomeprazole, Nelfinavir, Rabeprazole, Voriconazole
CYP2C19	Celexocib, Warfarin
CYP2D6	Aripiprazole, Atomoxetine, Carvedilol, Cevimeline, Clozapine, Codeine, Dextromethorphan and Quinidine, Doxepin, Fluoxetine, Fluoxetine and Olanzapine, Metoprolol, Propafenone, Propranolol, Protryptiline, Quinidine, Risperidone, Terbinafine, Tetrabenazine, Thioridazine, Timolol, Tiotropium, Tolterodine, Tramadol and Acetaminophen,Venlafaxine

Table 6. FDA-approved drugs with P450-related pharmacogenomic information in their labels (Taken from www.fda.gov, updated 2011, July).

Another result of pharmacogenetic knowledge is including pharmacogenomics into clinical trials. Carlquist and Anderson reported that this year until May, a total of 158 pharmacogenomic clinical trials were listed at http://www.clinicaltrials.gov. Of those trials the three leading disease areas for which pharmacogenetic guided intervention is sought were cancer (37%), psychiatric disorders (13%), and anticoagulation/thrombosis (9%) (Carlquist & Anderson, 2011).

In addition to pharmacogenetics, it has been also predicted that DNA methylation, histone modification and RNA-mediated regulation also affects gene expression. Until now, cancer is the only disease, where pharmacoepigenetics of drug metabolizing enzymes seems to be important. Epigenetic changes influence sensitivity to chemotherapeutic drugs suggesting that epigenetic factors could serve as molecular markers predicting the responsiveness of tumors and other diseases to therapy.

Ultimately, it could be concluded that pharmacogenetics and pharmacoepigenetics explains in large extent individual variation of drug metabolising enzymes and hopefully these two factors together will help to work out more specific dosing protocols for drugs.

5. References

Andersson, T.; Holmberg, J.; Rohss, K.; & Walan, A. (1998). Pharmacokinetics and effect on caffeine metabolism of the proton pump inhibitors, omeprazole, lansoprazole, and pantoprazole. *Br J Clin Pharmacol*, Vol. 45, pp. 369–375, ISSN 0306-5251

Andersson, T.; Miners, J.O.; Veronese, M.E. & Birkett, D.J. (1994). Diazepam metabolism by human liver microsomes is mediated by both S-mephenytoin hydroxylase and CYP3A isoforms. *Br J Clin Pharmacol*, Vol. 38, pp. 131–137, ISSN 0306-5251

Anttila, S.; Hakkola, J.; Tuominen, P.; Elovaara, E.; Husgafvel-Pursiainen, K.; Karjalainen, A.; Hirvonen, A. & Nurminen, T. (2003). Methylation of cytochrome P4501A1 promoter in the lung is associated with tobacco smoking. *Cancer Res*, Vol. 63, pp. 8623–8628, ISSN 0008-5472

Aoyama, N.; Tanigawara, Y.; Kita, T.; Sakai, T.; Shirakawa, K.; Shirasaka, D.; Kodama, F.; Okumura, K. & Kasuga, M. (1999). Sufficient effect of 1-week omeprazole and amoxicillin dual treatment for Helicobacter pylori eradication in cytochrome P450 2C19 poor metabolizers. *J Gastroenterol*, Vol. 34, pp. 80–83, ISSN 0944-1174

Assenat, E.; Gerbal-Chaloin, S.; Larrey, D.; Saric, J.; Fabre, J.M., Maurel, P.; Vilarem, M.J.; Pascussi, J.M. (2004). Interleukin 1beta inhibits CAR-induced expression of hepatic genes involved in drug and bilirubin clearance. *Hepatology*, Vol. 40, No. 4, pp. 951-60, ISSN 0169-5185

Berger, S.L.; Kouzarides, T.; Shiekhattar, R. & Shilatifard A. (2009). An operational definition of epigenetics. *Genes Dev*, Vol. 23, No. 7. pp. 781-3, ISSN 0890-9369

Bloomer, J.C.; Woods, F.R.; Haddock, R.E.; Lennard, M.S. & Tucker, G.T. (1992). The role of cytochrome P4502D6 in the metabolism of paroxetine by human liver microsomes. *Br J Clin Pharmacol*, Vol. 33, pp. 521–523, ISSN 0306-5251

Botto, F.; Seree, E.; el Khyari, S.; de Sousa, G.; Massacrier, A.; Placidi, M.; Cau, P.; Pellet, W.; Rahmani, R. & Barra, Y. (1994). Tissue-specific expression and methylation of the human CYP2E1 gene. *Biochem Pharmacol*, Vol. 48, No. 6, pp.1095-103, ISSN 0006-2952

Calcagno, A.M.; Fostel, J.M.; To, K.K., Salcido, C.D.; Martin, S.E., Chewning, K.J.; Wu, C.P.; Varticovski, L.; Bates, S.E.; Caplen, N.J. & Ambudkar, S.V. (2008). Single-step doxorubicin-selected cancer cells overexpress the ABCG2 drug transporter through epigenetic changes. *Br J Cancer*, Vol. 98, No. 9, pp.1515-1524, ISSN 0007-0920

Carlquist, J.F. & Anderson, J.L. (2011). Pharmacogenetic mechanisms underlying unanticipated drug responses. *Discov Med*, Vol. 11, No. 60, pp. 469-78, ISSN 1539-6509

Cooper, R.G.; Evans, D.A.P. & Whibley, E.J. (1984). Polymorphic hydroxylation of perhexiline maleate in man. *J Med Genet*, Vol. 21, pp. 27–33, ISSN 0022-2593

Daly, A.K. (2010). Pharmacogenetics and human genetic polymorphisms. *Biochem J*, Vol. 429, No. 3, pp. 435-49, ISSN 0264-6021

Dannenberg, L.O. & Edenberg, H.J. (2006). Epigenetics of gene expression in human hepatoma cells: expression profiling the response to inhibition of DNA methylation and histone deacetylation. *BMC Genomics*, Vol.19, No. 7, pp. 181, ISSN 1471-2164

Daigo, S.; Takahashi, Y.; Fujieda, M.; Ariyoshi, N.; Yamazaki, H.; Koizumi, W.; Tanabe, S.; Saigenji, K.; Nagayama, S.; Ikeda, K.; Nishioka, Y. & Kamataki, T. (2002). A novel mutant allele of the CYP2A6 gene (CYP2A6*11) found in a cancer patient who showed poor metabolic phenotype towards tegafur. Pharmacogenetics, Vol. 12, pp. 299–306, ISSN 0960-314X

De Smet, C.; Lurquin, C.; Lethe, B.; Martelange, V. & Boon, T. (1999). DNA methylation is the primary silencing mechanism for a set of germ line- and tumor-specific genes with a CpG-rich promoter. *Mol Cell Biol,* Vol. 19, No. 11, pp. 7327-7335, ISSN 0270-7306

Edler, D.; Stenstedt, K.; Ohrling, K.; Hallstrom, M.; Karlgren, M. & Ingelman-Sundberg, M. & Ragnhammar, P. (2009). The expression of the novel CYP2W1 enzyme is an independent prognostic factor in colorectal cancer - a pilot study. *Eur J Cancer,* Vol. 45, No. 4, pp. 705-712, ISSN 0014-2964

Eichelbaum, M.; Ingelman-Sundberg, M & Evans, W.E. (2006). Pharmacogenomics and individualized drug therapy. *Annu Rev Med,* Vol. 57, pp. 119-37, ISSN 0066-4219

Foster, A.; Wang, Z.; Usman, M.; Stirewalt, E. & Buckley, P. (2007). Pharmacogenetics of antipsychotic adverse effects: Case studies and a literature review for clinicians. *Neuropsychiatr Dis Treat,* Vol. 3, No. 6, pp. 965–973, ISSN 1176-6328

Fulco, P.P.; Zingone, M.M. & Higginson, R.T. (2008). Possible antiretroviral therapy-warfarin drug interaction. *Pharmacotherapy,* Vol. 28, No. 7, pp. 945-9, ISSN 0277-0008

Fuller, R.W.; Snoddy, H.D.; Krushinski, J.H. & Robertson, D.W. (1992). Comparison of norfluoxetine enantiomers as serotonin uptake inhibitors in vivo. *Neuropharmacology,* Vol. 31, pp. 997–1000, ISSN 0028-3908

Furuta, T.; Shirai, N.; Sugimoto, M.; Nakamura, A.; Hishida, A. & Ishizaki, T. (2005). Influence of CYP2C19 pharmacogenetic polymorphism on proton pump inhibitor-based therapies. *Drug Metab Pharmacokinet,* Vol. 20, No. 3, pp.153-67, ISSN 1347-4367

Futscher, B.W.; Oshiro, M.M.; Wozniak, R.J.; Holtan, N.; Hanigan, C.L.; Duan, H. & Domann, F.E. (2002). Role for DNA methylation in the control of cell type specific maspin expression. *Nat Genet,* Vol. 31, pp. 175–179, ISSN 1061-4036

Gardiner, S.J. & Begg, E.J. (2006). Pharmacogenetics, drug-metabolizing enzymes, and clinical practice. *Pharmacol Rev,* Vol. 58, No. 3, pp.521-90, ISSN 0031-6997

Gasche, Y.; Daali, Y.; Fathi, M.; Chiappe, A., Cottini, S., Dayer, P., Desmeules, J. (2004). Codeine intoxication associated with ultrarapid CYP2D6 metabolism. *N Engl J Med,* Vol. 351, pp. 2827–2831, ISSN 0028-4793

Ghanayem, B.I. & Hoffler, U. (2007). Investigation of xenobiotics metrabolism, genotoxicity and carcinogenicity using cyp2e1(-/-) mice. *Curr Drug Metab,* Vol. 8, pp. 728-749, ISSN 1389-2002

Gomez, A.; Karlgren, M.; Edler, D.; Bernal, M.L., Mkrtchian, S. & Ingelman-Sundberg, M. (2007). Expression of CYP2W1 in colon tumors: regulation by gene methylation. *Pharmacogenomics,* Vol. 8, No. 10, pp.1315-25, ISSN 1462-2416

Hirani, V.N.; Raucy, J.L. & Lasker, J.M. (2004) Conversion of the HIV protease inhibitor nelfinavir to a bioactive metabolite by human liver CYP2C19. *Drug Metab Dispos,* Vol. 32, No. 12, pp. 1462-7, ISSN 0090-9556

Ingelman-Sundberg, M. (2004a). Human drug metabolising cytochrome P450 enzymes: properties and polymorphisms. *Naunyn Schmiedebergs Arch. Pharmacol,* Vol. 369, pp. 89–104, ISSN 0003-9780

Ingelman-Sundberg, M. (2004b). Pharmacogenetics of cytochrome P450 and its applications in drug therapy: the past, present and future. *Trends Pharmacol Sci,* Vol. 25, No. 4, pp.193-200, ISSN 0165-6147

Ingelman-Sundberg, M.; Sim, S.C.; Gomez, A. & Rodriguez-Antona C. (2007). Influence of cytochrome P450 polymorphisms on drug therapies: pharmacogenetic, pharmacoepigenetic and clinical aspects. *Pharmacol Ther,* Vol. 116, No. 3, pp. 496-526, ISSN 0362-5486

Inomata, S.; Nagashima, A.; Itagaki, F.; Homma, M.; Nishimura, M.; Osaka, Y.; Okuyama, K.; Tanaka, E.; Nakamura, T.; Kohda, Y.; Naito, S.; Miyabe, M. & Toyooka, H. (2005). CYP2C19 genotype affects diazepam pharmacokinetics and emergence from general anesthesia. *Clin Pharmacol Ther,* Vol. 78, pp. 647–655, ISSN: 0009-9236

Jenuwein, T. & Allis, C.D. (2001). Translating the histone code. *Science,* Vol. 293, pp.1074-1080, ISSN 0193-3396

Jin, Y.; Desta, Z.; Stearns, V.; Ward, B.; Ho, H. ; Lee, K.H.; Skaar, T., Storniolo, A.M.; Li, L.; Araba, A.; Blanchard, R.; Nguyen, A.; Ullmer, L.; Hayden, J.; Lemler, S.; Weinshilboum, R.M.; Rae, J.M.; Hayes, D.F. & Flockhart, D.A. (2005). CYP2D6 genotype, antidepressant use, and tamoxifen metabolism during adjuvant breast cancer treatment. J Natl Cancer Inst, Vol. 97, pp. 30–39, ISSN 1052-6773

Jornil, J.; Jensen, K.G.; Larsen, F. & Linnet, K. (2010). Identification of cytochrome P450 isoforms involved in the metabolism of paroxetine and estimation of their importance for human paroxetine metabolism using a population-based simulator. *Drug Metab Dispos,* Vol. 38, No. 3, pp. 376-85, ISSN 0090-9556

Jung, F.; Richardson, T.H.; Raucy, R.L. & Johnson, E.F. (1997). Diazepam metabolism by cDNA-expressed human 2C P450s: identification of P4502C18 and P450 2C19 as low KM diazepam N-demethylases. *Drug Metab Dispos,* Vol. 25, pp. 133–139, ISSN: 0090-9556

Karlgren, M. & Ingelman-Sundberg, M. (2007). Tumour-specific expression of CYP2W1: its potential as a drug target in cancer therapy. *Expert Opin Ther Targets,* Vol. 11, No. 1, pp. 61-7, ISSN 1472-8222

Kellermann, G.; Shaw, C.R. & Luyten-Kellermann, M. (1973). Aryl hydrocarbon hydroxylase inducibility and bronchogenic carcinoma. *N Engl J Med,* Vol. 289, pp. 934-937, ISSN 0028-4793

Kirchheiner, J.; Meineke, I.; Freytag, G.; Meisel, C.; Roots, I. & Brockmoller, J. (2002). Enantiospecific effects of cytochrome P450 2C9 amino acid variants on ibuprofen pharmacokinetics and on the inhibition of cyclooxygenase 1 and 2. *Clin Pharmacol Ther,* Vol. 72, pp. 62–75, ISSN 0009-9236

Kircheiner, J. & Brockmoller, J. (2005). Clinical consequences of cytochrome P450 polymorphisms. *Clin Pharm Ther,* Vol. 77, pp. 1-16, ISSN 0009-9236

Kirchheiner, J.; Brøsen, K.; Dahl, M.L.; Gram, L.F.; Kasper, S.; Roots, I.; Sjöqvist, F.; Spina, E. & Brockmöller, J. (2001). CYP2D6 and CYP2C19 genotype-based dose recommendations for antidepressants: a first step towards subpopulation-specific dosages. *Acta Psychiatr Scand,* Vol. 104, No. 3, pp. 173-92, ISSN 0001-690X

Kirchheiner, J.; Nickchen, K.; Bauer, M.; Wong, M.L.; Licinio, J.; Roots, I. & Brockmöller, J. (2004). Pharmacogenetics of antidepressants and antipsychotics: the contribution of allelic variations to the phenotype of drug response. *Mol Psychiatry,* Vol. 9, No. 5, pp. 442-73, ISSN 1359-4184

Kosaki, K.; Tamura, K.; Sato, R.; Samejima, H.; Tanigawara, Y. & Takahashi, T. (2004). A major influence of CYP2C19 genotype on the steady-state concentration of N-desmethylclobazam. *Brain Dev,* Vol. 26, pp. 530-534, ISSN: 0387-7604

Kouzarides, T. (2007). Chromatin modifications and their function. *Cell,* Vol.128, pp.693-705, ISSN 0092-8674

Kroemer, H.K.; Funck-Brentano, C.; Silberstein, D.J.; Wood, A.J.J; Eichelbaum, M.; Woosley, R.L. & Roden, D.M. (1989a). Stereoselective disposition and pharmacologic activity of propafenone enantiomers. *Circulation,* Vol. 79, pp. 1068–1076, ISSN 0009-7322

Kroemer, H.K.; Mikus, G.; Kronbach, T.; Meyer, U.A. & Eichelbaum, M. (1989b). In vitro characterization of the human cytochrome P-450 involved in polymorphic oxidation of propafenone. *Clin Pharmacol Ther,* Vol. 45, pp. 28–33. ISSN 0009-9236

Labbe, L.; & Turgeon, J. (1999). Clinical pharmacokinetics of mexiletine. *Clin Pharmacokinet,* Vol. 37 pp. 361–384, ISSN 0312-5963

Laine, K.; Tybring, G.; Hartter, S.; Andersson, K.; Svensson, J.O.; Widen, J. & Bertilsson, L. (2001). Inhibition of cytochrome P4502D6 activity with paroxetine normalizes the ultrarapid metabolizer phenotype as measured by nortriptyline pharmacokinetics and the debrisoquin test. *Clin Pharmacol Ther,* Vol. 70, pp. 327–335, ISSN: 0009-9236

Lee, C.R.; Goldstein, J.A. & Pieper, J.A. (2002). Cytochrome P450 2C9 polymorphisms: a comprehensive review of the in-vitro and human data. *Pharmacogenetics,* Vol. 12, No. 3, pp. 251-63, ISSN 0960-314X

Lennard, M.S.; Jackson, P.R.; Freestone, S.; Ramsay, L.E.; Tucker, G.T. & Woods, H.F. (1984). The oral clearance and ß-adrenoceptor antagonist activity of propranolol after single dose are not related to debrisoquine oxidation phenotype. *Br J Clin Pharmacol,* Vol. 17, pp. 106S–107S, ISSN 0306-5251

Leppert W. (2011). CYP2D6 in the Metabolism of Opioids for Mild to Moderate Pain. *Pharmacology,* Vol. 87, No. 5-6, pp. 274-285, ISSN 0031-7012

Li, W.; Tang, Y.; Hoshino, T. & Neya, S. (2009). Molecular modeling of human cytochrome P450 2W1 and its interactions with substrates. *Mol Graph Model,* Vol. 28, No. 2, pp. 170-6, ISSN 1093-3263

Lim, L.P.; Lau, N.C.; Garrett-Engele, P.; Grimson, A.; Schelter, J.M.; Castle, J.; Bartel, D.P.; Linsley, P.S. & Johnson, J.M. (2005). Title microarray analysis shows that some microRNAs down regulate large numbers of target mRNAs. *Nature,* Vol. 433, No. 7027, pp.769–773, ISSN 0028-0836

Lundblad, M.S.; Ohlsson, S.; Johansson, P.; Lafolie, P. & Eliasson, E. (2006). Accumulation of celecoxib with a 7-fold higher drug exposure in individuals homozygous for CYP2C9*3. *Clin Pharmacol Ther,* Vol. 79, pp. 287–288, ISSN 0009-9236

Margolis, J.M.; O'Donnell, J.P.; Mankowski, D.C.; Ekins, S., & Obach, R.S. (2000). (R)-, (S)-, and racemic fluoxetine N-demethylation by human cytochrome P450 enzymes. *Drug Metab Dispos,* Vol. 28, pp. 1187–1191, ISSN 0090-9556

Martin, J.H.; Begg, E.J.; Kennedy, M.A.; Roberts, R. & Barclay, M.L. (2001). Is cytochrome P450 2C9 genotype associated with NSAID gastric ulceration? *Br J Clin Pharmacol,* Vol. 51, pp. 627–630, ISSN 0306-5251

McFadyen, M.C.; Breeman, S.; Payne, S.; Stirk, C.; Miller, I.D.; Melvin, W.T. & Murray, G.I. (1999). Immunohistochemical localization of cytochrome P450 CYP1B1 in breast cancer with monoclonal antibodies specific for CYP1B1. *J Histochem Cytochem,* Vol. 47, pp. 1457–64, ISSN 0022-1554

McGourty, J.C.; Silas, J.H.; Fleming, J.J.; McBurney, A. & Ward, J.W. (1985b). Pharmacokinetics and ß-blocking effects of timolol in poor and extensive metabolizers of debrisoquin. *Clin Pharmacol Ther,* Vol. 38, pp. 409–413, ISSN 0009-9236

McGourty, J.C.; Silas, J.H., Lennard, M.S.; Tucker, G.T. & Woods, H.F. (1985a). Metoprolol metabolism and debrisoquine metabolism — population and family studies. *Br J Clin Pharmacol*, Vol. 20, pp. 555–566, ISSN 0306-5251

Mikus, G.; Gross, A.S.; Beckmann, J.; Hertrampf, R.; Gundert-Remy, U. & Eichelbaum, M. (1989). The influence of the sparteine/debrisoquin phenotype on the disposition of flecainide. *Clin Pharmacol Ther*, Vol. 45, pp. 562–567, ISSN 0009-9236

Mohri, T.; Nakajima, M.; Fukami, T.; Takamiya, M.; Aoki, Y. & Yokoi, T. (2010). Human CYP2E1 is regulated by miR-378. *Biochem Pharmacol*, Vol. 79, No. 7, pp. 1045–1052, ISSN 0006-2952

Murray, G.I.; Taylor, M.C.; McFadyen, M.C.; MCMcKay, J.A.; Greenlee, W.F.; Burke, M.D. & Melvin, W.T. (1997). Tumor-specific expression of cytochrome P450 CYP1B1. *Cancer Res*, Vol. 57, pp. 3026–31, ISSN 0008-5472

Niemi, M.; Backman, J.T.; Fromm, M.F.; Neuvonen, P.J. & Kivistö, K.T. (2003). Pharmacokinetic interactions with rifampicin : clinical relevance. *Clin Pharmacokinet*, Vol. 42, No. 9, pp. 819-50, ISSN 0312-5963

Okino, S.T.; Pookot, D.; Li, L.C.; Zhao, H.; Urakami, S.; Shiina, H. & Dahiya, R. (2006). Epigenetic inactivation of the dioxin-responsive cytochrome P4501A1 gene in human prostate cancer. *Cancer Res*, Vol. 66, pp. 7420–7428, ISSN 0008-5472

Oldham, H.G. & Clarke, S.E. (1997). In vitro identification of the human cytochrome P450 enzymes involved in the metabolism of R(_)- and S(_)-carvedilol. *Drug Metab Dispos*, Vol. 25 pp. 970–977, ISSN 0090-9556

Pan, Y. Z.; Gao, W. & Yu, A.M. (2009). MicroRNAs regulate CYP3A4 expression via direct, indirect targeting. *Drug Metab Dispos*, Vol. 37, No. 10, pp. 2112–2117, ISSN 0090-9556

Pearce, R.E.; Rodrigues, A.D.; Goldstein, J.A. & Parkinson, A. (1996). Identification of the human P450 enzymes involved in lansoprazole metabolism. *J Pharmacol Exp Ther*, Vol. 277, pp. 805–816, ISSN 0022-3565

Rodriguez-Antona, C.; Gomez, A.; Karlgren, M.; Sim, S.C. & Ingelman-Sundberg, M. (2010). Molecular genetics and epigenetics of the cytochrome P450 gene family and its relevance for cancer risk and treatment. *Hum Genet*, Vol. 127, No. 1, pp. 1-17, ISSN 0340-6717

Rotger, M.; Colombo, S.; Furrer, H.; Bleiber, G.; Buclin, T.; Lee, B.L.; Keiser, O.; Biollaz, J.; Decosterd, L.A. & Telenti, A. (2005). Influence of CYP2B6 polymorphism on plasma and intracellular concentrations and toxicity of efavirenz and nevirapine in HIV infected patients. *Pharmacogenet Genomics*, Vol. 15, pp. 1–5. ISSN 1744-6872

Rountree, M.R.; Bachman, K.E.; Herman, J.G. & Baylin, S.B. (2001). DNA methylation, chromatin inheritance and cancer. *Oncogene*, Vol. 20, pp. 3156–3165, ISSN 0950-9232

Schnekenburger, M.; Peng, L. & Puga, A. (2007). HDAC1 bound to the Cyp1a1 promoter blocks histone acetylation associated with Ah receptor-mediated trans-activation. *Biochim Biophys Acta*, Vol. 1769, No. 9-10, pp. 569-78, ISSN 0006-3002

Simon, T.; Verstuyft, C.; Mary-Krause, M.; Quteineh, L.; Drouet, E.; Méneveau, N.; Steg, P.G.; Ferrières, J.; Danchin, N. & Becquemont, L. (2009). French Registry of Acute ST-Elevation and Non-ST-Elevation Myocardial Infarction (FAST-MI) Investigators. Genetic determinants of response to clopidogrel and cardiovascular events. *N Engl J Med*, Vol. 360, No. 4, pp. 363-75, ISSN 0028-4793

Siddoway, L.A.; Thompson, K.A.; McAllister, C.B.; Wang, T.; Wilkinson, G.R.; Roden, D.M. & Woosley, R.L. (1987). Polymorphism of propafenone metabolism and disposition in man: clinical and pharmacokinetic consequences. *Circulation,* Vol. 75, pp. 785–791, ISSN 0009-7322

Song, F.; Smith, J.F.; Kimura, M.T.; Morrow, A.D.; Matsuyama, T.; Nagase, H.& Held, W.A. (2005). Association of tissue-specific differentially methylated regions (TDMs) with differential gene expression. *Proc Natl Acad Sci USA,* Vol. 102, pp. 3336–3341, ISSN 0027-8424

Spear, B.B.; Heath-Chiozzi, M. & Huff, J. (2001). Clinical application of pharmacogenetics. *Trends Mol Med,* Vol. 7, pp. 201–204, ISSN 1471-4914

Spreafico, M.; Peyvandi, F.; Pizzotti, D.; Moia, M.; & Mannucci, P.M. (2002). Warfarin and acenocoumarol dose requirements according to CYP2C9 genotyping in North-Italian patients. *J Thromb Haemost,* Vol. 1, pp. 2252–2253, ISSN 1538-7933

Stein, R.; Razin, A. & Cedar, H. (1982). In vitro methylation of the hamster adenine phosphoribosyltransferase gene inhibits its expression in mouse L cells. *Proc Natl Acad Sci USA,* Vol. 79, pp. 3418–3422, ISSN 0027-8424

Stücker, I.; Jacquet, M.; de Waziers, I.; Cénée, S.; Beaune, P.; Kremers, P.; Hémon, D. (2000). Relation between inducibility of CYP1A1, GSTM1 and lung cancer in a French population. *Pharmacogenetics,* Vol. 10, pp. 617-627, ISSN 0960-314X

Takada, K.; Arefayene, M.; Desta, Z.; Yarboro, C.H.; Boumpas, D.T.; Balow J.E. Flockhart D.A., Illei, G.G. (2004). Cytochrome P450 pharmacogenetics as a predictor of toxicity and clinical response to pulse cyclophosphamide in lupus nephritis. Arthritis Rheum, Vol. 50, pp. 2202–2210, ISSN 0004-3591

Takahashi, H.; Kashima, T.; Nomoto, S.; Iwade, K.; Tainaka, H.; Shimizu, T.; Nomizo, Y.; Muramoto, N.; Kimura, S. & Echizen H. (1998). Comparisons between in-vitro and in-vivo metabolism of (S)-warfarin: catalytic activities of cDNA-expressed CYP2C9, its Leu359 variant and their mixture versus unbound clearance in patients with the corresponding CYP2C9 genotypes. *Pharmacogenetics,* Vol. 8, pp. 365–373, ISSN 0960-314X

Takagi, S.; Nakajima, M.; Mohri, T. & Yokoi, T. (2008). Post-transcriptional regulation of human pregnane X receptor by micro- RNA affects the expression of cytochrome P450 3A4. *J Biol Chem,* Vol. 283, No. 15, pp. 9674–9680, ISSN 0021-9258

Tamási, V.; Monostory, K.; Prough, R.A. & Falus, A. (2011) Role of xenobiotic metabolism in cancer: involvement of transcriptional and miRNA regulation of P450s. *Cell Mol Life Sci.* Vol. 68, No. 7, pp.1131-46, ISSN 1420-682X

Tamási, V.;Vereczkey, L.; Falus, A. & Monostory, K. (2003). Some aspects of interindividual variations in the metabolism of xenobiotics. *Inflamm Res,* Vol. 52, No. 8, pp. 322-33, ISSN 1023-3830

Tanigawara, Y.; Aoyama, N.; Kita, T.; Shirakawa, K.; Komada, F.; Kasuga, M. & Okumura, K. (1999). CYP2C19 genotype-related efficacy of omeprazole for the treatment of infection called by Helicobacter pylori. *Clin Pharmacol Ther,* Vol. 66, pp. 528–534, ISSN 0009-9236

Tate, P.H. & Bird, A.P. (1993). Effects of DNA methylation on DNA-binding proteins and gene expression. *Curr Opin Genet Dev,* Vol. 3, pp. 226–231, ISSN 0959-437X

Tokizane, T.; Shiina, H.; Igawa, M.; Enokida, H.; Urakami, S.; Kawakami, T.; Ogishima, T.; Okino, S.T.; Li, L.C.; Tanaka, Y.; Nonomura, N.; Okuyama, A. & Dahiya, R. (2005).

Cytochrome P450 1B1 is overexpressed and regulated by hypomethylation in prostate cancer. *Clin Cancer Res,* Vol. 11, pp. 5793–5801, ISSN 1078-0432

Toon, S.; Heimark, L.D.; Trager, W.F. & O'Reilly, R.A. (1985). Metabolic fate of phenprocoumon in humans. *J Pharm Sci,* Vol. 74, pp. 1037–1040, ISSN 0022-3549

Tsuchiya, Y.; Nakajima, M.; Takagi, S.; Taniya, T & Yokoi, T. (2006). MicroRNA regulates the expression of human cytochrome P450 1B1. *Cancer Res,* Vol. 66, No. 18, pp. 9090–9098, ISSN 0008-5472

Vangsted, A.J., Søeby, K., Klausen, T.W., Abildgaard, N., Andersen, N.F., Gimsing, P., Gregersen, H., Vogel, U., Werge, T. & Rasmussen, H.B. (2010). No influence of the polymorphisms CYP2C19 and CYP2D6 on the efficacy of cyclophosphamide, thalidomide, and bortezomib in patients with Multiple Myeloma. *BMC Cancer,* Vol. 4, No.10, pp. 40-4, ISSN 1471-2407

Varmus, H. (2010). Ten years on--the human genome and medicine. *N Engl J Med,* Vol. 362, No. 21, pp. 2028-9, ISSN 0028-4793

Vieira, I.; Pasanen, M.; Raunio, H. & Cresteil, T. (1998). Expression of CYP2E1 in human lung and kidney during development and in full-term placenta: a differential methylation of the gene is involved in the regulation process. *Pharmacol Toxicol,* Vol. 83, No. 5, pp. 183-7, ISSN 0901-9928

Vieira, I.; Sonnier, M. & Cresteil, T. (1996). Developmental expression of CYP2E1 in the human liver. Hypermethylation control of gene expression during the neonatal period. *Eur J Biochem,* Vol. 238, No. 2, pp. 476-83, ISSN 0014-2956

Wang, L., McLeod, H.L. & Weinshilboum, R.M. (2011). Genomics and drug response. *N Engl J Med,* Vol. 364, No. 12, pp. 1144-53, ISSN 0028-4793

Wang, L.; Oberg, A.L.; Asmann, Y.W.; Sicotte, H.; McDonnell, S.K.; Riska, S.M.; Liu, W.; Steer, C.J.; Subramanian, S.; Cunningham, J.M.; Cerhan, J.R. & Thibodeau, S.N. (2009). Genome-wide transcriptional profiling reveals microRNA-correlated genes and biological processes in human lymphoblastoid cell lines. *PLoS One,* Vol. 4, No. 6, e. 5878, ISSN 1932-6203

Weber, M.; Hellmann, I.; Stadler, M.B.; Ramos, L.; Paabo, S; Rebhan, M. & Schubeler, D. (2007) Distribution, silencing potential and evolutionary impact of promoter DNA methylation in the human genome. *Nat Genet,* Vol. 39, pp. 457–466, ISSN 1061-4036

Weinshilboum, R. (2003). Inheritance and drug response. *New Engl J Med* Vol. 348, pp. 529–537, ISSN 0028-4793

Wolf, C.R. & Smith, G. (1999). Pharmacogenetics. *Br Med Bull,* Vol. 55, No. 2, pp. 366-86, ISSN 0007-1420

Xie, Y.; Ke, S.; Ouyang, N.; He, J.; Xie, W.; Bedford, M.T. & Tian, Y. (2009). Epigenetic regulation of transcriptional activity of pregnane X receptor by protein arginine methyltransferase 1. *J Biol Chem,* Vol. 284, No. 14, pp. 9199-205, ISSN 0021-9258

Yoon, H.G.; Chan, D.W.; Reynolds, A.B.; Qin, J. & Wong, J. (2003). N-CoR mediates DNA methylation-dependent repression through a methyl CpG binding protein Kaiso. *Mol Cell,* Vol. 12, pp. 723-734, ISSN 1097-2765

7

Transcription Factors Potentially Involved in Regulation of Cytochrome P450 Gene Expression

Piotr Czekaj and Rafał Skowronek

Department of Histology, Medical University of Silesia in Katowice,
Poland

1. Introduction

Drug-metabolizing enzymes, including the cytochrome P450 (CYP) superfamily of enzymes, are subject to regulation by both exo- and endogenous factors, mostly hormones and cytokines (Monostory et al., 2009; Waxman & Chang, 2005). In this regulation transcription factors are the mediators. Among them, orphan nuclear receptors: CAR (*Constitutive Androstane Receptor*), PXR (*Pregnane X Receptor*), VDR (*Vitamin D Receptor*), FXR (*Farnesoid X Receptor*), LXR (*Liver X Receptor*), PPARα (*Peroxisome Proliferator-Activated Receptor α*) and RXR (*Retinoid X Receptor*) are the most important. They can create heterodimers in any configuration what, in conjunction with a broad spectrum of attached ligands, reflects the complexity of regulatory networks (Honkakoski & Negishi, 2000; Xu et al., 2005). Expression of some CYP isoforms is dependent on gender, which partly explains the metabolic difference between men and women in pharmacokinetics of drugs or, for instance, in susceptibility to carcinogens (Scandlyn et al., 2008). The main role in the sex-dependent regulation of CYP expression plays the growth hormone (GH) and to a lesser extent – other hormones. In principle, there are significant differences between genders in the daily profile of GH secretion into the bloodstream (Waxman & Chang, 2005). GH activates signaling pathway JAK-STAT (Lobie & Waxman, 2003). The main regulator of hepatic gene expression dependent on GH is transcription factor STAT5b which, together with other co-regulators (i.e. HNF-4α) can stimulate CYP genes directly by the binding to promoter sequences of target genes or indirectly by the activation of gene expressions of the gender-specific transcription factors (Park et al., 2006). As a result, in transactivation of cytochrome P450 genes, we can distinguish at least two pathways: (1) metabolic, dependent on the type of xeno- or endobiotic, mediated by several nuclear receptors and (2) signaling, associated with activation of numerous GH-dependent transcription factors. Therefore, some endocrine disorders may cause changes in the drug metabolism, as well as in the CYP-dependent metabolism of endogenous substrates.

2. Regulation of cytochrome P450 gene expression by the nuclear receptors

Cytoplasmic and nuclear receptors participate in the regulation of cytochrome P450 genes expression (table 1). Best known is the aryl hydrocarbon receptor (AhR), which being inactive in the cytosol remains associated with several co-chaperones: Hsp90 (*Heat shock protein-90*), XAP2 (*Hepatitis B virus X-associated Protein* 2) and the co-chaperone p23, regulating ligand-dependent nuclear import and protecting AhR from ubiquitination and further proteolysis (Monostory et al., 2009). Upon ligand binding to AhR, the cytosolic complex with chaperones dissociate, allowing the receptor phosphorylation by stimulated tyrosine kinase and translocation of AhR/ligand complex to the nucleus. In the nucleus, binding with ARNT (*AhR Nuclear Translocator*) protein into the heterodimer and interaction of the activated AhR/ARNT complex with the respective XRE (*Xenobiotic Response Element*) sequences located in the CYP genes, takes place (Honkakoski & Negishi, 2000; Monostory et al., 2009).

Nuclear receptors: CAR, PXR, RXR, VDR, FXR, LXR and PPARα participate in the complex regulation of CYP gene transcription, as transcription factors activated by ligand. Frequently they are activated in the cytoplasm and then translocated to the nucleus, where they form a heterodimer with RXR. These receptors are third class of nuclear hormone receptors, called xenoreceptors (XR) or xenosensors (Xu et al., 2005).

CAR binds to RXR into the heterodimer, which after binding to coactivators, interacts with the relevant regulatory sequences of target genes, mostly with the module sensitive to retinoic acid - RARE (*Retinoic Acid Response Element*). In the case of phenobarbital induction the formed heterodimer binds to the NR1 sequence (*Nuclear Receptor binding site 1*) being a part of PBRU (*Phenobarbital-Responsive enhancer Unit*) - multicomponent enhancer necessary to run the phenobarbital-dependent gene expression. In turn, the binding of CAR with natural ligand causes a loss of its activity (Czekaj, 2000).

PXR participates in the response to the numerous and structurally diverse xenobiotics. Dimeric complex PXR/RXR interacts with AGTTCA sequence in CYP3A1/2 genes separated by a trinucleotide spacer (DR3, *Direct Repeat-3*), and with XREM (*Xenobiotic-Response Enhancer Module*) and ER6 (*Everted Repeat with a 6-nucleotide spacer*) in the CYP3A4 gene. PXR gene polymorphism is probably one of the reasons for varied response to pharmacotherapy and the incidence of side effects in the population (Lamba & Schuetz, 2009).

VDR heterodimerizes with RXR and the formed complex can bind sequences of human CYP3A4 gene: pER6 (*proximal Everted Repeat with a 6-nucleotide spacer*) and dXREM (*distal Xenobiotic-Responsive Enhancer Module*), increasing its expression (K. Wang et al., 2008). Through the influence on CYP3A4 - the main enzyme metabolizing drugs in the intestine - VDR is a potential modulator of first-pass effect in the gastrointestinal tract. Moreover, it can be stimulated by bile acids and interact with FXR, as calcitriol inhibits transactivation of genes regulated by this receptor. VDR can form complexes with p65 subunit of NFκB factor (*Nuclear Factor kappa-light-chain-enhancer of activated B cells*) and thereby inhibit gene expression of proinflammatory proteins (Levi, 2011).

FXR regulates the expression of genes as a FXR/FXR homodimer or FXR/RXR heterodimer. FXR, through the CYP3A11 gene induction, CYP7A1 gene repression, and induction of expression of ileal bile acid binding protein (IBABP), inhibits the biosynthesis of bile acids and increases their transport from the intestine to the liver. High content of FXR in tissues associated with enterohepatic circulation makes it a regulator of drug distribution in the body (Gnerre et al., 2004; X. Wang et al., 2009).

Receptor		Natural ligands	Synthetic ligands	Response elements in CYP gene promoters (target sequence, spacer' orientation and length)	Cytochrome P450 genes regulated by receptor	Receptor-dependent function	References
Abbreviation (NRRNC symbol)	Full name (year of description)						
AhR	Aryl hydrocarbon Receptor (1992)	Tryptophan derivatives, bilirubin, metabolites of arachidonic acid, e.g.: prostaglandin G and lipoxin A4, carotenoids	Polycyclic and halogenated aromatic hydrocarbons	AHRE, DRE, XRE (*GCGTG*)	Human: *CYP1A1, CYP1A2, CYP1B1* Rat: *CYP1A1, CYP1A2, CYP1B1*	Xenobiotic metabolism, cell proliferation and differentiation	(Cui et al., 2009; Honkakoski & Negishi, 2000)
CAR (NR1I3)	Constitutive Androstane Receptor (1994)	Metabolites of 3α,5α-androstane: androstanol and androstenol (reverse agonists), DHEA	Phenobarbital, CITCO, TCPOBOP	CARE, RARE, PBRU (*AGGTCA*; DR3, DR4, DR5, ER6, ER8)	Human: *CYP2B6, CYP2C9, CYP2C19, CYP3A4, CYP3A5, CYP4A* Rat: *CYP2B1, CYP2B2*	Xenobiotic metabolism, regulation of lipid and energy metabolism, bile acid metabolism, heme synthesis, cholestasis, tumor promotion, hepatotoxicity	(Chen et al. 2010; Phillips et al., 2007; Xu et al, 2005)
PXR/SXR (NR1I2)	Pregnane X Receptor (rodent)/Steroid and Xenobiotic Receptor (human) (1998)	21-carbon steroids, so-called pregnans, e.g.: pregnenolone; progesterone, corticosteroids, estrogens, DHEA	Numerous xenobiotics, e.g.: phenobarbital, rifampicin, dexamethasone	XREM (*AGTTCA*; DR3, DR4, ER6, ER8, IR0)	Human: *CYP1A, CYP1B, CYP2A, CYP2B6, CYP2C8, CYP2C9, CYP2C19, CYP3A4, CYP3A5, CYP3A7, CYP4F* Rat: *CYP3A1, CYP3A2, CYP3A9, CYP3A18, CYP3A23*	Xenobiotic metabolism, regulation of lipid and bile acid metabolism, cholestasis, heme synthesis	(Honkakoski & Negishi, 2000; Takagi et al., 2008; Xu et al, 2005)
VDR (NR1I1)	Vitamin D Receptor (1988)	1,25 dihydroxyvitamin D3 - 1,25(OH)2D3, lithocholic acid, curcumin, polyunsaturated fatty acids,	Doxercalciferol, paricalcitol	VDRE, dXREM (*PuG(G/T)TCA*; DR3, DR4, DR5, DR6, pER6)	Human: *CYP2B6, CYP2C9, CYP3A4, CYP24, CYP27B1* Rat: *CYP24A1, CYP27A1, CYP27B1*	Calcium homeostasis, cell proliferation and differentiation, immunological response	(Honkakoski & Negishi, 2000; Levi, 2011; K. Wang et al., 2008; Zhang et al., 2010)

Table 1. Important receptors regulating cytochrome P450 expressions.

Receptor		Natural ligands	Synthetic ligands	Response elements in CYP gene promoters (target sequence, spacer orientation and length)	Cytochrome P450 genes regulated by receptors	Receptor-dependent function	References
Abbreviation (NRNC symbol)	Full name (year of description)						
FXR (NR1H4)	Farnesoid X Receptor/Bile Acids Receptor (1995)	Bile acids, e.g.: chenodeoxycholic acid	Farnesol, GW4064, INT-747	FXRE (*AGTTCAnTGAACT*; DR4, ER8, IR1, IR0)	Human: *CYP3A4, CYP7A1, CYP8B1* Rat: *CYP7A1*	Bile acid metabolism, regulation of lipid and carbohydrate metabolism	(Gnerre et al., 2004; Kemper et al., 2009; Thomas et al., 2008)
LXRα (NR1H3)	Liver X Receptor-α (1995)	Endogenous oxysterols: 22(R) and 24(S)-hydroxycholesterole, 24(S)-epoxycholesterole and 7 α-hydroxycholesterole	GW3965, DMHCA	LXRE (*AGTTCA*; DR4)	Human: *CYP7A1* Rat: *CYP7A1, CYP46A1, CYP51A1*	Cholesterol and bile acid metabolism	(Honkakoski & Negishi, 2000; Levi, 2011; Thomas et al., 2008; Wagner et al., 2011)
PPARα (NR1C1)	Peroxisome Proliferator-Activated Receptor-α (1990)	Polyunsaturated fatty acids and PFA derivatives: prostaglandins, eicosanoids and leukotrienes, DHEA	Fibrates, e.g.: fenofibrate, bezafibrate, clofibrate	PPRE (*AGGTCA*; DR1, DR2)	Human: *CYP1A, CYP2A, CYP2C, CYP2E, CYP4A, CYP7A1, CYP8B1, CYP27* Rat: *CYP4A1*	Cholesterol and bile acid metabolism, regulation of carbohydrate metabolism and inflammation	(Li & Chiang, 2009; Paumelle & Staels, 2007; Rigamonti et al., 2008; Zheng et al., 2010)
RARα (NR1B1)	Retinoic Acid Receptor-α (1987)	Vitamin A derivatives: all-trans (atRa) and 9-cis (9cRA) retinoic acid isomers, and other retinoids	Am 580, CD367	RARE (*PuG(G/T)TCA*; IP-8, DR1, DR2, DR5)	Human: *CYP26A1* Rat: *CYP1A, CYP2C7, CYP26*	Cell proliferation and differentiation, morphogenesis	(Alvarez et al., 2011; Honkakoski & Negishi, 2000)
RXRα (NR2B1)	Retinoid X Receptor-α (1990)	Vitamin A derivative: 9-cis (9cRA) retinoic acid isomer and other rexinoids, eicosanoids, phytanic acid	Methoprene, LGD1069, LG100268	RXRE (*AGGTCA*; DR1, DR2, DR3, DR4, DR5, IR0)	Genes dependent on nuclear receptors heterodimerizing with RXR	Cell proliferation, processes dependent on nuclear receptors heterodimerizing with RXR	(Chen et al. 2010; Perez et al., 2011; K. Wang et al., 2008; Xu et al., 2005)

Table 1. Important receptors regulating cytochrome P450 expressions (*Continuation*).

LXR, after joining the ligand, heterodimerization with RXR and binding of the complex with the promoter of CYP7 gene coding element of steroid 7α-hydroxylase, acts as a 'sensor' of cholesterol concentration, by stimulating its removal from the liver. Lack of LXR inhibits conversion of cholesterol into bile acids (Thomas et al., 2008; Wagner et al., 2011).

PPARα is most commonly associated with the mechanism of CYP4 gene family expression (Li & Chiang, 2009). After binding to ligand and heterodimerization with RXR, FXR, or LXR joins a PPRE (*Peroxisome Proliferator Response Element*) sequence, located in the promoter of target genes. PPARα is currently the subject of numerous pharmacological and pharmaceutical studies, as it is the target or it modulates the activity of many groups of commonly used hypolipemic and antidiabetic drugs: fibrates, glitazones and statins (Paumelle & Staels, 2007).

RXR, through the creation of numerous heterodimers, has a co-regulatory function as a nuclear auxiliary protein (NAP). There are two types of RXR heterodimers: a 'permissive', such as PPAR/RXR, LXR/RXR, FXR/RXR, activated freely by RXR ligands or his partner's ligands; and the 'nonpermissive' type, such as RAR/RXR, VDR/RXR and T₃R/RXR dimers, where only the ligands of bound orphan proteins are the activator (Xu et al., 2005). The fact that the receptors CAR, PXR, VDR, FXR, LXR and PPAR form heterodimers in any configuration with the same RXR protein related to the metabolism of endobiotics, makes him a 'connector' of various metabolic pathways in the body (the phenomenon of interference – 'cross-talk ') and gives a picture of a complex regulatory network.

Currently, intensively investigated are epigenetic modifications of cytoplasmic and nuclear receptors, which include DNA methylation, modifications of histones and regulation by microRNA (Klaassen et al., 2011). AhR is under the epigenetic regulation consisting of hypermethylation of promoter region of AhR gene (Cui et al., 2009). Such regulation occurs in acute lymphoblastic leukemia and impairs binding of the transcription factor Sp1 to the AhR promoter and, as a result, the initiation of transcription (Mulero-Navarro et al., 2006). In mouse models of obesity and diabetes type II increased acetylation of FXR protein can be observed (Kemper et al., 2009). MicroRNA (miRNA) may regulate signaling pathways of nuclear receptors on three levels, through direct interaction with 3'UTR mRNA sequence of: nuclear receptor, and/or co-regulators, or target genes (Pandey & Picard, 2009). It has been proven that the miR-148a causes post-transcriptional down regulation of PXR, which results in a lower induction of CYP3A4. Therefore, the levels of PXR mRNA and protein did not correlate with each other in normal human liver (Takagi et al., 2008). In the studies on the CAR receptor it has been shown that in precancerous, phenobarbital-induced lesions in the wild-type mice, disorders of gene methylation are present, in contrast to mice with silenced gene CAR (Philips et al., 2007). More and more evidences indicate the regulation of PPARα by miR-10b, depending on binding site in the 3'UTR sequence. miR-10b may be a new player in the pathogenesis of non-alcoholic fatty liver disease (NAFLD) and a new target for drugs in the treatment of this disease (Zheng et al., 2010). It has also been shown that expression of VDR, stimulated by ligand attachment - $1,25(OH)_2D_3$, is inhibited by miR-125b, miR-27b and mmu-miR- 298 (Mohri et al., 2009; Pan et al., 2009).

3. Regulation of cytochrome P450 gene expression dependent on the growth hormone

3.1 Growth hormone and the transduction of its signal

The main role in the sex-dependent regulation of CYP expression plays the growth hormone (GH) and to a lesser extent – other hormones. Growth hormone, also called somatotropic hormone (STH), is a 21.5 kDa protein secreted into the blood by acidic somatotrophs of the anterior pituitary. The release of this hormone is regulated by hypothalamic peptides, which means it is stimulated by somatotropin – GHRH (*Growth Hormone-Releasing Hormone*) and inhibited by somatostatin – GHIH (*Growth Hormone-Inhibiting Hormone; SST*). It is also regulated by other hormones and neurotransmitters, such as ghrelin (the strongest stimulator), leptin, sex hormones, corticosteroids, or dopamine (Veldhuis et al., 2006; Wójcikowski & Daniel, 2011). GH shows strong anabolic properties by stimulating the biosynthesis of proteins and nucleic acids, and insulin secretion, but also shows catabolic properties by stimulating lipolysis (Veldhuis et al., 2006).

In male rats the secretion of GH is a pulse type. Every 3.5–4 h the hormone concentration in blood reaches value up to 200 ng/ml, however outside these periods it is very low or even undetectable. To invoke the proper cellular response the impulse frequency, duration and amplitude are important. In females there is no clear pulsation and the average hormone concentration in serum is 30-60 ng/ml (Waxman & Chang, 2005).

The growth hormone receptor (GHR) is the integral cell membrane protein, by which GH has a direct impact on the cells of the liver, skeletal muscles, bones, brain, and adipose tissue (Rosenfeld & Hwa, 2009). On the surface of female hepatocytes there are much more GHRs, which probably play a role in different response to GH comparing to males (Waxman & Chang, 2005). Binding GH to the receptor causes its dimerization, and activation of JAK2 (*Janus-type Tyrosine Kinase-2*) tyrosine kinase initiating several signaling pathways. The main mechanism of GH-dependent transcriptional regulation is based on the JAK-STAT, pathway in which STAT (*Signal Transducers and Activators of Transcription*) proteins 1, 3, 5a and 5b are involved (Lobie & Waxman, 2003; Rosenfeld & Hwa, 2009). In addition, the small Ras (*Rat sarcoma viral oncogene*) proteins, the family of MAPK (*Mitogen-Activated Protein Kinases*), IRS-1-3 (*Insulin Receptor Substrates*) adapter proteins, GRB-2 (*Growth factor Receptor-bound protein 2*), SHC (*Src Homology/Collagen homology*); SOS (*Son of Sevenless*) protein, the protein kinase C (PKC) and phosphatidylinositol-3 kinase (PI 3-kinase) are activated. GH may also activate the epidermal growth factor receptor (EGFR) and non-receptor kinases: c-Src, c-Fyn and FAK (Lobie & Waxman, 2003). Indirectly, GH affects tissues through insulin-like growth factors: IGF-I and IGF-II, (GH/IGF axis), which are produced primarily in the liver (Veldhuis et al., 2006). In the external regulation of growth signal, CIS (*Cytokine-inducible SH2 protein*) and SOCS (*Suppressors of Cytokine Signaling*) proteins, are involved. They are regulated by proinflammatory interleukin 6 (IL-6) and concentration of these proteins increases in various pathological conditions, such as rheumatic diseases (MacRae et al., 2006).

3.2 Regulation of transcription factors gene expression dependent on the growth hormone

In 2008, sex-dependent genes expressed in the liver of hypophysectomized rats administered GH were examined by means of the DNA microarrays technique (Wauthier &

Waxman, 2008). Twenty four of 1032 genes were identified as early response genes, candidates for direct targets of GH action. 15 of them underwent induction and 9 - inhibition under the influence of GH (table 2). There were no cytochrome P450 genes among them, however, there were genes of transcription factors participating in their regulation, e.g. Bcl6, Cutl2, HNF-6 and PPARγ (described below), as well as Egr1, Myc and Nr0b2/SHP. It was also confirmed that GH maintains the hepatic sexual dimorphism, by means of both positive and negative regulatory mechanisms. In mouse liver, 88% of male-specific genes were subject to positive regulation by pituitary hormones, whereas in females, most genes (64%) were under negative regulation (Wauthier et al., 2010).

Gene symbol (alphabetical order)	Gene name	Response to GH	Sex-specific gene class	Involvement in CYP regulation
Asb9	Ankyrin repeat and SOCS box-containing protein 9	Suppression	none	no data
Bcl3	B-cell leukemia/lymphoma 3	Induction	none	no data
Bcl6	B-cell leukemia/lymphoma 6	Suppression	Male class IIA	yes
Cux2	Cutl2, Cut-like 2	Induction	Female class IA	yes
Egr1	Early growth response 1	Induction	none	yes
Etv6	Ets variant gene 6 (TEL oncogene)	Induction	none	no data
Foxq1	Forkhead box Q1; HFH-1	Induction	none	no data
Hhex	Hematopoietically expressed homeobox	Induction	none	no data
Jun	Jun oncogene	Induction	none	no data
Klf9	Kruppel-like factor 9	Induction	none	no data
Klf15	Kruppel-like factor 15	Suppression	none	no data
Lef1	Lymphoid enhancer binding factor 1	Suppression	none	no data
Lhx1	LIM homeobox protein 1	Suppression	none	no data

Gene symbol (alphabetical order)	Gene name	Response to GH	Sex-specific gene class	Involvement in CYP regulation
Msx1	Homeo box, msh-like 1	Induction	none	no data
Myc	Myelocytomatosis viral oncogene homolog (avian)	Induction	none	yes
Ncl	Nucleolin	Induction	Female class IB	no data
Nfyb	Nuclear transcription factor-Y beta	Induction	none	no data
Nr0b2	Nuclear receptor subfamily 0, group B, member 2; SHP	Suppression	none	yes
Onecut1	One cut domain, HNF6	Induction	Female class IB	yes
Pou3f3	POU domain, class 3, transcription factor 3	Induction	none	no data
Pparg	Peroxisome proliferator activated receptor gamma	Suppression	Male class IIB	yes
Tbx3	T-box 3	Suppression	none	no data
Zfp37	Zinc finger protein 37	Induction	Male class IA	no data
Zfp786	Zinc finger protein 786	Suppression	none	no data

Table 2. Early GH response genes of the DNA-binding proteins and transcription factors.

Well recognized examples of sex-specific transcription factors are: Tox (*Thymus high-mobility group box protein*), Cutl2 (*Cut-like 2*), and Trim 24 (*Tripartite motif-containing 24*). They undergo preferential expression in the liver of female rats, where their levels are accordingly 16, 125 and 73 times higher than those found in males. Both, Tox and Cutl2 belong to the GH response genes. Tox is a protein involved in the regulation of T lymphocytes maturation. Cutl2 (Cux2) is one of the early GH response genes and plays a role in the control of proliferation and differentiation of nervous tissue cells (Wauthier & Waxman, 2008). Trim 24 (TIF1α) participates in chromatin remodelling and thus controls its transcriptional activity. The expression of all three genes is increased, at least to the 'female' levels, in secondary feminized males (Laz et al., 2007).

Bcl6 (*B-cell leukemia/lymphoma 6 protein*) is a specific to males transcriptional repressor, whose binding with DNA increases significantly between GH pulsations, when the binding of the STAT5 factor is low. On the basis of studies on Bcl6, a new mechanism of GH-dependent sex specificity has been described (Meyer et al., 2009). The analysis of primary transcripts (hnRNA) showed that in females, in contrary to males, there comes to the dual block during the process of Bcl6 elongation: in the intron 4 and exon 5.

3.3 Regulation of cytochrome P450 gene expression by growth hormone

Sex-specific genes in rat liver were divided into two classes, depending on the character of the response to GH secretion pattern: class I genes, down-regulated in one, or both sexes after hypophysectomy and thus required pituitary hormones for full expression and class II genes, up-regulated in one or both sexes after hypophysectomy and thus suppressed by pituitary hormones (Wauthier & Waxman, 2008; Waxman & Chang, 2005; Waxman & Holloway, 2009). Additionally, these classes of genes were divided into subclasses. Male-specific genes into: class IA - down-regulated in males, but not in females; class IB - down-regulated in both males and females; class IC - down-regulated in males, but up-regulated in females; class IIA - selectively up-regulated in females; class IIB - up-regulated in both males and females. Female-specific genes into: class IA - down-regulated in females, but not in males; class IB - down-regulated in both males and females; class IC - down-regulated in females, but up-regulated in males; class IIA - selectively up-regulated in males; class IIB - up-regulated in both males and females (Wauthier & Waxman, 2008).

Class I, obligatorily dependent on GH pulsation includes 'male' CYP2C11 isoform (testosterone 2α- and 16α-hydroxylase). CYP2C11 expression does not occur in young animals and is induced only during sexual maturation. A similar dependence applies to CYP2A2, CYP2C13 and CYP3A18. Class I also includes 'female' CYP2C12 isoform (steroid sulfate 15α–hydroxylase), whose expression is similar in young rats of both sexes. However, in the progress of the sexual maturation the expression increases in females, whereas it is totally inhibited in males. The representative of class II is CYP3A2, whose expression in males occurs after reaching sexual maturation, whereas in females it is subject to selective suppression. In addition to the sex-specific isoforms, there are also isoforms which exist in both sexes, however they decisively prevail in one of them after reaching maturation. For example, in the liver of adult female rats the 'prevailing' isoforms are: CYP2C7, CYP3A9 and CYP2A1, because their expression is 3-10 times higher than in males. The best known model of sex-dependent hormonal regulation of cytochrome P450 expression is CYP2C11/12 expression in the rodent's liver. It is believed that similar regulatory mechanisms are responsible for sexual dimorphism of human cytochromes P450, such as CYP3A4, CYP1A2 and CYP2E1, however, this dimorphism is much less expressed (Scandlyn et al., 2008).

GH activates several signaling pathways of potential importance for the regulation of CYP expression. In females one of them is the cascade of arachidonic acid triggered by activated phospholipase A2 and enhanced by Ca^{2+} influx into the cell. As a result, it comes to CYP–dependent production of epoxide derivatives of arachidonic acid, which increases CYP2C12 expression (Gonzalez & Lee, 1996). In the liver, the key regulator of the GH-dependent cytochrome P450 gene expression is STAT5b transcription factor being a representative of STAT protein family (Buitenhuis et al., 2004). In male rats, in the period between GH pulsations, the STAT5b activity is negligible or undetectable. In females the continuous profile of GH secretion causes its constant activation at low, but detectable level. STAT5b, together with STAT5a, can activate CYP2C12 gene expression by binding sequences, which are unavailable in males (Tannenbaum et al., 2001). STAT5b contains sulfhydryl groups so it can bind to cytoplasmic domain of the GHR and undergo phosphorylation through the active GHR-JAK2 complex. Subsequently, STAT undergoes dimerization and then rapid translocation to the nucleus, where it activates transcription of target genes. It can regulate the expression of CYP genes directly, by binding their promoter sequences, or indirectly, by co-activation or co-repression of other transcription factors genes, which play the role of primary target (Lobie & Waxman, 2003). STAT5b has an influence to epigenetic regulatory mechanisms as well. It activates the genes silenced as a result of methylation, and strengthens the local conversion of chromatin to the transcriptionally active form (Waxman & O'Connor, 2006). On the other hand, it can inhibit binding of hepatocyte nuclear factors to CYP2C12 gene promoter. STAT5b is able to bind with the receptors of vitamin A derivatives, e.g. with retinoic acid receptor (RAR), however, it is not yet known if it is relevant in the hormone-dependent regulation of cytochrome P450. In the acute promyelocytic leukaemia, a fusion protein STAT5b-RARα has been described. It binds to RARE sequences both as a STAT5b-RARα/STAT5b-RARα homodimer and STAT5b-RARα/RXR heterodimer and inhibits the transcriptional activity of RARα/RXRα heterodimer (Dong & Tweardy, 2002).

In the process of the regulation of CYP gene expression, STAT proteins cooperate mostly with hepatocyte nuclear factors – HNFs (Park et al., 2006). HNFs representing this superfamily of proteins, such as HNF-1α, HNF-4α, HNF-3γ, HNF-3β and HNF-6, exist mainly in the liver. Some of them, e.g. HNF-6, are directly regulated by GH (Wauthier & Waxman, 2008). They take part in the differentiation of hepatocytes and regulation of gene expression associated with the fundamental metabolic pathways in the liver: glycolysis, gluconeogenesis, and the metabolism of lipoproteins, fatty acids and bile acids (Gonzalez, 2008). HNFs bind to DNA sequences as monomers, homodimers or RXR heterodimers.

A key role in the aspect of the sex-differentiated expression of hepatic proteins plays HNF-4α, binding GTTAAT sequence in target genes. HNF-3β and HNF-6 factors are the positive regulators of 'female' expression of CYP2C12 and the negative regulators of 'male' expression of CYP2C2, induced, in turn, by HNF-4α and HNF-3γ. In mice, HNF-4α is responsible for female-specific expression of Cyp3a41. Sex differences in the structure of chromatin - higher methylation and acetylation of respective binding sites in females, underlie this process (Bhadhprasit et al., 2011). HNF-4α is essential for the proper induction of CYP genes with participation of PXR (CYP2C9, CYP3A4) and CAR (CYP2C9) receptors (Tamási et al., 2011). It appeared that in humans, microRNA: miR-24 and miR-34a are responsible for the negative regulation of HNF-4α by degradation of its mRNA by miRNA/RISC complex (RNA-induced Silencing Complex) and/or translational repression (Takagi et al., 2010). Down-regulation of HNF-4α reduces the expression of CYP7A1 and CYP8B1 involved in the synthesis of bile acids. Because miR-24 and miR-34a are regulated by oxidative stress, it is considered that they play a negative role in the pathogenesis of liver diseases (Takagi et al., 2010). The fact that the natural HNF-4α ligand is linolenic acid, suggests the possibility of regulating its activity by the diet and pharmacological modulation (Gonzalez, 2008; Hwang-Verslues & Sladek, 2010; Jover et al., 2009).

GHNF (Growth Hormone-regulated liver Nuclear Factor) is another transcriptional factor regulated by GH, 'dominant' in females and having five binding sites in CYP2C12 gene promoter (Waxman et al., 1996). In turn, GABP (GA-binding Protein) is a protein, binding

DNA sequences rich in guanine and adenine. It is associated with sex-dependent regulation of CYP genes on the epigenetic level. Demethylation of CpG (*Cytosine-phosphate-Guanosine*) islands existing within the promoters of different genes allows binding of GABP and their transactivation (Waxman & O'Connor, 2006). Moreover, the representatives of Rsl (*Regulators of sex-limited proteins*) protein family – KRAB (*Krüppel-associated Box*) proteins, through the stabilization of the transcriptionally inactive heterochromatin, act as transcription repressors of genes specific to males in the liver of adult female rodents (Krebs et al., 2003).

4. Regulation of cytochrome P450 gene expression by other signaling pathways

In addition to already described factors, in the regulation of cytochrome P450 gene expression are involved numerous intracellular signaling cascades, until recently, not connected with this function. Among them are signaling pathways dependent on NF-κB, MAP kinases, and β-catenin (Braeuning, 2009; Murray et al., 2010; Zordoky & El-Kadi, 2009). Glucocorticoid receptor and GATA4, Nrf2 and C/EBP transcription factors also play important role in the transcriptional regulation of cytochromes P450 (Dvorak & Pavek, 2010; Jover et al., 2009; Mwinyi et al., 2010a; Yokota et al., 2011). It can not be excluded that there are significant functional dependencies allowing for the hormonal control of the mentioned signaling pathways. It is known that GH, the main hormone supervising CYP expression, directly regulates the gene of Nfkbiz (*Nuclear factor of kappa light polypeptide gene enhancer in B-cells inhibitor, zeta*), the inhibitor of transcription factor NF-κB (Wauthier & Waxman, 2008). In addition, the phenomenon of cross-talk was confirmed between the nuclear receptors of xenobiotics and multimodal transcription factors like glucocorticoid receptor and NF-κB (Dvorak & Pavek, 2010; Zordoky & El-Kadi, 2009).

NF-κB is a pleiotropic transcription factor, which regulates over 200 genes related to, among others, the immune response, apoptosis, osteoclastogenesis, and inflammatory processes (Zordoky & El-Kadi, 2009). Classical (canonical) NF-κB signaling pathway is the phosphorylation and subsequent degradation of IκB (*Inhibitory kappa B protein*) - cytoplasmic protein inhibiting translocation of NF-κB factor to the nucleus – by the activated I-κB kinase - IKK (*Inhibitory Kappa B protein Kinase*). The released NF-κB may bind to the corresponding DNA sequences in the nucleus. Three mechanisms regulating cytochrome P450 expression and activity, with the participation of NF-κB have been proposed: direct, by binding to promoter sequences of CYP1A1, CYP2B1/2, CYP2C11, CYP2D5, CYP2E1, CYP3A7 and CYP27B1 genes; indirect, through repression of receptors, such as AhR, CAR, GR, PXR, RXR, PPAR, FXR, and LXR; and by post-translational regulation including induction of heme oxygenase and/or an impact on the stability of CYP proteins (Willson & Kliewer, 2002; Zordoky & El-Kadi, 2009).

Growing evidence indicates that MAP kinases participate in regulating the expression of drug metabolizing enzymes of phase I and II (Murray et al., 2010). MAPK activators: sorbitol and EGF (*Epidermal Growth Factor*) inhibit constitutive and induced expression of CYP isoforms, however anisomycin does not cause such an effect or shows a weak stimulation effect (Bachleda et al., 2009). MAP kinases catalyze the phosphorylation of the complexes formed with the participation of transcription factors, including nuclear receptors, cytoplasmic receptors of AhR type and members of the AP-1 family (c-Fos, c-Jun), and because of that, they may affect their ability to transactivate target gens (Braeuning, 2009; Murray et al., 2010). MAPK-dependent pathways are crucial for regulating proliferation and differentiation of cells and their response to stress factors, exposure to chemicals present in the environment, and radiation (Murray et al., 2010). Activation of MAPKs by pro-inflammatory cytokines causes, among others, phosphorylation of JNK *(c-Jun N-terminus Kinase)* kinase, which in turn phosphorylates HNF-4α and inhibits transactivation of CYP7A1 and CYP8B1 genes (Riddick et al., 2004). In this way, MAPKs are involved in the feedback inhibition of CYP genes participating in the metabolism of endobiotics.

In the liver, drug metabolizing enzymes are characterized by zonal distibution with the predominance of expression in the perivenous zone (Braeuning & Schwarz, 2010a). EGF/Ras/MAPK and WNT/β-catenin/TCF signaling pathways participate in the regulation of such gene expression (Braeuning, 2009; Braeuning & Schwarz, 2010a). A model of antagonistic relationship between these pathways has been proposed: Ras-dependent pathway promotes the expression of genes in periportal zone (so called zone 1), whereas β-catenin-dependent pathway promotes expression in pericentral zone (zone 3), of liver acinus (Braeuning, 2009). This applies not only to genes encoding CYP apoprotein, but also to genes involved in heme biosynthesis, which is the prosthetic group of these enzymes (Braeuning & Schwarz, 2010b). Studies in a mouse model showed that β-catenin cooperates with AhR, activating a constitutive CYP1A1 expression and increasing its induction by AhR ligands, through strengthening AhR potential for transactivation (Brauning et al., 2011).

Glucocorticoid receptor (GR) is involved in the regulation of cytochrome P450 expression, through at least three mechanisms: direct binding of GR to specific promoter sequences called glucocorticoid response elements (GREs); indirect binding of GR to specific promoter sequences as a component of the multiprotein complex; and up or down-regulation of other transcription factors, AhR, or nuclear receptors: PXR, CAR and RXR. The final effect of glucocorticoids on CYP gene transcription is usually the result of several mechanisms (Dvorak & Pavek, 2010; Monostory et al., 2009).

GATA proteins belong to the group of transcription factors containing 'zinc finger domains', which recognize the DNA motif (A/T)GATA(A/G). They regulate the process of embryogenesis, especially heart development and the expression of detoxification enzymes and transporters. Binding sites of GATA-4, a main GATA protein in the liver, are located, among others, in the CYP2C19 and CYP2C9 gene. GATA-dependent expression is regulated by specific co-regulators, e.g. GATA-4-dependent activation of CYP2C19 gene transcription is inhibited by FOG-2 *(Friend of GATA-2)* (Mwinyi et al., 2010a, 2010b).

Transcription factor Nrf2 *(Nuclear factor-erythroid 2-related factor* or *NFE2-related factor 2)* is probably one of the main regulators of the antioxidant response (Nguyen et al., 2009). It belongs to the group of factors characterized by bZIP *(basic-leucine Zipper)* structure. It mostly regulates the expression of phase II enzymes of xenobiotic metabolism and phase III membrane-bound transporters, but it is also associated with the regulation of CYP2A5 and CYP2A6 genes through StRE *(Stress Response Elements)* and ARE *(Antioxidant Response Elements)* sequences (Abu-Bakar et al., 2007; Yokota et al., 2011). It has been suggested that there is interference between Nrf2 and other receptors regulating the expression of cytochrome P450, e.g. AhR, LXR and FXR. This may be important for individual susceptibility to the development of diseases, including lung cancer (Antiila et al., 2010; Kay et al., 2011).

C/EBP proteins *(CCAAT/Enhancer Binding Protein)* are transcription factors belonging to the group of LETF factors *(Liver-Enriched Transcription Factors)*. They bind to CCAAT regulatory sequence and TT/GNNGA/CAAT enhancer sequence (Ramji & Foka, 2002; Rodríguez-Antona et al., 2003). Just as Nrf2, they have a characteristic C-terminal domain responsible for DNA binding, characterized by the structure of basic-leucine zipper. C/EBP may participate in the transcriptional regulation of some cytochrome P450 genes, such as CYP2A6, CYP2B6, CYP2C9, CYP2D6, CYP3A4, CYP3A5 and CYP3A7 (Pitarque et al., 2005). In hepatocytes, this regulation takes place in cooperation with HNFs and other transcription factors. C/EBPα and HNF-3γ regulate CYP3A4 gene expression probably by chromatin remodeling (Rodríguez-Antona et al., 2003).

5. Clinical implications

Practical applications of the knowledge about signaling pathways regulating cytochrome P450 gene transcription are very attractive in the context of protection the body from the potential harmful action of xenobiotics and drugs, and retention of pathophysiological processes. Nuclear receptors important for transactivation of CYP genes play a key role in the pathogenesis of many diseases - mainly of metabolic origin – and they may represent valid therapeutic targets for these disorders. Their role in liver diseases, including cholestatic and fatty liver disease, drug-induced hepatotoxicity, viral hepatitis, fibrosis and neoplasmatic hiperplasia is well understood (Wagner et al., 2011). In the kidneys they play an important role in the mechanism of nephropathy, especially diabetic, as they regulate the intensity of cellular infiltration, apoptosis, secretion of inflammatory cytokines, intensity of oxidative and nitrosative stress, secretion of prothrombotic growth factors, fatty acids synthesis, and the accumulation of cholesterol and triglycerides. VDR, FXR and PPARs seem to play the main role in these processes (Levi, 2011). VDR shows a nephroprotective action, among others, by inhibition or antagonism in respect of the renin-angiotensin-aldosterone system (RAAS) and the NF-kB signaling pathway (Deb et al., 2009; Zhang et al., 2010). FXR inhibits expression of SREBP-1 *(Sterol Regulatory Element-Binding Protein 1)* and ChREBP *(Carbohydrate Response Element-Binding Protein)*, transcription factors that regulate gene expression of lipogenic and glycolytic enzymes, especially in the liver and adipose tissue (X. Wang et al., 2009). PPARα regulates renal fatty acid β-oxidation, preventing at the same time the accumulation of lipids and lipotoxicity phenomenon, and also controls the formation of foam cells (Rigamonti et al., 2008).

Increasingly, attempts are being made to modulate the expression of nuclear receptors through the creation of specific ligands (Perez et al., 2011; Levi et al., 2011). Unfortunately, at the present stage it is impossible to determine the correlation between the structure of the ligand and physiological response. The administration of non-selective rexinoids increases triglycerides concentration (as the result of SREBP-1c transactivation by LXR/RXR), inhibits the thyroid axis and causes hepatomegaly. It is desirable therefore to develop rexinoids selective for PPARγ/RXR and LXR/RXR heterodimers, the so-called SNuRMs *(Specific Nuclear Receptor Modulators)*, acting differently than the known PPARγ and LXR ligands (Perez et al., 2011). In the treatment of autoimmunological and neurodegenerative disorders, retinoids which are modulators of retinoic acid receptors can also be applied (Alvarez et al., 2011). Application of the agonists of: VDR (doxercalciferol), FXR (INT-747) and PPARs (fibrates) inhibits and even reverses the pathological changes observed in diabetic kidney injury (Levi, 2011; Thomas et al., 2008). Agonistic and antagonistic RXR ligands could be used in the treatment of obesity, type 2 diabetes and insulin resistance, i.e. the components of metabolic syndrome (Levi, 2011; Perez et al., 2011).

Some of cytochrome P450 and transcription factors genes are hormone-dependent. Sex differences in the expression of early GH response genes may be responsible for gender differences in predisposition to certain diseases. For example, 29 of these genes, specific to male mice, is a target for the Mef2 transcription factor (*Myocyte enhancer factor 2*), whose activation in hepatic stellate cells is associated with the process of liver fibrosis and cirrhosis, increasing the male' risk of developing hepatocellular carcinoma (Wauthier et al., 2010). Progress of the studies on this phenomenon is necessary for rational drug administration, a good example of what can be attempt to clinical use of NF-kB inhibitors. Significant changes in cytochrome P450 expression and activity caused by the activation of NF-κB are found in the states, in which increased secretion of inflammatory mediators and the excessive oxidative stress can be observed, e.g.: inflammatory bowel diseases, rheumatoid arthritis, chronic exposure to stress, diabetes, kidney diseases, congenital heart diseases, or during aging (Zordoky & El-Kadi, 2009). NF-κB is now seen as a factor linking inflammatory process, oxidative stress and cancer with the metabolism of xenobiotics (Assenat et al., 2006). The inflammatory process accompanying cancers, may, through NF-κB, disturb CYP expression and thereby alter the effectiveness of chemotherapy.

In addition, the role of glucocorticoid receptor in the regulation of expression of cytochromes P450 such as CYP1A1 or CYP1A2, is extremely important for clinical practice. On one hand - the use of glucocorticoids as drugs is commonplace in medicine and has many side effects including not always conscious interactions of drug-drug type. On the other hand - CYP1A subfamily is the main group of cytochrome P450 responsible for bioactivation of xenobiotics and production of harmful and carcinogenic derivatives (Dvorak & Pavek, 2010; Monostory et al., 2009). That results in serious medical implications, namely changes in susceptibility to xenobiotics and in pharmacokinetics and pharmacodynamics of drugs, which must be taken into account by physicians and lead to the control of pharmacotherapy.

6. Conclusion

In recent years there has been significant progress within the meaning of the mechanisms regulating cytochrome P450 expression. It was found that the main role in the regulation of sex-specific CYP expression plays the growth hormone, the effects of which are dependent on daily secretion pattern, different in males and females. Disorders of intrinsic mechanisms controlling hormone secretion may lead to the modulation of CYP genes expression.

Both GH-dependent and GH-independent signal transduction is strictly connected with activation of numerous DNA-binding proteins. It has been described a number of new factors and signaling pathways involved directly or indirectly in the regulation of expression, primarily on the stage of transcription. The ligands for nuclear receptors previously known as orphan have been identified (receptors deorphanisation).

In addition, drug-metabolizing enzymes, xenobiotic transporters and their targets appear to be under the epigenetic control, hence separation of the new discipline called pharmacoepigenetics. Although the effects of epigenetic modifications on drug metabolism were not examined extensively, they probably play an important role in determining the tissue-specific expression of CYP genes both in normal and cancer tissues. As a result, epigenetic modifiers may considerably alter the metabolism and/or disposition of many xenobiotics. Post-transcriptional regulation by microRNAs seems to be a key mechanism underlying the discrepancy between hepatic mRNA and protein expression of genes involved in drug metabolism.

Our knowledge of the regulatory mechanisms for cytochrome P450 expression represents the base of understanding the cross-talk between endobiotic and xenobiotic metabolism. On the other hand, there are large inter-individual variations in the expression of CYP genes in humans and the genotypic and phenotypic variability of the key regulators of the CYP gene transcription significantly influences individual response to xenobiotics, including drugs. A major future challenge will be to explain the role of co-activators and co-repressors of cytochrome P450 gene transcription into current pathogenic and therapeutic concepts for the diseases. More population-based studies should be conducted, because they may help physicians predicting the results of therapy and adverse drug effects, including drug-drug interactions.

7. References

Abu-Bakar, A., Lämsä, V., Arpiainen, S., Moore, M.R., Lang, M.A. & Hakkola, J. (2007). Regulation of CYP2A5 gene by the transcription factor nuclear factor (erythroid-derived 2)-like 2. *Drug Metabolism and Disposition*. Vol.35, No.5, (May 2010), pp. 787-794, ISSN 0090-9556

Alvarez, S., Bourguet, W., Gronemeyer, H. & de Lera, AR. (2011). Retinoic acid receptor modulators: a perspective on recent advances and promises. *Expert Opinion on Therapeutic Patents*, Vol.21, No.1, (January 2011), pp. 55-63, ISSN 1354-3776

Anttila, S., Raunio, H. & Hakkola, J. (2010). Cytochrome P450 Mediated Pulmonary Metabolism of Carcinogens: Regulation and Cross-talk in Lung Carcinogenesis. *American Journal of Respiratory Cell and Molecular Biology*. Vol.44, No.5, (May 2010), pp. 583-590. ISSN 1044-1549

Assenat, E., Gerbal-Chaloin, S., Maurel, P., Vilarem, M.J. & Pascussi, J.M. (2006). Is nuclear factor kappa-B the missing link between inflammation, cancer and alteration in hepatic drug metabolism in patients with cancer? *European Journal of Cancer*. Vol.42, No.6, (April 2006), pp. 785-792, ISSN 0959-8049

Bachleda, P., Vrzal, R. & Dvořák, Z. (2009). Activation of MAPKs influences the expression of drug-metabolizing enzymes in primary human hepatocytes. *General Physiology and Biophysics*. Vol.28, No.3, (September 2009), pp. 316-320, ISSN 0231-5882

Bhadhprasit, W., Sakuma, T., Kawasaki, Y. & Nemoto, N. (2011). Hepatocyte nuclear factor 4α regulates expression of the mouse female-specific Cyp3a41 gene in the liver. *Drug Metabolism and Disposition*. Vol.39, No.3, (March 2011), pp. 490-497, ISSN 0090-9556

Braeuning, A. (2009). Regulation of cytochrome P450 expression by Ras- and beta-catenin-dependent signaling. *Current Drug Metabolism*. Vol.10, No.2, (February 2009), pp. 138-158, ISSN 1389-2002

Braeuning, A. & Schwarz, M. (2010). beta-Catenin as a multilayer modulator of zonal cytochrome P450 expression in mouse liver. *Biological Chemistry*. Vol.391, No.2-3, (February-March 2010), pp. 139-148, ISSN 1431-6730

Braeuning, A. & Schwarz, M. (2010). Zonation of heme synthesis enzymes in mouse liver and their regulation by b-catenin and Ha-ras. *Biological Chemistry*. Vol.391, No.11, (November 2010), pp. 1305–1313, ISSN 1431-6730

Braeuning, A., Köhle, C., Buchmann, A. & Schwarz, M. (April 2011). Coordinate Regulation of Cytochrome P450 1A1 Expression in Mouse Liver by the Aryl Hydrocarbon Receptor and the {beta}-Catenin Pathway, In: *Toxicological Sciences*, 20.07.2011, Available from

http://toxsci.oxfordjournals.org/content/early/2011/04/16/toxsci.kfr080.long

Buitenhuis, M., Coffer, P.J. & Koenderman, L. (2004). Signal transducer and activator of transcription 5 (STAT5). *International Journal of Biochemistry & Cell Biology*. Vol.36, No.11, (November 2004), pp. 2120-2124, ISSN 1357-2725

Chen, S., Wang, K. & Wan, Y.J. (2010). Retinoids activate RXR/CAR-mediated pathway and induce CYP3A. *Biochemical Pharmacology*. Vol. 79, No.2, (January 2010), pp. 270-276, ISSN 0006-2952

Cui, Y.J., Yeager, R.L., Zhong, X.B. & Klaassen, C.D. (2009). Ontogenic expression of hepatic Ahr mRNA is associated with histone H3K4 di-methylation during mouse liver development. *Toxicology Letters*. Vol.189, No.3, (September 2009), pp. 184-190, ISSN 0378-4274

Czekaj, P. (2000). Phenobarbital-induced expression of cytochrome P450 genes. *Acta Biochimica Polonica*. Vol.47, No.4, (October 2000) pp. 1093-1105, ISSN 0001-527X

Deb, D.K., Chen, Y., Zhang, Z., Zhang, Y., Szeto, F.L., Wong, K.E., Kong, J. & Li, Y.C. (2009). 1,25-Dihydroxyvitamin D3 suppresses high glucose-induced angiotensinogen expression in kidney cells by blocking the NF-{kappa}B pathway. *American Journal of Physiology - Renal Physiology*. Vol.296, No.5, (May 2009), pp. F1212-F1218, ISSN 0363-6127

Dong, S. & Tweardy, D.J. (2002). Interactions of STAT5b-RARalpha, a novel acute promyelocytic leukemia fusion protein, with retinoic acid receptor and STAT3 signaling pathways. *Blood*. Vol.99, No.8, (April 2001), pp. 2637-2646, ISSN 0006-4971

Dvorak, Z. & Pavek, P. (2010). Regulation of drug-metabolizing cytochrome P450 enzymes by glucocorticoids. *Drug Metabolism Reviews*. Vol.42, No.4, (November 2010), pp. 621-635, ISSN 0360-2532

Gnerre, C., Blattler, S., Kaufmann, M.R., Looser, R. & Meyer, U. A. (2004). Regulation of CYP3A4 by the bile acid receptor FXR: evidence for functional binding sites in the CYP3A4 gene. *Pharmacogenetics*. Vol.14, No.10, (October 2004), pp. 635-645, ISSN 0960-314X

Gonzalez, F.J. (2008). Regulation of Hepatocyte Nuclear Factor 4α-mediated Transcription. *Drug metabolism and pharmacokinetics*. Vol.23, No.1, (January 2008), pp. 2-7, ISSN 1347-4367

Gonzalez, F.J. & Lee, Y.H. (1996). Constitutive expression of hepatic cytochrome P450 genes. *FASEB Journal*. Vol.10, (August 1996), pp. 1112-1117, ISSN 0892-6638

Honkakoski, P. & Negishi, M. (2000). Regulation of cytochrome P450 (CYP) genes by nuclear receptors. *Biochemical Journal*, Vol.347, No.2, (April 2000), pp. 321-337, ISSN 0264-6021

Hwang-Verslues, W.W. & Sladek, F.M. (2010). HNF4α - role in drug metabolism and potential drug target? *Current Opinion in Pharmacology*. Vol.10, No.6, (December 2010), pp. 698-705, ISSN 1471-4892

Jover, R., Moya, M. & Gomez-Lechon, M.J. (2009). Transcriptional regulation of cytochrome P450 genes by the nuclear receptor hepatocyte nuclear factor 4-alpha. *Current Drug Metabolism.* Vol.10, No.5, (June 2009), pp. 508-519, ISSN 1389-2002

Kay, H.Y., Kim, W.D., Hwang, S.J., Choi, H.S., Gilroy, R.K., Wan, Y.J. & Kim, S.G. (June 2011). Nrf2 Inhibits LXRα-Dependent Hepatic Lipogenesis by Competing with FXR for Acetylase Binding, In: *Antioxidants & Redox Signaling,* 20.07.2011, Available from http://www.liebertonline.com/doi/abs/10.1089/ars.2010.3834

Kemper, J.K., Xiao, Z., Ponugoti, B., Miao, J., Fang, S., Kanamaluru, D., Tsang, S., Wu, S.Y., Chiang, C.M. & Veenstra, T.D. (2009). FXR acetylation is normally dynamically regulated by p300 and SIRT1 but constitutively elevated in metabolic disease states. *Cell Metabolism.* Vol.10, No.5, (November 2009), pp. 392-404, ISSN 1550-4131

Klaassen, C.D., Lu, H. & Yue Cu J. (2011). Epigenetic regulation of drug processing genes. *Toxicology Mechanisms and Methods.* Vol.21, No.4, (May 2011), pp. 312-324, ISSN 1537-6516

Krebs, C.J., Larkins, L.K., Price, R., Tullis, K.M., Miller, R.D. & Robins, D.M. (2003). Regulator of sex-limitation (Rsl) encodes a pair of KRAB zinc-finger genes that control sexually dimorphic liver gene expression. *Genes & Develeopment.* Vol.17, No.21, (November 2003), pp. 2664-2674, ISSN 0890-9369

Lamba, J. & Schuetz, E.G. (2009). Genetic Variants of Xenobiotic Receptors and Their Implications in Drug Metabolism and Pharmacogenetics, In: *Nuclear receptors in drug metabolism,* W. Xie, (Ed.), 241-273, Wiley, ISBN 978-0-470-08679-7, New Jersey, USA

Laz, E.V., Holloway, M.G., Chen, C.S. & Waxman, D.J. (2007). Characterization of three growth hormone-responsive transcription factors preferentially expressed in adult female liver. *Endocrinology.* Vol.148, No.7, (July 2007), pp. 3327-3337, ISSN 0013-7227

Levi M. (2011). Nuclear receptors in renal disease. *Biochimica et Biophysica Acta.* Vol.1812, No.8, (August 2011), pp. 1061-1067, ISSN 0006-3002

Levi, M., Wang, X. & Choudhury D. (2011). Nuclear hormone receptors as therapeutic targets. *Contributions to Nephrology.* Vol.170, (June 2011), pp. 209-216, ISSN 0302-5144

Li, T. & Chiang, J.Y.L. (May 2009). Regulation of Bile Acid and Cholesterol Metabolism by PPARs, In: *PPAR Research,* 20.07.2011, Available from http://www.hindawi.com/journals/ppar/2009/501739

Lobie, P.E. & Waxman, D.J. (2003). Growth Hormone (GH), In: *Encyclopedia of Hormones,* H.L. Henry & A.W. Norman, (Ed.), 208-216, Academic Press, ISBN 978-0123411037, San Diego, USA

MacRae, V.E., Farquharson, C. & Ahmed, S.F. (2006). The pathophysiology of the growth plate in juvenile idiopathic arthritis. *Rheumatology.* Vol.45, No.1, (January 2006), pp. 11-19, ISSN 1462-0332

Meyer, R.D., Laz, E.V., Su, T. & Waxman, D.J. (2009). Male-specific hepatic Bcl6: growth hormone-induced block of transcription elongation in females and binding to target genes inversely coordinated with STAT5. *Molecular Endocrinology.* Vol.23, No.11, (November 2009), pp. 1914-1926, ISSN 0888-8809

Mohri, T., Nakajima, M., Takagi, S., Komagata, S. & Yokoi, T. (2009). MicroRNA regulates human vitamin D receptor. *International Journal of Cancer.* Vol.125, No.6, (September 2009), pp. 1328-1333, ISSN 0020-7136

Monostory, K., Pascussi, J.M., Kobori, L. & Dvorak, Z. (2009). Hormonal regulation of CYP1A expression. *Drug Metabolism Reviews*, Vol.41, No.4, (November 2009), pp. 547-572, ISSN 0360-2532

Mulero-Navarro, S., Carvajal-Gonzalez, J.M., Herranz, M., Ballestar, E., Fraga, M.F., Ropero, S., Esteller, M. & Fernandez-Salguero, P.M. (2006). The dioxin receptor is silenced by promoter hypermethylation in human acute lymphoblastic leukemia through inhibition of Sp1 binding. *Carcinogenesis*. Vol.27, No.5, (May 2006), pp. 1099-1104, ISSN 0143-3334

Murray, M., Cui, P.H. & Zhou, F. (2010). Roles of mitogen-activated protein kinases in the regulation of CYP genes. *Current Drug Metabolism*. Vol.11, No.10, (December 2010), pp. 850-858, ISSN 1389-2002

Mwinyi, J., Hofmann, Y., Pedersen, R.S., Nekvindová, J., Cavaco, I., Mkrtchian, S. & Ingelman-Sundberg, M. (2010). The transcription factor GATA-4 regulates cytochrome P4502C19 gene expression. *Life Sciences*. Vol.86, No.19-20, (May 2010), pp. 699–706, ISSN 0024-3205

Mwinyi, J., Nekvindová, J., Cavaco, I., Hofmann, Y., Pedersen, R.S., Landman, E., Mkrtchian, S. & Ingelman-Sundberg, M. (2010). New insights into the regulation of CYP2C9 gene expression: the role of the transcription factor GATA-4. *Drug Metabolism and Disposition*. Vol.38, No.3, (March 2010), pp. 415-421, ISSN 0090-9556

Nguyen,T., Nioi, P. & Pickett, C.B. (2009). The Nrf2-antioxidant response element signaling pathway and its activation by oxidative stress. *Journal of Biological Chemistry*. Vol.284, No.20, (May 2009), pp. 13291–13295, ISSN 0021-9258

Pan, Y.Z., Gao, W., & Yu A.M. (2009). MicroRNAs regulate CYP3A4 expression via direct and indirect targeting. *Drug Metabolism and Disposition*. Vol.37, No.10, (October 2009), pp. 2112-2117, ISSN 0090-9556

Pandey, D.P. & Picard, D. (2009). miR-22 inhibits estrogen signaling by directly targeting the estrogen receptor α mRNA. *Molecular and Cellular Biology*. Vol.29, (July 2009), pp. 3783-3790, ISSN 0270-7306

Park, S.H., Wiwi, C.A. & Waxman, D.J. (2006). Signalling cross-talk between hepatocyte nuclear factor 4α and growth-hormone-activated STAT5b. *Biochemical Journal*, 2006; Vol.397, No.1, (July 2006), pp. 159-168, ISSN 0264-6021

Paumelle, R. & Staels, B. (2007). Peroxisome Proliferator-Activated Receptors Mediate Pleiotropic Actions of Statins. *Circulation Research*. Vol.100, No.10, (May 2007), pp. 1394-1395, ISSN 0009-7300

Pérez, E., Bourguet, W., Gronemeyer, H. & de Lera, A.R. (April 2011). Modulation of RXR function through ligand design, In: *Biochimica et Biophysica Acta*, 20.07.2011, Available from http://www.sciencedirect.com /science/article/pii/ S13881981110 0461

Pitarque, M., Rodríguez-Antona, C., Oscarson, M., Ingelman-Sundberg, M. (2005). Transcriptional regulation of the human CYP2A6 gene. *Journal of Pharmacology and Experimental Therapeutics*. Vol.313, No.2, (May 2005), pp. 814-822, ISSN 0022-3565

Phillips, J.M., Yamamoto, Y., Negishi, M., Maronpot, R.R. & Goodman, J.I. (2007). Orphan nuclear receptor constitutive active/androstane receptor mediated alterations in DNA methylation during phenobarbital promotion of liver tumorigenesis. *Toxicological Sciences*. Vol.96, No.1, (March 2007), pp. 72-82, ISSN 1096-6080

Ramji, D.P. & Foka, P. (2002). CCAAT/enhancer-binding proteins: structure, function and regulation. *Biochemical Journal*. Vol.365, No.3, (August 2002), pp. 561-575, ISSN 0264-6021

Riddick, D.S., Lee, C., Bhathena, A., Timsit, Y.E., Cheng, P.Y., Morgan, E.T., Prough, R.A., Ripp, S.L., Miller, K.K.M., Jahan, A. & Chiang, J.Y.L. (2004). Transcriptional suppression of cytochrome p450 genes by endogenous and exogenous chemicals. *Drug Metabolism and Disposition*. Vol.32, No.4, (April 2004), pp. 367–375, ISSN 0090-9556

Rigamonti, E., Chinetti-Gbaguidi, G. & Staels, B. (2008). Regulation of macrophage functions by PPAR-alpha, PPAR-gamma, and LXRs in mice and men. *Arteriosclerosis, Thrombosis, and Vascular Biology*. Vol.28, No.6, (June 2008), pp. 1050-1059, 1079-5642

Rodríguez-Antona, C., Bort, R., Jover, R., Tindberg, N., Ingelman-Sundberg, M., Gómez-Lechón, M.J. & Castell, J.V. (2003). Transcriptional regulation of human CYP3A4 basal expression by CCAAT enhancer-binding protein alpha and hepatocyte nuclear factor-3 gamma. *Molecular Pharmacology*. Vol.63, No.5, (May 2003), pp. 1180-1189, ISSN 0026-895X

Rosenfeld, R.G. & Hwa, V. (2009). The Growth Hormone Cascade and Its Role in Mammalian Growth. *Hormone Research*. Vol.71, suppl.2, (April 2009), pp. 36–40, ISSN 0301-0163

Scandlyn, M.J., Stuart, E.C. & Rosengren R.J. (2008). Sex-specific differences in CYP450 isoforms in humans. *Expert Opinion on Drug Metabolism & Toxicology*, Vol.4, No.4, (April 2008), pp. 413-424, ISSN 1742-5255

Takagi, S., Nakajima, M., Takagi, S., Taniya, T. & Yokoi, T. (2008). Post-transcriptional regulation of human pregnane X receptor by micro-RNA affects the expression of cytochrome P450 3A4. *Journal of Biological Chemistry*. Vol.283, No.15, (April 2008), pp. 9674-9680, ISSN 0021-9258

Takagi, S., Nakajima, M., Kida, K., Yamaura, Y., Fukami, T. & Yokoi, T. (2010). MicroRNAs regulate human hepatocyte nuclear factor 4alpha, modulating the expression of metabolic enzymes and cell cycle. *Journal of Biological Chemistry*. Vol.285, No.7, (February 2010), pp. 4415-4422, ISSN 0021-9258

Tamási, V., Monostory, K., Prough, R.A. & Falus, A. (2011). Role of xenobiotic metabolism in cancer: involvement of transcriptional and miRNA regulation of P450s. *Cellular and Molecular Life Sciences*. Vol.68, No.7, (April 2011), pp. 1131-1146, ISSN 1420-682X

Tannenbaum, G.S., Choi, H.K., Gurd, W. & Waxman D.J. (2001). Temporal Relationship Between the Sexually Dimorphic Spontaneous GH Secretory Profiles and Hepatic STAT5 Activity. *Endocrinology*. Vol.142, No.11, (November 2001), pp. 4599-4606, ISSN 0013-7227

Thomas, C., Pellicciari, R., Pruzanski, M., Auwerx, J. & Schoonjans, K. (2008). Targeting bile-acid signalling for metabolic diseases. *Nature Reviews Drug Discovery*. Vol.7, No.8, (August 2008), pp. 678-693, ISSN 1474-1776

Veldhuis, J.D., Roemmich, J.N., Richmond, E.J. & Bowers, C.Y. (2006). Somatotropic and gonadotropic axes linkages in infancy, childhood, and the puberty-adult transition. *Endocrine Reviews*. Vol.27, No.2, (April 2006), pp. 101-140, ISSN 0163769X

Wagner, M., Zollner, G. & Trauner, M. (2011). Nuclear receptors in liver disease. *Hepatology*. Vol.53, No.3, (March 2011), pp. 1023-1034, ISSN 0270-9139

Wang, K., Chen, S., Xie, W. & Wan, Y.J. (2008). Retinoids induce cytochrome P450 3A4 through RXR/VDR-mediated pathway. *Biochemical Pharmacology*. Vol.75, No.11, (June 2008), pp. 2204-2213, ISSN 0006-2952

Wang, X., Jiang, T., Shen, Y., Adorini, L., Pruzanski, M., Gonzalez, F.J., Scherzer, P., Lewis, L., Miyazaki-Anzai, S. & Levi, M. (2009). The farnesoid X receptor modulates renal lipid metabolism and diet-induced renal inflammation, fibrosis, and proteinuria.

American Journal of Physiology - Renal Physiology. Vol.297, No.6, (December 2009), pp. F1587-F1596, ISSN 0363-6127

Wauthier, V. & Waxman, D.J. (2008). Sex-specific early growth hormone response genes in rat liver. *Molecular Endocrinology.* Vol.22, No.8, (August 2008), pp. 1962-1974, ISSN 0888-8809

Wauthier, V., Sugathan, A., Meyer, R.D., Dombkowski, A.A. & Waxman, D.J. (2010). Intrinsic sex differences in the early growth hormone responsiveness of sex-specific genes in mouse liver. *Molecular Endocrinology.* Vol.24, No.3, (March 2010), pp. 667-678, ISSN 0888-8809

Waxman, D.J., Zhao, S. & Choi, H.K. (1996). Interaction of a Novel Sex-dependent, Growth Hormone-regulated Liver Nuclear Factor with CYP2C12 Promoter. *Journal of Biological Chemistry.* Vol.271, No.47, (November 1996), pp. 29978-29987, ISSN 0021-9258

Waxman, D.J. & Chang, T.K.H. (2005). Hormonal Regulation of Liver Cytochrome P450 Enzymes, In: *Cytochrome P450: Structure, Mechanism and Biochemistry,* P.R. Ortiz de Montellano, (Ed.), 347-376, Kluwer Academic/Plenum Publishers, ISBN 0-306-48324-6, New York, USA

Waxman, D.J. & O'Connor, C. (2006). Growth hormone regulation of sex-dependent liver gene expression. *Molecular Endocrinology.* Vol.20, No.11, (November 2006), pp. 2613-2629, ISSN 0888-8809

Waxman, D.J. & Holloway, M.G. (2009). Sex differences in the expression of hepatic drug metabolizing enzymes. *Molecular Pharmacology.* Vol.76, No.2, (August 2009), pp. 215-228, ISSN 0026-895X

Willson, T.M. & Kliewer, S.A. (2002). PXR, CAR and drug metabolism. *Nature Reviews Drug Discovery.* Vol.1, No.4, (April 2002) pp. 259-266, ISSN 1474-1776

Wójcikowski, J. & Daniel W.A. (February). The role of the nervous system in the regulation of liver cytochrome p450. *Current Drug Metabolism.* Vol.12, No.2, (February 2011), pp. 124-38, ISSN 1389-2002

Xu, Ch., Yong-Tao, Li, Ch. & Kong, A.T. (2005). Induction of Phase I, II and III Drug Metabolism/Transport by Xenobiotics. *Archives of Pharmacal Research,* Vol.28, No.3, (March 2005), pp. 249-268, ISSN 0253-6269

Yokota, S., Higashi, E., Fukami, T., Yokoi, T. & Nakajima, M. (2011). Human CYP2A6 is regulated by nuclear factor-erythroid 2 related factor 2. *Biochemical Pharmacology.* Vol.81, No.2, (January 2011), pp. 289-294, ISSN 0006-2952

Zhang, J., Kong, J., Deb, D.K., Chang, A. & Li, Y.C. (2010). Vitamin D receptor attenuates renal fibrosis by suppressing the renin-angiotensin system. *Journal of the American Society of Nephrology.* Vol. 21, No.6, (June 2010), pp. 966-973, ISSN 1046-6673

Zheng, L., Lv, G.C., Sheng, J. & Yang, Y.D. (2010). Effect of miRNA-10b in regulating cellular steatosis level by targeting PPAR-alpha expression, a novel mechanism for the pathogenesis of NAFLD. *Journal of Gastroenterology and Hepatology.* Vol.25, No.1, (January 2010), pp. 156-163, ISSN 0815-9319

Zordoky, B.N & El-Kadi, A.O. (2009). Role of NF-kappaB in the regulation of cytochrome P450 enzymes. *Current Drug Metabolism.* Vol.10, No.2, (February 2009), pp. 164-178, ISSN 1389-2002

8

Determination of Cytochrome P450 Metabolic Activity Using Selective Markers

Jan Jurica and Alexandra Sulcova

Masaryk University, Brno, CEITEC - Central European Institute of Technology,
Faculty of Medicine, Department of Pharmacology,
Czech Republic

1. Introduction

Cytochrome P450 enzymes (CYP) play a pivot role in phase I of xenobiotic biotransformation. Many of CYP enzymes are known to be polymorphic, with many allelic variants. As a consequence of huge number of possible allele combinations, a wide range of metabolic activity can be observed among patients in population. Individual CYP activity may be also affected by various xenobiotics – either induction or inhibition of distinct CYP isoenzyme may cause failure or toxicity of pharmacotherapy. Due to this, some prediction of metabolic activity is worthwhile in clinical practice. This chapter is going to briefly summarize the possibilities of *in vivo* and *in vitro* CYP metabolic activity assessments of CYP1A2, CYP2C9, CYP2C19, CYP2D6 and CYP3A4 enzymes.

2. *In vivo* enzyme activity assessment

2.1 Clinical need for CYP phenotyping

It is useful to assess CYP metabolic activity prior to or during the pharmacotherapy and to adjust the individual dosage according to the patient's phenotype at least in some cases.

The best studied CYP enzyme concerning polymorphisms, enzyme inhibition and dosage individualization according to phenotype is probably CYP2D6, followed by CYP2C9 and CYP2C19. These enzymes are highly polymorphic, contrary to CYP3A4, where the metabolic activity may vary due to differences in CYP3A4 gene expression and pharmacokinetic interactions [Ingelman-Sundberg 2004]. Nevertheless, any shift in metabolic capacity of individual CYP enzyme may result either in decreased or increased therapeutic response or intensity of adverse effects. For example, after paroxetine administration to the patients on tamoxifen, a decrease in plasma levels of active metabolite of tamoxifen was detected [Stearns et al. 2003]. This can be crucially important in breast cancer treatment. On the other hand, CYP2D6 ultrarapid metabolizer phenotype may cause failure of pharmacotherapy due to the very low and thus ineffective drug plasma levels [Corruble 2008]. In antipsychotic treatment, an association has been observed between extrapyramidal adverse effects and CYP2D6 genotype [Fleeman et al. 2011]. Significant clinical consequences of CYP2D6 genotype or enzyme inhibition were described also in beta-blockers, antianginal, antiarrythmic drugs, antihistamines and antiemetics. The clinical impact of enzyme polymorphism or changes due to inhibition or induction usually depends on the contribution of other CYP forms to the total drug's elimination. By this, the relative therapeutic potency of the parent drug or any of its metabolites may be altered [Zhou 2009].

Methodological approaches such as assessment of metabolic ratio of specific substrate to metabolite(s) in saliva, plasma / serum or urine are most widely used to assess metabolic activity *in vivo*. Besides determination of the concentrations of probe and metabolite in biological fluids, specific substrates are used in various breath tests. Rarely some other approaches are used, e.g. the pupilometry after opioid administration.

It is essentially important to differentiate between *in vivo* and *in vitro* metabolic activity assessments, as they show very often discrepant results.

One of the greatest advantages of genotype assessment is that it does not need to be repeated because it does not change with time or under the simultaneous influences of drugs and other factors. On the other side the disadvantage of the pharmacogenetic testing is, that genotype does not always correlate with observed metabolic activity recorded using probe drug(s). This discrepancy may be caused by various epigenetic factors as well as by inhibition or induction of enzyme metabolic activity caused by other xenobiotics coadministered.

2.2 Conventional probe substrates for *in vivo* metabolic activity assessment

Metabolic activity of various CYP enzymes is most often assessed using selective substrate of distinct CYP enzyme ("marker of metabolic activity"), i.e. a drug (or substance) which is ideally metabolized by the single CYP enzyme [Pelkonen et al. 1998, Pelkonen et al. 2008]. Ideal marker should be a non-toxic substance, with regard to its possible usage *in vivo*. Moreover, such ideal marker should be easily available substance (i.e. registered as a therapeutic drug), which is assessable in biological fluids together with its main metabolite(s). Pharmacokinetics of ideal marker should be determined by metabolism and not by intensity of liver perfusion, protein binding or elimination of unchanged drug [Frank et al. 2007, Kivisto & Kroemer 1997, Pelkonen et al. 1998]. Phenotype classification *in vivo* is based on the drug to metabolite concentration ratio in biological fluids (metabolic ratio): MR = $[c_{drug}/c_{metabolite}]$. With regard to the phenotype (or MR), metabolizers can be classified into 4 different categories – poor metabolizers (PM), intermediate metabolizers (IM), extensive metabolizers (EM) and ultrarapid metabolizers (UM) [Zanger et al. 2004]. Bimodal or trimodal distribution of log-transformed MR is observed in some probe substrates. Histograms of log-transformed MR may refer to cut-off values of MR which distinguish EM from UM, PM or IM.. Doses of medication may be adjusted according to the current phenotype, following the principles of personalized medicine. Probe drugs with unimodal distribution of their MRs cannot reflect genetically encoded differences in the metabolism. Despite this, such probe substrates have also been used for CYP metabolic activity prognosis, but with varying degree of predictive success [Benet 2005]. Some of the probe drugs are metabolized by multiple CYPs, as observed in warfarin or caffeine [Kaminsky & Zhang 1997, Tassaneeyakul et al. 1994]. Moreover, metabolic fate of some substrates may be enantiomer specific: *R*-warfarin is primarily metabolized by CYP1A2 and CYP3A4, *S*-warfarin by CYP2C9 [Kaminsky & Zhang 1997]. Despite this, the major metabolic pathway may serve as a tool for distinct isoenzyme metabolic activity assessment (*S*-warfarin for CYP2C9 phenotype assessment). Phenotype expressed as MR is basically determined by the genotype, but may be also influenced by age [Kamali et al. 2004], sex [Nafziger et al. 1998], habits [Bozikas et al. 2004], co-medication and/or liver disease [Rost et al. 1995].

The above mentioned principles are also utilized in drug development, where drugs are evaluated concerning their CYP-mediated interactions prior to the registration and launch on the basis of the enzyme-specific reaction [Zlokarnik et al. 2005].

2.2.1 CYP1A2

Many substrates have been tried for CYP1A2 metabolic activity assessment, but caffeine is the most widely used one, although other enzymes are involved in biotransformation of caffeine and its metabolites (xanthinoxidase, N-acetyl transferase and with lesser extent also CYP2E1, CYP2A6, CYP3A4, CYP3A5) [Dorne et al. 2001, Tassaneeyakul et al. 1994]. Many metabolic ratios were used in phenotyping studies, with "caffeine metabolic ratio" (CMR) as the well determined marker of CYP1A2 metabolic activity [Hakooz 2009]. On the other hand, simple paraxanthine to caffeine molar concentration ratio assessed in serum/plasma or saliva is also used [van Troostwijk et al. 2003]. Other substrates are used much rarely in phenotyping studies. Probes for CYP1A2 metabolic activity assessment are summarized in Table 1. Moreover, various concentration ratios of caffeine and its metabolites are also used for determination of NAT2 (arylamine N-acetyltransferase), CYP2A6 and xanthinoxidase metabolic activities [Begas et al. 2007, Hakooz 2009, Nyeki et al. 2001].

Probe	CYP1A2-specific reaction
caffeine	N-demethylation
phenacetine	O-deethylation
theophylline	N-demethylation

Table 1. Probes for CYP1A2 metabolic activity assessment [Ou-Yang et al. 2000, Takata et al. 2006]

2.2.2 CYP2C9

CYP2C9 is known to be polymorphic, with more than 40 alleles identified [Ingelman-Sundberg et al. 2011]. Ten years ago it was thought that with CYP2C9 genotyping it will be possible to avoid adverse reactions in patients receiving warfarin [Ma et al. 2002]. These expectations were mostly calmed by reality, that CYP2C19 genotype is not the single major factor influencing warfarin toxicity.

Most often used CYP2C9-specific reactions are summarized in the Table 2. Diclofenac 4'-hydroxylation and tolbutamide methylhydroxylation [Zhou et al. 2009] seem to be the most frequently used, however, tolbutamide methylhydroxylation is also catalyzed by CYP2C19 [Wester et al. 2000]. Phenotyping with the use of substrates with low therapeutic index (phenytoin, oral anticoagulants) would be unsafe since the enzyme activity in CYP2C9*3 homozygotes is nearly absent, and these subjects could suffer from drug toxicities or adverse drug reactions [Zhou et al. 2009]. *In vivo* biotransformation of celecoxib, a cyclooxygenase (COX)-2 inhibitor, is affected by CYP2C9 polymorphisms [Guengerich 2005] and thus is object of interest as a potential probe substrate. CYP2C9 protein levels correlate with hexobarbital C3-hydroxylation activity [Kato et al. 1992] and Rendic mentions hexobarbital among CYP2C9 probe substrates [Rendic 2002] .

Probe	CYP2C9-specific reaction
diclofenac	4'-hydroxylation
losartan	oxidation
phenytoin	4'-hydroxylation
S-flurbiprofen	4'-hydroxylation
S-warfarin	7-hydroxylation
tolbutamide	methylhydroxylation

Table 2. Probes for CYP2C9 metabolic activity assessment [Zhou et al. 2009]

2.2.3 CYP2C19

Folowing CYP2D6 and CYP2C9, CYP2C19 is the third well investigated polymorphic drug-metabolizing enzyme. CYP2C19 metabolizes many psychoactive drugs. Many of them are able to inhibit CYP2C19 metabolic activity. Probes for CYP2C19 metabolic activity assessment are summarized in Table 3.

Probe	CYP2C19-specific reaction
chloroguanine (proguanil)	conversion to cycloguanine
omeprazole	5-hydroxylation
S-mephenytoin	4'- hydroxylation

Table 3. Probes for CYP2C19 metabolic activity assessment [FDA 2006, Nolin & Frye 2003, Tenneze et al. 1999]

2.2.4 CYP2D6

Suitable substrates for *in vivo* CYP2D6 phenotyping are listed in the Table 4. Among them, bufuralol and dextromethorphan are the most preferred substrates for *in vitro* preclinical studies [Zhou 2009]. Tramadol is metabolized to O-demethyltramadol (M1) by CYP2D6, but in studies *in vitro* was shown that M1 formation is mediated also by CYP2B6 in high extent. Moreover, correlation of tramadol/M1 metabolic ratio with MR of dextromethorphan/dextrorphan is modest and therefore tramadol use as a probe substrate is limited [Frank et al. 2007]. Since debrisoquine and sparteine are currently not available as registered drugs, dextromethorphan remains the most widely used probe drug for CYP2D6 metabolic activity assessment *in vivo* [Zhou 2009].

Probe	CYP2D6-specific reaction
codeine	O-demethylation
debrisoquine	4-hydroxylation
dextromethorphan	O-demethylation
metoprolol	α-hydroxylation
sparteine	dehydrogenation
tramadol	O-demethylation

Table 4. Probes for CYP2D6 metabolic activity assessment [Rasmussen et al. 1998, Rendic 2002, Zanger et al. 2004, Zhou 2009].

2.2.5 CYP3A4

CYP3A4 is the predominant enzyme of CYP3A subfamily and plays the pivot role in drug metabolism [Guengerich 2005]. Hepatic CYP3A4 metabolizes about 50 % of clinically used drugs [Guengrich 1999] and CYP3A4 is the most abundant intestinal CYP enzyme [Guengerich 2005]. CYP3A4 is not supposed to be polymorphic as e.g. CYP2D6, but CYP3A4 activity may vary among individuals from 5 up to 50 fold [Ma et al. 2002]. Metabolic activity of CYP3A4 (expressed as log MR) has unimodal distribution; variation is probably a consequence of both genetic and non-genetic factors [Guengrich 1999, Ozdemir et al. 2000, Shimada et al. 1994, Wilkinson 1996]. Common probes for CYP3A4 metabolic ativity assessment are listed in the Table 5.

Probe	CYP3A4-specific reaction
alfentanil	demethylation
alprazolam	4-hydroxylation
codeine	O-demethylation
cortisol	6-β hydroxylation
dapsone	N-hydroxylation
dextromethorphan	N-demethylation
erythromycin	N-demethylation
lidocaine	N-deethylation
midazolam	1-hydroxylation
nifedipine	oxidation
quinidine	3-hydroxylation / N-oxidation
testosterone	6-β hydroxylation
triazolam	1-hydroxylation

Table 5. Probes for CYP3A4 metabolic activity assessment [Liu et al. 2007, Rasmussen et al. 1998, Rendic 2002, Wennerholm et al. 2005]

Since none of suggested probes for CYP3A4 phenotyping is metabolized uniquely by this enzyme, and the active site of CYP3A4 is thought to be large and able to bind multiple substrates simultaneously, it is recommended to use at least 2 structurally unrelated probe substrates for precise enzyme activity evaluation [Ekroos & Sjogren 2006, Foti et al. 2010, Liu et al. 2007]. The apparent metabolic activity of CYP3A4 (assessed using probe substrates) may be affected by P-glycoprotein mediated decrease of availability of probe substrates [Guengerich 2005].

By this, some authors suggest that there are no useful CYP3A4 substrates for accurate prediction of its metabolic activity [Benet 2005].

2.3 Differentiation between poor and extensive metabolizers: MR cut-off values

2.3.1 CYP1A2

Caffeine is the most frequently used probe drug and several metabolic ratios are used for CYP1A2 phenotyping. Urinary MR of (AFMU + 1U + 1X)/17U (also named as caffeine metabolic ratio, CMR) is probably mostly utilized [Campbell et al. 1987], followed by urinary MR of (17X + 17U)/137X [Muscat et al. 2008, Schrenk et al. 1998], salivary and plasmatic MR of 17X /137X [Fuhr et al. 1996, Simon et al. 2001] or MR of (AFMU + 1U + 1X + 17U + 17X)/137X in serum [Aklillu et al. 2003]. Due to several MRs used, there is not the only one, clear, and widely accepted MR cut-off value distinguishing poor and extensive metabolizers. Furthermore, bimodal or trimodal distribution of MR may be observed depending on the kind of ratio used [Muscat et al. 2008]. Using MR of (AFMU + 1U + 1X + 17U + 17X)/137X in serum, log MR of 0.96 (corresponding MR = 9.12) was found to distinguish PM from EM [Aklillu et al. 2003]. Other authors assessed CYP1A2 phenotype using molar ratio of 17X/137X in the 4 h urine samples, and observed a bimodal distribution with a cut point of 1.85 separating poore and extensive phenotypes [Muscat et al. 2008]. Histograms of serum 17X/137X ratio indicated the antimode of 0.16 [Han et al. 2001].

Metabolic ratio of AFMU/(AFMU +1U +1X) with an apparent antimode at 0.25 may serve for NAT2 phenotyping - subjects with metabolic ratios < 0.25 were then classified as slow acetylators and those with metabolic ratios > 0.25 as fast acetylators [Begas et al. 2007, Bendriss et al. 2000]. Some other authors suggest and use antimode of 0.34 of the same ratio [Nyeki et al. 2001, Tang et al. 1991].

Total salivary caffeine assessment (TOSCA) as a measure of general liver function was used for identification of patients with liver cirrhosis, with a cut-off value of 4.2 µg/ml, but TOSCA was not used for CYP1A2 phenotyping [Tarantino et al. 2006].

*abbreviations
137X   = 1,3,7 trimethylxanthine or caffeine
17X   = 1,7-dimethylxanthine or paraxanthine
AFMU   = 5-acetylamino-6-formylamino-3-methyluracil
1U   = 1-methyluric acid
1X   = 1-methylxanthine
17U   = 1,7-dimethyluric acid

2.3.2 CYP2C9

Phenytoin: Phenytoin hydroxylation index (amount of phenytoin administered/0-32 hr urinary output of hydroxyphenytoin) seems to be bimodaly distributed in population [Horsmans et al. 1997]. MR of 4-hydroxyphenytoin/phenytoin reveals a bimodal distribution although substantial overlap of this MR was seen between genetic variants of CYP2C9 [Aynacioglu et al. 1999]. Nevertheless, clear cut-off MR values are not suggested.

Tolbutamide: Tolbutamide metabolism appears to be depend on CYP2C9 genotype [Lee et al. 2005], but there was not suggested a clear MR (tolbutamide/4-hydroxytolbutamide) cut-off value to distinguish poor and extensive metabolizers.

2.3.3 CYP2C19

Omeprazole: Omeprazole is hydroxylated in position 5 to form 5-hydroxyomeprazole. A bimodal distribution of omeprazole to 5-hydroxyomeprazole metabolic ratio histograms and probit plots is observed. Using above mentioned MR, there was found antimode of 5.6 to distinguish between poor and extensive metabolizers in Chinese population [Wang et al. 2007]. Different antimode of 12.0 distinguishing poor and extensive metabolizers was found when used MR of omeprazole + omeprazole sulfone /5'-hydroxyomeprazole [Rost et al. 1995].

Mephenytoin: Both urinary 4-hydroxymephenytoin and the S/R enantiomer ratio of mephenytoin are able to discriminate between extensive and poor metabolizers [Wedlund et al. 1984]. In Chinese population sample, when S/R mephenytoin ratio was analyzed, probit plot suggested antimode of 0.8 distinguishing poor and extensive metabolizers [Demorais et al. 1995]. Antimode of 2 % of dose excreted as 4-hydroxymephenytoin has been used to distinguish poor and extensive metabolizers [Demorais et al. 1995]. An antimode of 1.0 in the log-mephenytoin hydroxylation index [log10 (μmol dose S-mephenytoin/μmol 4'-hydroxymephenytoin excreted in 8-h urine], was used to classify the extensive and poor metabolizers [Yin et al. 2004].

Proguanil: Bimodal distribution of proguanil/cycloguanil MR was observed in Polynesian population with antimode of 10.0 [Wanwimolruk et al. 1998]. The same antimode was reported by Australian study [Coller et al. 1997].

2.3.4 CYP2D6

Dextromethorphan: Eight-hour urinary MR of dextromethorphan to dextrorphan (conjugated + unconjugated) with 0.3 as a cut-off value is well established and used to differentiate between extensive and poor metabolizers [Chladek et al. 2000, Ito et al. 2010, Lotsch et al. 2009, O'Mathuna et al. 2008]. Urinary metabolic ratios based on free compounds (with an antimode of 4.0) also correlated with the conventional MR [Yeh et al. 2003]. Collection of urine during 8 hour (sometimes also 24 h) interval could be demanding process. Therefore alternative procedures have been developed for easier phenotyping. In addition to urine, saliva or plasma samples can also be used for the determination of MR [Chladek et al. 1997]. The serum $MR_{DEM/DOR}$ may serve as alternative tool for CYP2D6 phenotyping as also our results indicate tight correlation (r2 = 0.87) exists between $MR_{DEM/DOR}$ measured in serum (3h postdose) and $MR_{DEM/DOR}$ measured in urine (0-8 h postdose). Another approach has been tried for CYP2D6 phenotyping [Hu et al. 1998], in which a single or multiple-dose controlled-release dextromethorphan tablets were administered. It has been demonstrated that there is a good correlation between MR after single-dose and multiple-dose dextromethorphan as well as between MRs assessed in various kinds of samples [Hu et al. 1998, Yeh et al. 2003]. Plasmatic (or serum) 3, 4 or 6 hour MRs and salivary 2, 3, 4, 5, 6 hour MRs were investigated regarding possibility to discriminate EM from PM and alternatively also from IM [Frank et al. 2007]. However, only 3 studies have determined the cut-off values for plasma or serum MR, namely those of Shiran et al. who determined the value of 0.1 for differentiating between EM and PM (using 3-hour postdose $MR_{DEM/DOR}$)[Shiran et al. 2003]. The others, observed antimode of 2.0 to delineate EM from IM (using any time point in steady state) [Yeh et al. 2003], and Kohler et al. found the intercept separating EM from PM to be 0.126 (1-hour postdose $MR_{DEM/DOR}$) [Kohler et al. 1997]. These results are in accordance with our results showing a cut-off found for serum $MR_{DEM/DOR}$ to discriminate between poor metabolizers from either extensive or extensive+intermediate metabolizers, but not for serum $MR_{DEM/DOR}$ to discriminate extensive metabolizers from intermediate metabolizers. On the other hand, it has been suggested, that it is not possible to delineate EM from IM using plasma MR [Hu et al. 1998]. In conclusion, there is a lack of evidence for clear plasma/serum or saliva dextromethorphan MR cut-off values. As the most used and best proved remains the urinary 0 - 8 h dextromethorphan to dextrorphan MR [Frank et al. 2007], but alternative procedures for phenotyping may be usefull in some groups of patients.

Debrisoquine: MR of debrisoquine/4-OH debrisoquine in urine collected for 8 hours serves as a well proved determinant of metabolic status: a bimodal distribution was observed in Caucasian population with antimode of 12.6 separating EM (MR < 12.6) from PM (MR > 12.6) [Eiermann et al. 1998, Sachse et al. 1997]. For debrisoquine, there is not recommended any other sampling interval or other way of phenotypization except of urine 0 - 8h MR.

Sparteine: MR of sparteine/sum of dehydrosparteines in urine collected 0 - 6 h post-dose is used for phenotype assessment, with 20.0 as the conventional cut-off point between PM and EM subjects [Basci et al. 1994, Paar et al. 1997]. This value was suggested to be slightly modified to 14.0 in another study [Halling et al. 2005].

2.3.5 CYP3A4

There is a lack of evidence for existence of a bimodal distribution of CYP3A4 activity and therefore there is no consensus for antimode or cut-off values in any of used probe substrates.

2.4 Breath tests and other approaches for CYP enzyme activity assessment

Erythromycine breath test (EBT) is probably one of the best proved models for CYP3A4 activity assessment. The hepatic CYP3A4 catalyzes *N*-demethylation of $[^{14}C]$-erythromycin with subsequent formation of CO_2, and therefore the metabolic activity of this enzyme may be expressed as the amount of the expired $^{14}CO_2$ [Liu et al. 2007, Watkins 1994].

Similar breath tests detecting radiolabeled metabolites (or ratio of $^{14}CO_2$ or $^{13}CO_2$ to $^{12}CO_2$) were designed for phynotyping CYP2C19 with use of $[^{13}C]$ pantoprazole [Furuta et al. 2009], and CYP1A2 with the use of $[^{14}C]$ caffeine [Kalow & Tang 1993]. Multiple CYP metabolic activities (CYP2C19, 1A2, 3A4, and 2C9) were evaluated with $[^{13}C]$-aminophenazone ("aminopyrine breath test") [Kodaira et al. 2011]. CYP2E1 activity in rats was measured using $[^{14}C]$ nitrosodimethylamine as a probe substrate [Bastien & Villeneuve 1998].

2.5 Miotic response to opioids

Significant correlations were observed between alfentanil pharmacokinetic parameters and its induced miotic kinetic parameters either under ambient or dark conditions. This means that pupillary response after alfentanil administration may be used as noninvasive measure of CYP3A4 metabolic activity [Baririan et al. 2005, Kharasch et al. 2004, Klees et al. 2005].

O-demethylation of tramadol has been tried as a probe reaction for CYP2D6 phenotyping [Frank et al. 2007]. Pharmacokinetic parameters of its metabolite, *O*-demethyltramadol (M1) correlates well with pupillary constriction after tramadol administration. Since intrinsic efficacy of M1 is higher than of tramadol, higher pupillary constriction was observed in EM subjects [Slanar et al. 2007]. Interestingly, it was observed not only different patterns of miotic response between PM and EM groups, but also difference in the kinetic parameters (median time to reach max. miosis) between heterozygous and homozygous EM [Slanar et al. 2007]. It seems possible to discriminate EM from PM on the basis of the miotic response after tramadol administration [Slanar et al. 2007].

2.6 Cocktail approaches

In early phase of drug development, there are utilized so called "high-throughput" methods increasing the efficiency and effectiveness of assay to assess metabolic activity of many CYP enzymes in short time [Smith et al. 2007, Testino & Patonay 2003, Zlokarnik et al. 2005]. Investigative methodologies for CYP enzymes often utilize so-called "cocktail" of markers to assess the metabolic activity of multiple CYP forms in one session [Asimus et al. 2007, Frye et al. 1997, Kumar et al. 2007, Smith et al. 2007, Tanaka et al. 2003, Yao, M. et al. 2007, Yao, Y.M. et al. 2007]. This approach is used either for *in vivo* or *in vitro* metabolic assessment. The markers of metabolic activity and their enzyme-specific metabolites can be assessed either simultaneously or separately [Blakey et al. 2004, Sharma et al. 2004]. A well known advantage of the cocktail approach is obtaining information of multiple CYP enzymes in a single experimental session [Tanaka et al. 2003]. Several different cocktails of markers have been used for this purpose (Table 6) [Asimus et al. 2007, Dierks et al. 2001, Sharma et al. 2004, Zhou et al. 2004]; as a "cocktail" is sometimes called any combination of at least 2 probe drugs, but generally from three up to six probes have been tried for *in vivo* CYP phenotyping [Zhou et al. 2004]. Among the most frequently used is e.g. "Pitsburgh cocktail": caffeine, chlorzoxazone, dapsone, debrisoquine, and mephenytoin for the combined assessment of CYP1A2, CYP2E1, CYP2D6, CYP2C19, CYP3A and N-acetyltransferase activities [Zhou et al. 2004]. Unfortunately, the disadvantages of cocktail approach are also well defined: the frequent occurrence of adverse effects due to various pharmacodynamic-based interactions, more sample consumption (collection) for analysis and more complicated analytical methods [Tanaka et al. 2003]. After developing precise analytical methods, the cocktail approach became widely used and is now one of the basic analytical tools in early drug development (*in vitro* cocktails) [Zlokarnik et al. 2005]. Methods utilizing reaction with a marker and subsequent chromatographic analysis are recommended by the FDA in initial drug evaluations for investigating pharmacokinetic interactions with CYP enzymes [FDA 2006] (in contrast to some other high throughput methods). On the other hand, a "cocktail" approach can open a further question - can one marker influence the biotransformation rate of the other one? In some of these "cocktails", it was proved that the rates of biotransformation of single substrates are not affected by other drugs coadministered, but there are some examples that one probe substrate may affect the biotransformation rate of another one. Namely, there were reported an inhibition of midazolam metabolism by chlorzoxazone in humans [Palmer et al. 2001], inhibition of nifedipine aromatization and sparteine dehydrogenation by quinidine in humans [Schellens et al. 1991], increase in phenacetin deethylation by tolbutamide in rats [Jurica et al. 2009]. Therefore, such assay may provide invalid (or at least inaccurate) results [Palmer et al. 2001]. Review of cocktails used *in vivo* is given in the Table 6. Except of these, only few other combinations of probe substrates have been used, e.g. assessment of CYP2A6 metabolic activity (coumarin) with CYP2D6 (dextromethorphan) and CYP2C19 (mephenytoin) [Endres et al. 1996].

3. *In vitro* CYP activity assessment

The specific probe substrates for CYP activity assessment and inhibition studies are used in the preclinical drug development as well as for clinical purpose. Research in this field is carried out on various models (human liver microsomes, recombinant CYP enzymes, hepatocytes, precision-cut human liver slices, organ perfusions etc.) which enables use of wide range of techniques and model substrates (e.g. luminometric, fluorometric,

Note	CYP1A2	CYP2C9	CYP2C19	CYP2D6	CYP2E1	CYP3A4	Ref.
GW cocktail	caffeine	diclofenac	mephenytoin	debrisoquine	chlorzoxazone	midazolam	[Scott et al. 1999]
	caffeine	diclofenac	mephenytoin	debrisoquine		midazolam	[Palmer et al. 2001]
Karolinska cocktail	caffeine	losartan	omeprazole			quinine	[Christensen et al. 2003]
	caffeine	warfarin + vit. K	mephenytoin	debrisoquine	chlorzoxazone	dapsone	[Frye et al. 1997]
Coperstown 5+1 cocktail	caffeine		omeprazole	dextromethorphan		midazolam	[Shelepova et al. 2003]
	caffeine	tolbutamide		dextromethorphan		midazolam	[Bruce et al. 2001, Gorski et al. 2000, Wang et al. 2001]
	caffeine	tolbutamide	mephenytoin			midazolam	[Tomalik-Scharte et al. 2005]
Coperstown cocktail	caffeine		omeprazole	dextromethorphan		midazolam	[Streetman et al. 2000]
	caffeine	tolbutamide	omeprazole	dextromethorphan		dapsone	[Gupta et al. 2011]
	caffeine	tolbutamide		dextromethorphan		midazolam	[Zhang et al. 2010]
	theophylline	tolbutamide		dextromethorphan		midazolam	[Ardjomand-Woelkart et al. 2011]
used in rats	caffeine	phenytoin	mephenytoin	debrisoquine		lidocaine	[Tanaka et al. 1995]
used in rats	caffeine		mephenytoin			dapsone	[Black et al. 1992]
				dextromethorphan	trimethadione	lidocaine	[Tanaka et al. 1994]
							[Brockmoller & Roots 1994]
	caffeine	flurbiprofen	mephenytoin	metoprolol		dapsone	[Setiabudy et al. 1995]
			omeprazole				[Jenkins et al. 2010]

Table 6. Probe substrate combinations for *in vivo* CYP activity assessment (adapted from [Tanaka et al. 2003, Zhou et al. 2004])

radiolabeled etc.). *In vitro* methods are mostly used in preclinical drug development to predict possible CYP-mediated pharmacokinetic interactions. Unfortunately, there is a consensus that a prediction of *in vivo* interactions from *in vitro* data is not reliable. Moreover, as some authors hypothesize, in case of CYP3A4, any inductive or inhibitory effect observed in study with one probe CYP3A4 substrate can not accurately predict the extent of the *in vivo* interaction for another CYP3A4 substrate [Benet 2005]. FDA recommends suitable probe substrates for *in vitro* experiments in the drug development [FDA 2006]. These substrates are also mentioned in the appropriate tables below.

3.1 Conventional probe substrates used *in vitro*

3.1.1 CYP1A2

Simple *in vitro* spectrophotometric methods like ethoxyresorufin *O*-deethylation (EROD) and methoxyresorufin *O*-demethylation (MROD) are frequently utilized in CYP1A metabolic activity assessment. These probe substrates were used in various models with liver microsomes from human, monkey, rat and mouse [FDA 2006, Hanioka et al. 2000, Chun et al. 1999]. Besides these, conventional probe substrates (registered drugs) are used *in vitro* as well (Table 7).

Probe	CYP1A2-specific reaction
acetanilide	C$_4$- hydroxylation
7-ethoxyresorufin	*O*-deethylation
7-methoxyresorufin	*O*-demethylation
caffeine	*N*-demethylation
phenacetine	*O*-deethylation
tacrine	1-hydroxylation
theophylline	*N*-demethylation

Table 7. *In vitro* probes for CYP1A2 metabolic activity assessment [Henderson et al. 2000, Rendic 2002, Yuan et al. 2002]

3.1.2 CYP2C9

Despite that probe substrates are in general supposed to be highly specific and selective towards individual CYP forms, it was reported that with use of (*S*)-warfarin as a CYP2C9 probe, significantly lower Ki values were obtained when compared to diclofenac, flurbiprofen, phenytoin or tolbutamide [Foti et al. 2010, Kumar et al. 2006]. Selective probe substrates for CYP2C9 *in vitro* activity assessment are summarized in the Table 8.

3.1.3 CYP2C19

Probe substrates for CYP2C19 activity assessment are summarized in the Table 9. As in the case of CYP2C9, also in CYP2C19 there were reported different sensitivities of probe substrates to inhibitors. (*S*)-mephenytoin was the most sensitive to a set of inhibitors when compared to (*S*)- or (*R*)-omeprazole or (*S*)-fluoxetine [Foti & Wahlstrom 2008, Foti et al. 2010].

Probe	CYP2C9-specific reaction
celecoxib	methyl hydroxylation
diclofenac	4'-hydroxylation
losartan	oxidation
naproxen	O-demethylation
Ppenytoin	4'-hydroxylation
S-flurbiprofen	4'-hydroxylation
S-warfarin	7-hydroxylation
tolbutamide	methylhydroxylation

Table 8. *In vitro* probes for CYP2C9 metabolic activity assessment [Hummel et al. 2004, Rendic 2002, Tang et al. 2000, Yuan et al. 2002]

Probe	CYP2C19-specific reaction
R-omeprazole	5-hydroxylation
S-fluoxetine	O-dealkylation
S-mephenytoin	4'-hydroxylation
S-omeprazole	5-hydroxylation

Table 9. *In vitro* probes for CYP2C19 metabolic activity assessment [FDA 2006, Yuan et al. 2002]

3.1.4 CYP2D6

In vitro CYP2D6 metabolic activity may be evaluated using the same substrates as *in vivo*. Except of these, bufuralol, and some fluorogenic probes were used to evaluate CYP2D6 activity *in vitro* [Wang et al. 2009] (Table 10). Bufuralol is also metabolized via CYP2C19 [Mankowski 1999] and CYP1A2 [Yamazaki et al. 1994], therefore its specificity for CYP2D6 may be decreased. Nevertheless, bufuralol is the most preferred *in vitro* probe substrate (60 % of *in vitro* studies) followed by dextromethorphan (30 % of *in vitro* studies) [Zhou 2009]. FDA recommends to use bufuralol, dextromethorphan or debrisoquine for *in vitro* experiments [FDA 2006].

Probe	CYP2D6-specific reaction
bufuralol	1-hydroxylation
debrisoquine	4-hydroxylation
carteolol	C_8-hydroxylation
dextromethorphan	O-demethylation
metoprolol	α-hydroxylation
sparteine	dehydrogenation
tramadol	O-demethylation

Table 10. *In vitro* probes for CYP2D6 metabolic activity assessment [FDA 2006, Frank et al. 2007, Kudo & Odomi 1998, Rendic 2002, Zhou 2009]

3.1.5 CYP3A4

Besides probe drugs used *in vivo*, some other conventional substrates are also used *in vitro* (listed in Table 11). As it was already mentioned above, it is strongly recommended to use at least 2 structurally urelated probe substrates for CYP3A4 meabolic activity evaluation.

Standard inhibitors are used in preclinical drug development for evaluation of the inhibitory potency of new chemical entity or to identify individual CYP enzymes responsible for a drug's metabolism, and to determine the relative contribution of an individual CYP enzyme to biotransformation of evaluated chemical entity (Table 12).

Probe	CYP3A4-specific reaction
alfentanil	demethylation
alprazolam	4-hydroxylation
benzyloxyresorufin	O-dealkylation
cortisol	6-β hydroxylation
cyclosporine	oxidation
dextromethorphan	N-demethylation
diazepam	N-demethylation
erythromycin	N-demethylation
ethylmorphine	N-demethylation
midazolam	1-hydroxylation
nifedipine	oxidation
quinidine	3-hydroxylation / N-oxidation
terfenadine	C-hydroxylation
testosterone	6-β hydroxylation
triazolam	1-hydroxylation

Table 11. *In vitro* probes for CYP3A4 metabolic activity assessment [FDA 2006, Meyer et al. 2010, Yuan et al. 2002]

CYP enzyme	Inhibitor	Ki (μM)
CYP1A2	α-naphthoflavone	0.01
	furafylline	0.6 - 0.73
CYP2C9	fluconazole	7
	fluvoxamine	6.4 - 19
	fluoxetine	18 - 41
	sulfaphenazole	0.3
CYP2C19	nootkatone	0.5
	ticlopidine	1.2
CYP2D6	quinidine	0.027 - 0.4
CYP3A4	itraconazole	0.27; 2.3
	ketoconazole	0.0037 - 0.18

Table 12. Inhibitors of CYP enzymes recommended by FDA for *in vitro* use (adapted from [FDA 2006])

3.2 High throughput methods for CYP metabolic activity assays

In past two decades, the role of *in vitro* drug metabolism and toxicity studies is slightly changing. Absorption, distribution, metabolism, excretion and toxicity studies (ADMET) have formerly been performed with a few compounds in the late stages of drug development. The number of compounds entering the drug discovery is increasing what requires to perform ADMET studies at earlier stages in the drug development [Atterwill & Wing 2002, Trubetskoy et al. 2005].

Therefore, there is a need for new generation of assays with higher throughput capability, sensitivity and reproducibility. These assays are often automated and miniaturized. Plate-scanning readers and handling robots, multi-channel analyzers, high-density assay plates together with automated LC-MS systems are mostly mentioned as the major support for such high throughput methods [Zlokarnik et al. 2005]. Thanks to these techniques, these approaches are also cheaper than standard procedures, maintaining sufficient selectivity, sensitivity and precision, and enable testing of large sets of compounds.

3.2.1 Radiolabeled substrates

Detection of $^{13/14}C$ or ^3H metabolites ($H^{13/14}CHO$ and/or $^{13/14}CO_2$) of radiolabeled substrates (erythromycin, caffeine, cyclosporine, aminophenazone, diazepam etc.) is used in some *in vitro* studies to assess metabolic activity of CYP3A4 [Grand et al. 2002, Kenworthy et al. 1999]. Metabolites may be detected radiochemically, ^{14}C-formaldehyde may be extracted and detected by radioluminescence in a microplate scintillation counter [Zlokarnik et al. 2005]. In general, detection of radiolabeled substrates and metabolites seems to provide better limits of detection, accuracy and sensitivity than other conventional methods. Other advantage (over fluorogenic and luminogenic probe substrates) of this approach is ability to use common probe substrates with well known specificity, kinetic parameters and solubility [Zlokarnik et al. 2005].

3.2.2 Fluorogenic substrates

Fluorogenic substrates are used *in vitro* very often. In general, these substrates are structurally modified fluorogenic compounds which are metabolized via various CYP forms to generate a fluorescent dye. These substrates are commercially available and widely used in preclinical drug development. Due to insufficient selectivity towards single CYP enzyme, these substrates are mostly used in recombinant CYP enzymes [Foti et al. 2010]. On the other hand, some of the fluorogenic substrates seem to be isoform-specific in lower concentrations, such as 3-O-methylfluorescein, which was evaluated for selectivity towards CYP2C19 [Sudsakorn et al. 2007].

These difficulties are pronounced in many probe substrates - the most widely used fluorogenic substrate for assessment of CYP2C9 activity *in vitro* is 7-methoxy-4-trifluoromethylcoumarin (MFC) [Crespi & Stresser 2000]. Despite this, some controversy about the selectivity of MFC towards CYP2C9 (the participation of several CYP enzymes in MFC O-demethylation) was also reported [Porrogi et al. 2008]. Nevertheless, MFC-based fluorometric CYP2C9 assays are described as "rapid with a high-throughput screening capacity, easy to perform, and amenable to automation" [Zhou et al. 2009]. Overview of fluorogenic substrates for individual CYP enzymes is given in the Table 13.

CYP enzyme	Probe substrate	Product / commercial name
CYP1A2	3-cyano-7-ethoxycoumarin (CEC)	3-cyano-7-hydroxycoumarin (CHC)
	7-ethoxy-methyloxy-3-cyanocoumarin (EOMCC)	Vivid Blue
CYP2C9	7-methoxy-4-(trifluoromethyl)-coumarin (7-MFC)	7-hydroxy-4-(trifluoromethyl)-coumarin (HFC)
	dibenzylfluorescein (DBF)	fluorescein
	7-benzyloxy-methyloxy-3-cyanocoumarin (BOMCC)	Vivid Blue
	N-octyloxymethyl-resorufin (OOMR)	Vivid Red
	benzyloxy-methyl-fluorescein (BOMF)	Vivid Green
CYP2C19	3-cyano-7-ethyoxycoumarin (CEC)	3-cyano-7-hydroxycoumarin (CHC)
	dibenzylfluorescein (DBF)	fluorescein
	3-O-methylfluorescein (OMF)	fluorescein
	7-ethoxy-methyloxy-3-cyanocoumarin (EOMCC)	Vivid Blue
CYP2D6	7-methoxy-4-(aminomethyl)-coumarin (MAMC)	7-hydroxy-4-(aminomethyl)-coumarin (HAMC)
	3-[2-(N,N diethyl-N-methylammonium)ethyl]-7-methoxy-4-methylcoumarin (AMMC)	3-[2-(diethylamino)-ethyl]-7-hydroxy-4-methylcoumarin (AHMC)
	7- p-methoxy-benzyloxy-4-trifluorocoumarin (MOBFC)	Vivid Cyan
	7-ethoxy-methyloxy-3-cyanocoumarin (EOMCC)	Vivid Blue
CYP3A4	7-benzyloxy-trifluoromethylcoumarin (BFC)	7-hydroxy-4-(trifluoromethyl)-coumarin (HFC)
	7-benzyloxyquinoline (7-BQ)	quinolinol
	benzylresorufin	resorufin
	di(benzyloxymethoxy)fluorescein (DBF)	fluorescein
	benzyloxy-methyl-resorufin (BOMR)	Vivid Red
	dibenzylmethylfluorescein (DBOMF)	Vivid Green
	7-benzyloxy-methyloxy-3-cyanocoumarin (BOMCC)	Vivid Blue
	7-benzyloxy-methyloxy-4-(trifluoromethyl)-coumarin (BOMFC)	Vivid Cyan

Table 13. Fluorogenic substrates for *in vitro* CYP enzyme activity assessment (adapted from Foti et. al. [FDA 2006, Foti et al. 2010])

Some of disadvantages (background fluorescence of unmetabolized substrate, low aqueous solubility, and low signal-to-noise ratio) which may limit the use of fluorescent substrates [Trubetskoy et al. 2005] were resolved by structurally related derivatives (e.g.

oxyphenylmethyl- , oxymethyl-, octyloxymethyl-) of commonly available substrates such as resorufin (red), coumarin (blue and cyan) and fluorescein (green). Currently (2011), there are available 8 modified fluorescent substrates for CYP1A2, CYP2B6, CYP2C9, CYP2C19, CYP2D6, CYP2E1, CYP3A4, CYP3A5 metabolic activities assessment [Makings & Zlokarnik 2011]. Similarly to other common fluorogenic substrates, these derivatives were synthetized as "blocked" fluorophores with negligible background fluorescence (lower than in common fluorogenic probes). Fluorescence signal is triggered after isoenzyme specific biotransformation (Fig. 1) [Marks et al. 2003]. Moreover, these modified (Vivid®) substrates exhibit higher aqueous solubility and their molecule contains 2 potential cleavage sites [Marks et al. 2003]. Fluorogenic assays may be performed in miniaturized form in microplates.

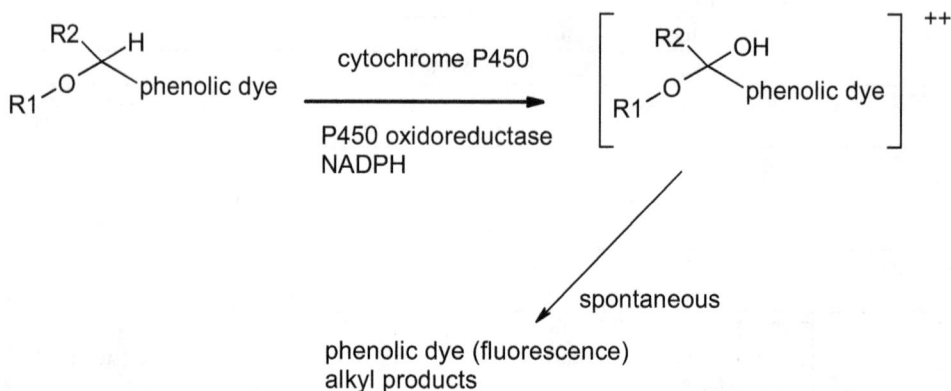

Fig. 1. Illustrative reaction of fluorescent CYP probe substrate (adapted from [Makings & Zlokarnik 2011].

3.2.3 Luminometric substrates

Luminometric substrate probes are used for CYP activity assessment since 2003. These probes are derivatives of luciferin, substrate for the firefly luciferase which generates light. The derivatives have to be metabolized by CYP enzymes to form luciferin prior to the reaction with luciferase and light emission [Cali et al. 2003]. Then, recorded luminiscence is proportional to the amount of metabolite what is dependent on activity of the CYP enzyme. Illustrative example of reaction is given in Figure 2.

Various bioluminometric probe substrates (derivatives of luciferin) to test CYP1A1, CYP1A2, CYP2C9, CYP2C19, CYP2D6, CYP3A4, MAO-A and MAO-B activity are available. Luciferin 6´ chloroethyl ether (Luciferin –CEE) is a substrate for CYP1A1 and CYP1B1, luciferin 6´ methyl ether (Luciferin-ME) for CYP1A2 and CYP2C8, 6´ deoxyluciferin (luciferin-H) for CYP2C9, ethylene glycol ester of luciferin 6'-methyl ether (Luciferin-ME EGE) for CYP2D6, 6-deoxyluciferin ethyleneglycol ester (Luciferin-H EGE) for CYP2C19, luciferin 6´ benzyl ether (Luciferin –BE) and luciferin 6´ pentafluorobenzyl ether (Luciferin-PFBE) for CYP3A4 and CYP3A7, luciferin phenylpiperazine xylene ether (Luciferin-PPXE) and the latest one developed, luciferin isopropylacetal (Luciferin-IPA) for CYP3A4.

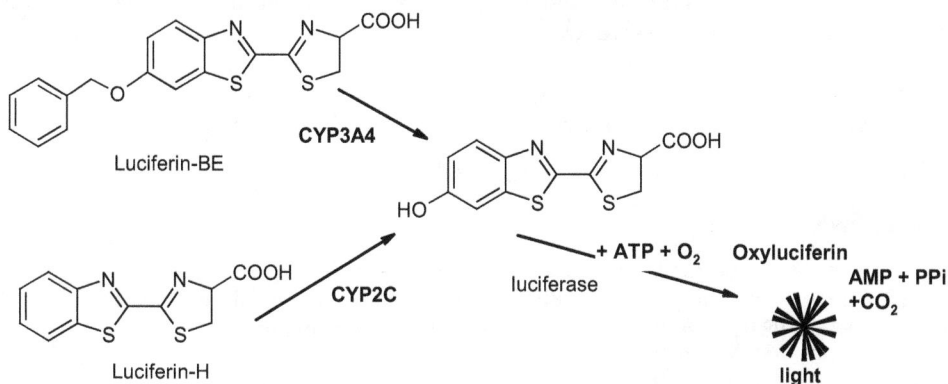

Fig. 2. Examples of CYP – mediated activation of luciferin (adapted from [Cali et al. 2011])

These methods may be also automated, miniaturized and used in "high-throughput" mode, in 3 or 6 µl 1536-well plates and low volume 384- well plates. The signal half-life of over 2 hours enables batch processing of plates [Cali et al. 2008].

4. Conclusion

The selection of probe drug for either assessment of CYP metabolic activity *in vitro* or *in vivo* phenotyping is crucial for results of CYP metabolic activity assessment. Despite undeniable selectivity of probe substrates it seems that selection of distinct probe substrate may influence results obtained either *in vitro* or *in vivo* [Kumar et al. 2006, Stein et al. 1996]. The selection of appropriate probe drugs also depends on the system used - for *in vivo* phenotyping are used only conventional substrates (the registered drugs or endogenous substrate). A wide scale of substrates may be chosen for various *in vitro* systems such as human liver microsomes, recombinant CYP enzymes, hepatocytes, tissue slices and isolated organ perfusions. Conventional probe substrates mimics well the properties of other drugs, but the metabolites have to be analyzed by HPLC, mostly with MS, UV, fluorescence or electrochemical detection, or occasionally also with capillary electrophoretic methods [Konecny et al. 2007].

In addition, in CYP3A4 it is recommended to use at least 2 structurally unrelated probe substrates because of presence of multiple substrate binding domains within CYP3A4 protein [Khan et al. 2002, Korzekwa et al. 1998, Schrag & Wienkers 2001, Tucker et al. 2001]. Published crystal structures of CYP enzymes confirmed the ability of individual CYP enzyme to metabolize a wide range of substrates or to bind multiple substrate/inhibitor molecules simultaneously [Ekroos & Sjogren 2006, Foti et al. 2010].

In some CYP forms, it seems that polymorphisms may have variable consequences in different substrates, as was shown in the case of CYP2D6 and CYP2C19. This phenomenon is also described as allele-dependent differences of substrates [Benet 2005]. In detail, this means that in the case of polymorphism CYP2D6*17, the rate of metabolism depends on the substrate used [Bogni et al. 2005, Zhou 2009].

Fluorogenic and bioluminometric probe substrates proved sufficiently their usability in early stages of drug development; these methods of CYP metabolic activity assessment are reproducible, robust and sensitive. On the other hand, since there is occasionally reported lack of correlation in specificity and sensitivity between fluorogenic and conventional probes (mostly in CYP3A4), follow-up studies with conventional probe substrates are strictly recommended to be performed in the clinical phase of new drug development [Cohen et al. 2003].

5. Acknowledgement

This chapter was supported by the project of Ministry of Health of Czech Republic: NS 9676-4/2008 and by the project "CEITEC - Central European Institute of Technology" (CZ.1.05/1.1.00/02.0068) from European Regional Development Fund.

6. References

Aklillu, E., J.A. Carrillo, E. Makonnen, K. Hellman, M. Pitarque, L. Bertilsson&M. Ingelman-Sundberg, (2003), Genetic polymorphism of CYP1A2 in ethiopians affecting induction and expression: Characterization of novel haplotypes with single-nucleotide polymorphisms in intron 1. *Molecular Pharmacology*, Vol. 64, No 3, pp. 659-669, 0026-895X.

Ardjomand-Woelkart, K., M. Kollroser, L. Li, H. Derendorf, V. Butterweck&R. Bauer, (2011), Development and validation of a LC-MS/MS method based on a new 96-well Hybrid-SPE (TM)-precipitation technique for quantification of CYP450 substrates/metabolites in rat plasma. *Analytical and Bioanalytical Chemistry*, Vol. 400, No 8, pp. 2371-2381, 1618-2642.

Asimus, S., D. Elsherbiny, T.N. Hai, B. Jansson, N.V. Huong, M.G. Petzold, U.S.H. Simonsson&M. Ashton, (2007), Artemisinin antimalarials moderately affect cytochrome P450 enzyme activity in healthy subjects. *Fundamental & Clinical Pharmacology*, Vol. 21, No 3, pp. 307-316, 0767-3981.

Atterwill, C.K.&M.G. Wing, (2002), In vitro preclinical lead optimisation technologies (PLOTs) in pharmaceutical development. *Toxicology Letters*, Vol. 127, No 1-3, pp. 143-151, 0378-4274.

Aynacioglu, A.S., J. Brockmoller, S. Bauer, C. Sachse, P. Guzelbey, Z. Ongen, M. Nacak&I. Roots, (1999), Frequency of cytochrome P450CYP2C9 variants in a Turkish population and functional relevance for phenytoin. *British Journal of Clinical Pharmacology*, Vol. 48, No 3, pp. 409-415, 0306-5251.

Baririan, N., Y. Horsmans, J.P. Desager, R. Verbeeck, R. Vanbinst, P. Wallemacq&L. Van Obbergh, (2005), Alfentanil-induced miosis clearance as a liver CYP3A4 and 3A5 activity measure in healthy volunteers: Improvement of experimental conditions. *Journal of Clinical Pharmacology*, Vol. 45, No 12, pp. 1434-1441, 0091-2700.

Basci, N.E., K. Brosen, A. Bozkurt, A. Isimer, A. Sayal&S.O. Kayaalp, (1994), S-Mephenytoin, Sparteine and Debrisoquine Oxidation - Genetic Polymorphisms in a Turkish Population. *British Journal of Clinical Pharmacology*, Vol. 38, No 5, pp. 463-465, 0306-5251.

Bastien, M.C.&J.P. Villeneuve, (1998), Characterization of cytochrome P450 2E1 activity by the [C-14]nitrosodimethylamine breath test. *Canadian Journal of Physiology and Pharmacology*, Vol. 76, No 7-8, pp. 756-763, 0008-4212.

Begas, E., E. Kouvaras, A. Tsakalof, S. Papakosta&E.K. Asprodini, (2007), In vivo evaluation of CYP1A2 CYP2A6, NAT-2 and xanthine oxidase activities in a Greek population sample by the RP-HPLC monitoring of caffeine metabolic ratios. *Biomedical Chromatography*, Vol. 21, No 2, pp. 190-200, 0269-3879.

Bendriss, E.K., N. Markoglou&I.W. Wainer, (2000), Liquid chromatographic method for the simultaneous determination of caffeine and fourteen caffeine metabolites in urine. *Journal of Chromatography B*, Vol. 746, No 2, pp. 331-338, 0378-4347.

Benet, L.Z., (2005), There are no useful CYP3A probes that quantitatively predict the in vivo kinetics of other CYP3A substrates and no expectation that one will be found. *Molecular Interventions*, Vol. 5, No 2, pp. 79-+, 1534-0384.

Black, C., M.E. Csuka, S. Lupoli, G.R. Wilkinson&R.A. Branch, (1992), Activity of Oxidative Routes of Metabolism of Debrisoquin, Mephenytoin, and Dapsone Is Unrelated to the Pathogenesis of Vinyl-Chloride Induced Disease. *Clinical Pharmacology & Therapeutics*, Vol. 52, No 6, pp. 659-667, 0009-9236.

Blakey, G.E., J.A. Lockton, J. Perrett, P. Norwood, M. Russell, Z. Aherne&J. Plume, (2004), Pharmacokinetic and pharmacodynamic assessment of a five-probe metabolic cocktail for CYPs 1A2, 3A4, 2C9, 2D6 and 2E1. *British Journal of Clinical Pharmacology*, Vol. 57, No 2, pp. 162-169, 0306-5251.

Bogni, A., M. Monshouwer, A. Moscone, M. Hidestrand, M. Ingelman-Sundberg, T. Hartung&S. Coecke, (2005), Substrate specific metabolism by polymorphic cytochrome P450 2D6 alleles. *Toxicology in Vitro*, Vol. 19, No 5, pp. 621-629, 0887-2333.

Bozikas, V.P., M. Papakosta, L. Niopas, A. Karavatos&V. Mirtsou-Fidani, (2004), Smoking impact on CYP1A2 activity in a group of patients with schizophrenia. *European Neuropsychopharmacology*, Vol. 14, No 1, pp. 39-44, 0924-977X.

Brockmoller, J.&I. Roots, (1994), Assessment of Liver Metabolic Function - Clinical Implications. *Clinical Pharmacokinetics*, Vol. 27, No 3, pp. 216-248, 0312-5963.

Bruce, M.A., S.D. Hall, B.D. Haehner-Daniels&J.C. Gorski, (2001), In vivo effect of clarithromycin on multiple cytochrome P450S. *Drug Metabolism and Disposition*, Vol. 29, No 7, pp. 1023-1028, 0090-9556.

Cali, J.J., S. Frackman, S. Ho, D.P. Ma, D. Simpson, W. Daily&D.H. Klaubert, (2003), Luminescent cytochrome P450 assays that utilize beetle luciferin derivatives as probe substrates. *Drug Metabolism Reviews*, Vol. 35, No pp. 44-44, 0360-2532.

Cali, J.J., D. Klaubert, W. Daily, S.K.S. Ho, S. Frackman, E. Hawkins&K.V. Wood, *Luminiscence-based methods and probes for measuring cytochrome P450 activity.* 2011, Promega Corp.: USA. p. 1-27.

Cali, J.J., A. Niles, M.P. Valley, M.A. O'Brien, T.L. Riss&J. Shultz, (2008), Bioluminescent assays for ADMET. *Expert Opinion on Drug Metabolism & Toxicology*, Vol. 4, No 1, pp. 103-120, 1742-5255.

Campbell, M.E., S.P. Spielberg&W. Kalow, (1987), A Urinary Metabolite Ratio That Reflects Systemic Caffeine Clearance. *Clinical Pharmacology & Therapeutics*, Vol. 42, No 2, pp. 157-165, 0009-9236.

Cohen, L.H., M.J. Remley, D. Raunig&A.D.N. Vaz, (2003), In vitro drug interactions of cytochrome P450: An evaluation of fluorogenic to conventional substrates. *Drug Metabolism and Disposition*, Vol. 31, No 8, pp. 1005-1015, 0090-9556.

Coller, J.K., A.A. Somogyi&F. Bochner, (1997), Association between CYP2C19 genotype and proguanil oxidative polymorphism. *British Journal of Clinical Pharmacology*, Vol. 43, No 6, pp. 659-660, 0306-5251.

Corruble, E., (2008), Non-response to consecutive antidepressant therapy caused by CYP2D6 ultrarapid metabolizer phenotype. *International Journal of Neuropsychopharmacology*, Vol. 11, No 5, pp. 727-728, 1461-1457.

Crespi, C.L.&D.M. Stresser, (2000), Fluorometric screening for metabolism-based drug-drug interactions. *Journal of Pharmacological and Toxicological Methods*, Vol. 44, No 1, pp. 325-331, 1056-8719.

Demorais, S.M.F., J.A. Goldstein, H.G. Xie, S.L. Huang, Y.Q. Lu, H. Xia, Z.S. Xiao, N. Ile&H.H. Zhou, (1995), Genetic-Analysis of the S-Mephenytoin Polymorphism in a Chinese Population. *Clinical Pharmacology & Therapeutics*, Vol. 58, No 4, pp. 404-411, 0009-9236.

Dierks, E.A., K.R. Stams, H.K. Lim, G. Cornelius, H.L. Zhang&S.E. Ball, (2001), A method for the simultaneous evaluation of the activities of seven major human drug-metabolizing cytochrome P450s using an in vitro cocktail of probe substrates and fast gradient liquid chromatography tandem mass spectrometry. *Drug Metabolism and Disposition*, Vol. 29, No 1, pp. 23-29, 0090-9556.

Dorne, J.L.C.M., K. Walton&A.G. Renwick, (2001), Uncertainty factors for chemical risk assessment: human variability in the pharmacokinetics of CYP1A2 probe substrates. *Food and Chemical Toxicology*, Vol. 39, No 7, pp. 681-696, 0278-6915.

Eiermann, B., P.O. Edlund, A. Tjernberg, P. Dalen, M.L. Dahl&L. Bertilsson, (1998), 1- and 3-hydroxylations, in addition to 4-hydroxylation, of debrisoquine are catalyzed by cytochrome P450 2D6 in humans. *Drug Metabolism and Disposition*, Vol. 26, No 11, pp. 1096-1101, 0090-9556.

Ekroos, M.&T. Sjogren, (2006), Structural basis for ligand promiscuity in cytochrome P450 3A4. *Proceedings of the National Academy of Sciences of the United States of America*, Vol. 103, No 37, pp. 13682-13687, 0027-8424.

Endres, H.G.E., L. Henschel, U. Merkel, M. Hippius&A. Hoffmann, (1996), Lack of pharmacokinetic interaction between dextromethorphan, coumarin and mephenytoin in man after simultaneous administration. *Pharmazie*, Vol. 51, No 1, pp. 46-51, 0031-7144.

FDA, *Guidance for Industry: Drug Interaction Studies - Study Design, Data Analysis, and Implications for Dosing and Labeling; Draft Guidance*, in *Drug Information Branch (HFD-210), Center for Drug Evaluation and Research (CDER), Online URL: http://www.fda.gov/cder/Guidance/6695dft.htm*. 2006, FDA. p. 1-55.

FDA (2006) *Guidance for Industry: Drug Interaction Studies - Study Design, Data Analysis, and Implications for Dosing and Labeling; Draft Guidance*. Drug Information Branch, Center for Drug Evaluation and Research (CDER) Volume, 1-55

FDA (2006) *Guidance for Industry: Drug Interaction Studies - Study Design, Data Analysis, and Implications for Dosing and Labeling;*. Drug Information Branch, Center for Drug Evaluation and Research (CDER) Volume, 1-55

Fleeman, N., Y. Dundar, R. Dickson, A. Jorgensen, S. Pushpakom, C. McLeod, M. Pirmohamed&T. Walley, (2011), Cytochrome P450 testing for prescribing antipsychotics in adults with schizophrenia: systematic review and meta-analyses. *Pharmacogenomics Journal*, Vol. 11, No 1, pp. 1-14, 1470-269X.

Foti, R.S.&J.L. Wahlstrom, (2008), CYP2C19 inhibition: The impact of substrate probe selection on in vitro inhibition profiles. *Drug Metabolism and Disposition*, Vol. 36, No 3, pp. 523-528, 0090-9556.

Foti, R.S., L.C. Wienkers&J.L. Wahlstrom, (2010), Application of Cytochrome P450 Drug Interaction Screening in Drug Discovery. *Combinatorial Chemistry & High Throughput Screening*, Vol. 13, No 2, pp. 145-158, 1386-2073.

Frank, D., U. Jaehde&U. Fuhr, (2007), Evaluation of probe drugs and pharmacokinetic metrics for CYP2D6 phenotyping. *European Journal of Clinical Pharmacology*, Vol. 63, No 4, pp. 321-333, 0031-6970.

Frye, R.F., G.R. Matzke, A. Adedoyin, J.A. Porter&R.A. Branch, (1997), Validation of the five-drug "Pittsburgh cocktail" approach for assessment of selective regulation of drug-metabolizing enzymes. *Clinical Pharmacology & Therapeutics*, Vol. 62, No 4, pp. 365-376, 0009-9236.

Fuhr, U., K.L. Rost, R. Engelhardt, M. Sachs, D. Liermann, C. Belloc, P. Beaune, S. Janezic, D. Grant, U.A. Meyer&A.H. Staib, (1996), Evaluation of caffeine as a test drug for CYPIA2, NAT2 and CYP2E1 phenotyping in man by in vivo versus in vitro correlations. *Pharmacogenetics*, Vol. 6, No 2, pp. 159-176, 0960-314X.

Furuta, T., C. Kodaira, M. Nishino, M. Yamade, M. Sugimoto, M. Ikuma, A. Hishida, H. Watanabe&K. Umemura, (2009), [C-13]-pantoprazole breath test to predict CYP2C19 phenotype and efficacy of a proton pump inhibitor, lansoprazole. *Alimentary Pharmacology & Therapeutics*, Vol. 30, No 3, pp. 294-300, 0269-2813.

Gorski, J.C., S.D. Hall, P. Becker, M.B. Affrime, D.L. Cutler&B. Haehner-Daniels, (2000), In vivo effects of interleukin-10 on human cytochrome P450 activity. *Clinical Pharmacology & Therapeutics*, Vol. 67, No 1, pp. 32-43, 0009-9236.

Grand, F., I. Kilinc, A. Sarkis&J. Guitton, (2002), Application of isotopic ratio mass Spectrometry for the in vitro determination of demethylation activity in human liver microsomes using N-methyl-C-13-labeled substrates. *Analytical Biochemistry*, Vol. 306, No 2, pp. 181-187, 0003-2697.

Guengerich, P.F., *Human cytochrome P450 enzymes*, in *Cytochrome P450: Structure, Mechanism, and Biochemistry*, P.O. Montellano, Editor. 2005, Kluwer Academic/Plenum Publishers. p. 473-535.

Guengrich, F.P., (1999), Cytochrome P-450 3A4: Regulation and role in drug metabolism. *Annual Review of Pharmacology and Toxicology*, Vol. 39, No pp. 1-17, 0362-1642.

Gupta, S.K., K. Kolz&D.L. Cutler, (2011), Effects of multiple-dose pegylated interferon alfa-2b on the activity of drug-metabolizing enzymes in persons with chronic hepatitis C. *European Journal of Clinical Pharmacology*, Vol. 67, No 6, pp. 591-599, 0031-6970.

Hakooz, N.M.K., (2009), Caffeine Metabolic Ratios for the In Vivo Evaluation of CYP1A2, N-acetyltransferase 2, Xanthine Oxidase and CYP2A6 Enzymatic Activities. *Current Drug Metabolism*, Vol. 10, No 4, pp. 329-338, 1389-2002.

Halling, J., M. Petersen, P. Damkier, F. Nielsen, P. Grandjean, P. Weihe, S. Lundgren, M. Lundblad&K. Brosen, (2005), Polymorphism of CYP2D6, CYP2C19, CYP2C9 and

CYP2C8 in the Faroese population. *European Journal of Clinical Pharmacology*, Vol. 61, No 7, pp. 491-497, 0031-6970.

Han, X.M., D.S. Ou-Yang, P.X. Lu, C.H. Jiang, Y. Shu, X.P. Chen, Z.R. Tan&H.H. Zhou, (2001), Plasma caffeine metabolite ratio (17X/137X) in vivo associated with G-2964A and C734A polymorphisms of human CYP1A2. *Pharmacogenetics*, Vol. 11, No 5, pp. 429-435, 0960-314X.

Hanioka, N., N. Tatarazako, H. Jinno, K. Arizono&M. Ando, (2000), Determination of cytochrome P450 1A activities in mammalian liver microsomes by high-performance liquid chromatography with fluorescence detection. *Journal of Chromatography B*, Vol. 744, No 2, pp. 399-406, 0378-4347.

Henderson, M.C., C.L. Miranda, J.F. Stevens, M.L. Deinzer&D.R. Buhler, (2000), In vitro inhibition of human P450 enzymes by prenylated flavonoids from hops, Humulus lupulus. *Xenobiotica*, Vol. 30, No 3, pp. 235-251, 0049-8254.

Horsmans, Y., V. VandenBerge, A. Bouckaert&J.P. Desager, (1997), Phenytoin hydroxylation in a healthy Caucasian population: Bimodal distribution of hydroxyphenytoin urinary excretion. *Pharmacology & Toxicology*, Vol. 81, No 6, pp. 276-279, 0901-9928.

Hu, O.Y.P., H.S. Tang, H.Y. Lane, W.H. Chang&T.M. Hu, (1998), Novel single-point plasma or saliva dextromethorphan method for determining CYP2D6 activity. *Journal of Pharmacology and Experimental Therapeutics*, Vol. 285, No 3, pp. 955-960, 0022-3565.

Hummel, M.A., L.J. Dickmann, A.E. Rettie, R.L. Haining&T.S. Tracy, (2004), Differential activation of CYP2C9 variants by dapsone. *Biochemical Pharmacology*, Vol. 67, No 10, pp. 1831-1841, 0006-2952.

Chladek, J., G. Zimova, M. Beranek&J. Martinkova, (2000), In-vivo indices of CYP2D6 activity: comparison of dextromethorphan metabolic ratios in 4-h urine and 3-h plasma. *European Journal of Clinical Pharmacology*, Vol. 56, No 9-10, pp. 651-657, 0031-6970.

Christensen, M., K. Andersson, P. Dalen, R.A. Mirghani, G.J. Muirhead, A. Nordmark, G. Tybring, A. Wahlberg, U. Yasar&L. Bertilsson, (2003), The Karolinska cocktail for phenotyping of five human cytochrome P450 enzymes. *Clinical Pharmacology & Therapeutics*, Vol. 73, No 6, pp. 517-528, 0009-9236.

Chun, Y.J., M.Y. Kim&F.P. Guengerich, (1999), Resveratrol is a selective human cytochrome P450 1A1 inhibitor. *Biochemical and Biophysical Research Communications*, Vol. 262, No 1, pp. 20-24, 0006-291X.

Ingelman-Sundberg, M., (2004), Human drug metabolising cytochrome P450 enzymes: properties and polymorphisms. *Naunyn-Schmiedebergs Archives of Pharmacology*, Vol. 369, No 1, pp. 89-104, 0028-1298.

Ingelman-Sundberg, M., A.K. Daly&D.W. Nebert, *Home Page of the Human Cytochrome P450 (CYP) Allele Nomenclature Committee* 2011.

Ito, T., M. Kato, K. Chiba, O. Okazaki&Y. Sugiyama, (2010), Estimation of the Interindividual Variability of Cytochrome 2D6 Activity from Urinary Metabolic Ratios in the Literature. *Drug Metabolism and Pharmacokinetics*, Vol. 25, No 3, pp. 243-253, 1347-4367.

Jenkins, J., D. Williams, Y.L. Deng, D.A. Collins&V.S. Kitchen, (2010), Eltrombopag, an oral thrombopoietin receptor agonist, has no impact on the pharmacokinetic profile of probe drugs for cytochrome P450 isoenzymes CYP3A4, CYP1A2, CYP2C9 and

CYP2C19 in healthy men: a cocktail analysis. *European Journal of Clinical Pharmacology*, Vol. 66, No 1, pp. 67-76, 0031-6970.

Jurica, J., M. Kyr, E.M. Hadasova&J. Tomandl, (2009), Evaluation of the activity of P450 enzymes in rats: use of the single marker or combined drug administration. *Neuroendocrinology Letters*, Vol. 30, No pp. 92-95, 0172-780X.

Kalow, W.&B.K. Tang, (1993), The Use of Caffeine for Enzyme Assays - a Critical-Appraisal. *Clinical Pharmacology & Therapeutics*, Vol. 53, No 5, pp. 503-514, 0009-9236.

Kamali, F., T.I. Khan, B.P. King, R. Frearson, P. Kesteven, P. Wood, A.K. Daly&H. Wynne, (2004), The impact of patient age and genetic polymorphism of CYP2C9 on warfarin dose requirements. *British Journal of Clinical Pharmacology*, Vol. 57, No 5, pp. 668-668, 0306-5251.

Kaminsky, L.S.&Z.Y. Zhang, (1997), Human P450 metabolism of warfarin. *Pharmacology & Therapeutics*, Vol. 73, No 1, pp. 67-74, 0163-7258.

Kato, R., Y. Yamazoe&T. Yasumori, (1992), Polymorphism in stereoselective hydroxylations of mephenytoin and hexobarbital by Japanese liver samples in relation to cytochrome P-450 human-2 (IIC9). *Xenobiotica*, Vol. 22, No 9-10, pp. 1083-1092, 0049-8254 (Print) 0049-8254 (Linking).

Kenworthy, K.E., J.C. Bloomer, S.E. Clarke&J.B. Houston, (1999), CYP3A4 drug interactions: correlation of 10 in vitro probe substrates. *British Journal of Clinical Pharmacology*, Vol. 48, No 5, pp. 716-727, 0306-5251.

Khan, K.K., Y.Q. He, T.L. Domanski&J.R. Halpert, (2002), Midazolam oxidation by cytochrome P450 3A4 and active-site mutants: an evaluation of multiple binding sites and of the metabolic pathway that leads to enzyme inactivation. *Molecular Pharmacology*, Vol. 61, No 3, pp. 495-506, 0026-895X.

Kharasch, E.D., A. Walker, C. Hoffer&P. Sheffels, (2004), Intravenous and oral alfentanil as in vivo probes for hepatic and first-pass cytochrome P450 3A activity: Noninvasive assessment by use of pupillary miosis. *Clinical Pharmacology & Therapeutics*, Vol. 76, No 5, pp. 452-466, 0009-9236.

Kivisto, K.T.&H.K. Kroemer, (1997), Use of probe drugs as predictors of drug metabolism in humans. *Journal of Clinical Pharmacology*, Vol. 37, No 1, pp. S40-S48, 0091-2700.

Klees, T.M., P. Sheffels, O. Dale&E.D. Kharasch, (2005), Metabolism of alfentanil by cytochrome P4503A (CYP3A) enzymes. *Drug Metabolism and Disposition*, Vol. 33, No 3, pp. 303-311, 0090-9556.

Kodaira, C., S. Uchida, M. Yamade, M. Nishino, M. Ikuma, N. Namiki, M. Sugimoto, H. Watanabe, A. Hishida&T. Furuta, (2011), Influence of different proton pump inhibitors on activity of cytochrome P450 assessed by [13C]-aminopyrine breath test. *The Journal of Clinical Pharmacology*, Vol. XX, No XX, pp. XX-XX,

Kohler, D., S. Hartter, K. Fuchs, W. Sieghart&C. Hiemke, (1997), CYP2D6 genotype and phenotyping by determination of dextromethorphan and metabolites in serum of healthy controls and of patients under psychotropic medication. *Pharmacogenetics*, Vol. 7, No 6, pp. 453-461, 0960-314X (Print) 0960-314X (Linking).

Konecny, J., J. Jurica, J. Tomandl&Z. Glatz, (2007), Study of recombinant cytochrome P4502C9 activity with diclofenac by MEKC. *Electrophoresis*, Vol. 28, No 8, pp. 1229-1234, 0173-0835.

Korzekwa, K.R., N. Krishnamachary, M. Shou, A. Ogai, R.A. Parise, A.E. Rettie, F.J. Gonzalez&T.S. Tracy, (1998), Evaluation of atypical cytochrome P450 kinetics with two-substrate models: Evidence that multiple substrates can simultaneously bind to cytochrome P450 active sites. *Biochemistry*, Vol. 37, No 12, pp. 4137-4147, 0006-2960.

Kudo, S.&M. Odomi, (1998), Involvement of human cytochrome P450 3A4 in reduced haloperidol oxidation. *European Journal of Clinical Pharmacology*, Vol. 54, No 3, pp. 253-259, 0031-6970.

Kumar, A., H.J. Mann&R.P. Remmel, (2007), Simultaneous analysis of cytochrome P450 probes - dextromethorphan, flurbiprofen and midazolam and their major metabolites by HPLC-mass-spectrometry/fluorescence after single-step extraction from plasma. *Journal of Chromatography B-Analytical Technologies in the Biomedical and Life Sciences*, Vol. 853, No 1-2, pp. 287-293, 1570-0232.

Kumar, V., J.L. Wahlstrom, D.A. Rock, C.J. Warren, L.A. Gorman&T.S. Tracy, (2006), CYP2C9 inhibition: Impact of probe selection and pharmacogenetics on in vitro inhibition profiles. *Drug Metabolism and Disposition*, Vol. 34, No 12, pp. 1966-1975, 0090-9556.

Lee, C.R., R.L. Hawke&J.A. Pieper, (2005), Twenty-four hour tolbutamide plasma concentration as a phenotypic measure of CYP2C9 activity. *European Journal of Clinical Pharmacology*, Vol. 61, No 4, pp. 315-316, 0031-6970.

Liu, Y.T., H.P. Hao, C.X. Liu, G.J. Wang&H.G. Xie, (2007), Drugs as CYP3A probes, inducers, and inhibitors. *Drug Metabolism Reviews*, Vol. 39, No 4, pp. 699-721, 0360-2532.

Lotsch, J., M. Rohrbacher, H. Schmidt, A. Doehring, J. Brockmoller&G. Geisslinger, (2009), Can extremely low or high morphine formation from codeine be predicted prior to therapy initiation? *Pain*, Vol. 144, No 1-2, pp. 119-124, 0304-3959.

Ma, M.K., M.H. Woo&H.L. McLeod, (2002), Genetic basis of drug metabolism. *American Journal of Health-System Pharmacy*, Vol. 59, No 21, pp. 2061-2069, 1079-2082.

Makings, L.R.&G. Zlokarnik, *US patent No. 6514687: Optical molecular sensors for cytochrome P450 activity*, in *http://www.patentgenius.com/patent/6514687.html*. 2011: USA. p. 1-24.

Mankowski, D.C., (1999), The role of CYP2C19 in the metabolism of (plus /-) bufuralol, the prototypic substrate of CYP2D6. *Drug Metabolism and Disposition*, Vol. 27, No 9, pp. 1024-1028, 0090-9556.

Marks, B.D., T.A. Goossens, H.A. Braun, M.S. Ozers, R.W. Smith, C. Lebakken&O.V. Trubetskoy, (2003), High-throughput screening assays for CYP2B6 metabolism and inhibition using fluorogenic vivid substrates. *Aaps Pharmsci*, Vol. 5, No 2, pp. -, 1522-1059.

Meyer, R.P., C.E. Hagemeyer, C. Burck, R. Schwab&R. Knoth, (2010), 7-Benzyloxyresorufin-O-dealkylase activity as a marker for measuring cytochrome P450 CYP3A induction in mouse liver. *Analytical Biochemistry*, Vol. 398, No 1, pp. 104-111, 0003-2697.

Muscat, J.E., B. Pittman, W. Kleinman, P. Lazarus, S.D. Stellman&J.P. Richie, (2008), Comparison of CYP1A2 and NAT2 phenotypes between black and white smokers. *Biochemical Pharmacology*, Vol. 76, No 7, pp. 929-937, 0006-2952.

Nafziger, A.N., A.D.M. Kashuba, A. James, G.L. Kearns, J.S. Leeder, R. Gotschall&J.S. Bertino, (1998), The influence of sex and menstrual cycle (MC) on CYP1A2, NAT2 and xanthine oxidase (XO) activity. *Clinical Pharmacology & Therapeutics*, Vol. 63, No 2, pp. 216-216, 0009-9236.

Nolin, T.D.&R.F. Frye, (2003), Stereoselective determination of the CYP2C19 probe drug mephenytoin in human urine by gas chromatography-mass spectrometry. *Journal of Chromatography B-Analytical Technologies in the Biomedical and Life Sciences*, Vol. 783, No 1, pp. 265-271, 1570-0232.

Nyeki, A., J. Biollaz, U.W. Kesselring&L.A. Decosterd, (2001), Extractionless method for the simultaneous high-performance liquid chromatographic determination of urinary caffeine metabolites for N-acetyltransferase 2, cytochrome P450 1A2 and xanthine oxidase activity assessment. *Journal of Chromatography B*, Vol. 755, No 1-2, pp. 73-84, 0378-4347.

O'Mathuna, B., M. Farre, A. Rostami-Hodjegan, J. Yang, E. Cuyas, M. Torrens, R. Pardo, S. Abanades, S. Maluf, G.T. Tucker&R. de la Torre, (2008), The consequences of 3.4-methylenedioxymethamphetamine induced CYP2D6 inhibition in humans. *Journal of Clinical Psychopharmacology*, Vol. 28, No 5, pp. 525-531, 0271-0749.

Ou-Yang, D.S., S.L. Huang, W. Wang, H.G. Xie, Z.H. Xu, Y. Shu&H.H. Zhou, (2000), Phenotypic polymorphism and gender-related differences of CYP1A2 activity in a Chinese population. *British Journal of Clinical Pharmacology*, Vol. 49, No 2, pp. 145-151, 0306-5251.

Ozdemir, V., W. Kalow, B.K. Tang, A.D. Paterson, S.E. Walker, L. Endrenyi&A.D.M. Kashuba, (2000), Evaluation of the genetic component of variability in CYP3A4 activity: a repeated drug administration method. *Pharmacogenetics*, Vol. 10, No 5, pp. 373-388, 0960-314X.

Paar, W.D., S. Poche, J. Gerloff&H.J. Dengler, (1997), Polymorphic CYP2D6 mediates O-demethylation of the opioid analgesic tramadol. *European Journal of Clinical Pharmacology*, Vol. 53, No 3-4, pp. 235-239, 0031-6970.

Palmer, J.L., R.J. Scott, A. Gibson, M. Dickins&S. Pleasance, (2001), An interaction between the cytochrome P450 probe substrates chlorzoxazone (CYP2E1) and midazolam (CYP3A). *British Journal of Clinical Pharmacology*, Vol. 52, No 5, pp. 555-561, 0306-5251.

Pelkonen, O., J. Maenpaa, P. Taavitsainen, A. Rautio&H. Raunio, (1998), Inhibition and induction of human cytochrome P450 (CYP) enzymes. *Xenobiotica*, Vol. 28, No 12, pp. 1203-1253, 0049-8254.

Pelkonen, O., M. Turpeinen, J. Hakkola, P. Honkakoski, J. Hukkanen&H. Raunio, (2008), Inhibition and induction of human cytochrome P450 enzymes: current status. *Archives of Toxicology*, Vol. 82, No 10, pp. 667-715, 0340-5761.

Porrogi, P., L. Kobori, K. Kohalmy, J. Gulyas, L. Vereczkey&K. Monostory, (2008), Limited applicability of 7-methoxy-4-trifluoromethylcoumarin as a CYP2C9-selective substrate. *Pharmacological Reports*, Vol. 60, No 6, pp. 972-979, 1734-1140.

Rasmussen, E., B. Eriksson, K. Oberg, U. Bondesson&A. Rane, (1998), Selective effects of somatostatin analogs on human drug-metabolizing enzymes. *Clinical Pharmacology & Therapeutics*, Vol. 64, No 2, pp. 150-159, 0009-9236.

Rendic, S., (2002), Summary of information on human CYP enzymes: human P450 metabolism data. *Drug Metab Rev*, Vol. 34, No 1-2, pp. 83-448, 0360-2532 (Print) 0360-2532 (Linking).

Rost, K.L., J. Brockmoller, F. Esdorn&I. Roots, (1995), Phenocopies of Poor Metabolizers of Omeprazole Caused by Liver-Disease and Drug-Treatment. *Journal of Hepatology*, Vol. 23, No 3, pp. 268-277, 0169-5185.

Sachse, C., J. Brockmoller, S. Bauer&I. Roots, (1997), Cytochrome P450 2D6 variants in a Caucasian population: Allele frequencies and phenotypic consequences. *American Journal of Human Genetics*, Vol. 60, No 2, pp. 284-295, 0002-9297.

Scott, R.J., J. Palmer, I.A.S. Lewis&S. Pleasance, (1999), Determination of a 'GW cocktail' of cytochrome P450 probe substrates and their metabolites in plasma and urine using automated solid phase extraction and fast gradient liquid chromatography tandem mass spectrometry. *Rapid Communications in Mass Spectrometry*, Vol. 13, No 23, pp. 2305-2319, 0951-4198.

Setiabudy, R., M. Kusaka, K. Chiba, I. Darmansjah&T. Ishizaki, (1995), Dapsone N-Acetylation, Metoprolol Alpha-Hydroxylation, and S-Mephenytoin 4-Hydroxylation Polymorphisms in an Indonesian Population - a Cocktail and Extended Phenotyping Trial (Vol 56, Pg 142, 1994). *Clinical Pharmacology & Therapeutics*, Vol. 57, No 1, pp. 66-66, 0009-9236.

Sharma, A., S. Pilote, P.M. Belanger, M. Arsenault&B.A. Hamelin, (2004), A convenient five-drug cocktail for the assessment of major drug metabolizing enzymes: a pilot study. *British Journal of Clinical Pharmacology*, Vol. 58, No 3, pp. 288-297, 0306-5251.

Shelepova, T., A.N. Nafziger, J. Victory, A.D. Kashuba, E. Rowland, Y. Zhang, E. Sellers, G.L. Kearns, S. Leeder, A. Gaedigk&J.S. Bertino, (2003), Effect of oral contraceptives (OCs) on drug metabolizing enzymes (DMEs) as measured by the validated cooperstown 5+1 cocktail (5+1). *Clinical Pharmacology & Therapeutics*, Vol. 73, No 2, pp. P14-P14, 0009-9236.

Shimada, T., H. Yamazaki, M. Mimura, Y. Inui&F.P. Guengerich, (1994), Interindividual Variations in Human Liver Cytochrome-P-450 Enzymes Involved in the Oxidation of Drugs, Carcinogens and Toxic-Chemicals - Studies with Liver-Microsomes of 30 Japanese and 30 Caucasians. *Journal of Pharmacology and Experimental Therapeutics*, Vol. 270, No 1, pp. 414-423, 0022-3565.

Shiran, M.R., J. Chowdry, A. Rostami-Hodjegan, S.W. Ellis, M.S. Lennard, M.Z. Iqbal, O. Lagundoye, N. Seivewright&G.T. Tucker, (2003), A discordance between cytochrome P450 2D6 genotype and phenotype in patients undergoing methadone maintenance treatment. *British Journal of Clinical Pharmacology*, Vol. 56, No 2, pp. 220-224, 0306-5251.

Schellens, J.H.M., H. Ghabrial, H.H.F. Vanderwart, E.N. Bakker, G.R. Wilkinson&D.D. Breimer, (1991), Differential-Effects of Quinidine on the Disposition of Nifedipine, Sparteine, and Mephenytoin in Humans. *Clinical Pharmacology & Therapeutics*, Vol. 50, No 5, pp. 520-528, 0009-9236.

Schrag, M.L.&L.C. Wienkers, (2001), Covalent alteration of the CYP3A4 active site: Evidence for multiple substrate binding domains. *Archives of Biochemistry and Biophysics*, Vol. 391, No 1, pp. 49-55, 0003-9861.

Schrenk, D., D. Brockmeier, K. Morike, K.W. Bock&M. Eichelbaum, (1998), A distribution study of CYP1A2 phenotypes among smokers and non-smokers in a cohort of healthy Caucasian volunteers. *European Journal of Clinical Pharmacology*, Vol. 53, No 5, pp. 361-367, 0031-6970.

Simon, T., L. Becquemont, B. Hamon, E. Nouyrigat, Y. Chodjania, J.M. Poirier, C. Funck-Brentano&P. Jaillon, (2001), Variability of cytochrome P450 1A2 activity over time in young and elderly healthy volunteers. *British Journal of Clinical Pharmacology*, Vol. 52, No 5, pp. 601-604, 0306-5251.

Slanar, O., M. Nobilis, J. Kvetina, R. Mikoviny, T. Zima, J.R. Idle&F. Perlik, (2007), Miotic action of tramadol is determined by CYP2D6 genotype. *Physiological Research*, Vol. 56, No 1, pp. 129-136, 0862-8408.

Smith, D., N. Sadagopan, M. Zientek, A. Reddy&L. Cohen, (2007), Analytical approaches to determine cytochrome P450 inhibitory potential of new chemical entities in drug discovery. *Journal of Chromatography B-Analytical Technologies in the Biomedical and Life Sciences*, Vol. 850, No 1-2, pp. 455-463, 1570-0232.

Stearns, V., M.D. Johnson, J.M. Rae, A. Morocho, A. Novielli, P. Bhargava, D.F. Hayes, Z. Desta&D.A. Flockhart, (2003), Active tamoxifen metabolite plasma concentrations after coadministration of tamoxifen and the selective serotonin reuptake inhibitor paroxetine. *Journal of the National Cancer Institute*, Vol. 95, No 23, pp. 1758-1764, 0027-8874.

Stein, C.M., M.T. Kinirons, T. Pincus, G.R. Wilkinson&A.J.J. Wood, (1996), Comparison of the dapsone recovery ratio and the erythromycin breath test as in vivo probes of CYP3A activity in patients with rheumatoid arthritis receiving cyclosporine. *Clinical Pharmacology & Therapeutics*, Vol. 59, No 1, pp. 47-51, 0009-9236.

Streetman, D.S., J.F. Bleakley, J.S. Kim, A.N. Nafziger, J.S. Leeder, A. Gaedigk, R. Gotschall, G.L. Kearns&J.S. Bertino, (2000), Combined phenotypic assessment of CYP1A2, CYP2C19, CYP2D6, CYP3A, N-acetyltransferase-2, and xanthine oxidase with the "Cooperstown cocktail". *Clinical Pharmacology & Therapeutics*, Vol. 68, No 4, pp. 375-383, 0009-9236.

Sudsakorn, S., J. Skell, D.A. Williams, T.J. O'Shea&H.L. Liu, (2007), Evaluation of 3-O-methylfluorescein as a selective fluorometric substrate for CYP2C19 in human liver microsomes. *Drug Metabolism and Disposition*, Vol. 35, No 6, pp. 841-847, 0090-9556.

Takata, K., J. Saruwatari, N. Nakada, M. Nakagawa, K. Fukuda, F. Tanaka, S. Takenaka, S. Mihara, T. Marubayashi&K. Nakagawa, (2006), Phenotype-genotype analysis of CYP1A2 in Japanese patients receiving oral theophylline therapy. *European Journal of Clinical Pharmacology*, Vol. 62, No 1, pp. 23-28, 0031-6970.

Tanaka, E., A. Ishikawa&S. Misawa, (1994), Changes in Caffeine, Lidocaine and Trimethadione Metabolism in Carbon Tetrachloride-Intoxicated Rats as Assessed by a Cocktail Study. *Pharmacology & Toxicology*, Vol. 75, No 3-4, pp. 150-153, 0901-9928.

Tanaka, E., A. Ishikawa&S. Misawa, (1995), Changes in the Metabolism of 3 Model Substrates Catalyzed by Different P450 Isozymes When Administered as a Cocktail to the Carbon Tetrachloride-Intoxicated Rat. *Xenobiotica*, Vol. 25, No 10, pp. 1111-1118, 0049-8254.

Tanaka, E., N. Kurata&H. Yasuhara, (2003), How useful is the 'cocktail approach' for evaluating human hepatic drug metabolizing capacity using cytochrome P450 phenotyping probes in vivo? *Journal of Clinical Pharmacy and Therapeutics*, Vol. 28, No 3, pp. 157-165, 0269-4727.

Tang, B.K., D. Kadar, L. Qian, J. Iriah, J. Yip&W. Kalow, (1991), Caffeine as a Metabolic Probe - Validation of Its Use for Acetylator Phenotyping. *Clinical Pharmacology & Therapeutics*, Vol. 49, No 6, pp. 648-657, 0009-9236.

Tang, C.Y., M.G. Shou&A.D. Rodrigues, (2000), Substrate-dependent effect of acetonitrile on human liver microsomal cytochrome P4502C9 (CYP2C9) activity. *Drug Metabolism and Disposition*, Vol. 28, No 5, pp. 567-572, 0090-9556.

Tarantino, G., P. Conca, D. Capone, A. Gentile, G. Polichetti&V. Basile, (2006), Reliability of total overnight salivary caffeine assessment (TOSCA) for liver function evaluation in compensated cirrhotic patients. *European Journal of Clinical Pharmacology*, Vol. 62, No 8, pp. 605-612, 0031-6970.

Tassaneeyakul, W., D.J. Birkett, M.E. Mcmanus, W. Tassaneeyakul, M.E. Veronese, T. Andersson, R.H. Tukey&J.O. Miners, (1994), Caffeine Metabolism by Human Hepatic Cytochromes P450 - Contributions of 1a2, 2e1 and 3a Isoforms. *Biochemical Pharmacology*, Vol. 47, No 10, pp. 1767-1776, 0006-2952.

Tenneze, L., C. Verstuyft, L. Becquemont, J.M. Poirier, G.R. Wilkinson&C. Funck-Brentano, (1999), Assessment of CYP2D6 and CY2C19 activity in vivo in humans: A cocktail study with dextromethorphan and chloroguanide alone and in combination. *Clinical Pharmacology & Therapeutics*, Vol. 66, No 6, pp. 582-588, 0009-9236.

Testino, S.A.&G. Patonay, (2003), High-throughput inhibition screening of major human cytochrome P450 enzymes using an in vitro cocktail and liquid chromatography-tandem mass spectrometry. *Journal of Pharmaceutical and Biomedical Analysis*, Vol. 30, No 5, pp. 1459-1467, 0731-7085.

Tomalik-Scharte, D., A. Jetter, M. Kinzig-Schippers, A. Skott, F. Sorgel, T. Klaassen, D. Kasel, S. Harlfinger, O. Doroshyenko, D. Frank, J. Kirchheiner, M. Brater, K. Richter, T. Gramatte&U. Fuhr, (2005), Effect of propiverine on cytochrome p450 enzymes: A cocktail interaction study in healthy volunteers. *Drug Metabolism and Disposition*, Vol. 33, No 12, pp. 1859-1866, 0090-9556.

Trubetskoy, O.V., J.R. Gibson&B.D. Marks, (2005), Highly miniaturized formats for in vitro drug metabolism assays using Vivid((R)) fluorescent substrates and recombinant human cytochrome P450 enzymes. *Journal of Biomolecular Screening*, Vol. 10, No 1, pp. 56-66, 1087-0571.

Tucker, G.T., J.B. Houston&S.M. Huang, (2001), Optimizing drug development: strategies to assess drug metabolism/transporter interaction potential - towards a consensus. *British Journal of Clinical Pharmacology*, Vol. 52, No 1, pp. 107-117, 0306-5251.

van Troostwijk, L.J.A.E.D., R.P. Koopmans, H.D.B. Vermeulen&H.J. Guchelaar, (2003), CYP1A2 activity is an important determinant of clozapine dosage in schizophrenic patients. *European Journal of Pharmaceutical Sciences*, Vol. 20, No 4-5, pp. 451-457, 0928-0987.

Wang, B., L.P. Yang, X.Z. Zhang, S.Q. Huang, M. Bartlam&S.F. Zhou, (2009), New insights into the structural characteristics and functional relevance of the human cytochrome P450 2D6 enzyme. *Drug Metabolism Reviews*, Vol. 41, No 4, pp. 573-643, 0360-2532.

Wang, J.H., P.Q. Li, Q.Y. Fu, Q.X. Li&W.W. Cai, (2007), Cyp2c19 genotype and omeprazole hydroxylation phenotype in Chinese Li population. *Clinical and Experimental Pharmacology and Physiology*, Vol. 34, No 5-6, pp. 421-424, 0305-1870.

Wang, Z.Q., C. Gorski, M.A. Hamman, S.M. Huang, L.J. Lesko&S.D. Hall, (2001), The effects of St John's wort (Hypericum perforatum) on human cytochrome P450 activity. *Clinical Pharmacology & Therapeutics*, Vol. 70, No 4, pp. 317-326, 0009-9236.

Wanwimolruk, S., S. Bhawan, P.F. Coville&S.C.W. Chalcroft, (1998), Genetic polymorphism of debrisoquine (CYP2D6) and proguanil (CYP2C19) in South Pacific Polynesian populations. *European Journal of Clinical Pharmacology*, Vol. 54, No 5, pp. 431-435, 0031-6970.

Watkins, P.B., (1994), Noninvasive Tests of Cyp3a Enzymes. *Pharmacogenetics*, Vol. 4, No 4, pp. 171-184, 0960-314X.

Wedlund, P.J., W.S. Aslanian, C.B. Mcallister, G.R. Wilkinson&R.A. Branch, (1984), Mephenytoin Hydroxylation Deficiency in Caucasians - Frequency of a New Oxidative Drug-Metabolism Polymorphism. *Clinical Pharmacology & Therapeutics*, Vol. 36, No 6, pp. 773-780, 0009-9236.

Wennerholm, A., A. Allqvist, J.O. Svensson, L.L. Gustafsson, R.A. Mirghani&L. Bertilsson, (2005), Alprazolam as a probe for CYP3A using a single blood sample: pharmacokinetics of parent drug, and of alpha- and 4-hydroxy metabolites in healthy subjects. *European Journal of Clinical Pharmacology*, Vol. 61, No 2, pp. 113-118, 0031-6970.

Wester, M.R., J.M. Lasker, E.F. Johnson&J.L. Raucy, (2000), CYP2C19 participates in tolbutamide hydroxylation by human liver microsomes. *Drug Metabolism and Disposition*, Vol. 28, No 3, pp. 354-359, 0090-9556.

Wilkinson, G.R., (1996), Cytochrome P4503A (CYP3A) metabolism: Prediction of in vivo activity in humans. *Journal of Pharmacokinetics and Biopharmaceutics*, Vol. 24, No 5, pp. 475-490, 0090-466X.

Yamazaki, H., Z.Y. Guo, M. Persmark, M. Mimura, K. Inoue, F.P. Guengerich&T. Shimada, (1994), Bufuralol Hydroxylation by Cytochrome-P450 2d6 and 1a2 Enzymes in Human Liver-Microsomes. *Molecular Pharmacology*, Vol. 46, No 3, pp. 568-577, 0026-895X.

Yao, M., M.S. Zhu, M.W. Sinz, H.J. Zhang, W.G. Humphreys, A.D. Rodrigues&R. Dai, (2007), Development and full validation of six inhibition assays for five major cytochrome P450 enzymes in human liver microsomes using an automated 96-well microplate incubation format and LC-MS/MS analysis. *Journal of Pharmaceutical and Biomedical Analysis*, Vol. 44, No 1, pp. 211-223, 0731-7085.

Yao, Y.M., W. Cao, Y.J. Cao, Z.N. Cheng, D.S. Ou-Yang, Z.Q. Liu&H.H. Zhou, (2007), Effect of sinomenine on human cytochrome P450 activity. *Clinica Chimica Acta*, Vol. 379, No 1-2, pp. 113-118, 0009-8981.

Yeh, G.C., P.L. Tao, H.O. Ho, Y.J. Lee, J.Y.R. Chen&M.T. Sheu, (2003), Analysis of pharmacokinetic parameters for assessment of dextromethorphan metabolic phenotypes. *Journal of Biomedical Science*, Vol. 10, No 5, pp. 552-564, 1021-7770.

Yin, O.Q.R., B. Tomlinson, A.H.L. Chow, M.M.Y. Waye&M.S.S. Chow, (2004), Omeprazole as a CYP2C19 marker in Chinese subjects: Assessment of its gene-dose effect and intrasubject variability. *Journal of Clinical Pharmacology*, Vol. 44, No 6, pp. 582-589, 0091-2700.

Yuan, R., S. Madani, X.X. Wei, K. Reynolds&S.M. Huang, (2002), Evaluation of cytochrome P450 probe substrates commonly used by the pharmaceutical industry to study in vitro drug interactions. *Drug Metabolism and Disposition*, Vol. 30, No 12, pp. 1311-1319, 0090-9556.

Zanger, U.M., S. Raimundo&M. Eichelbaum, (2004), Cytochrome P450 2D6: overview and update on pharmacology, genetics, biochemistry. *Naunyn-Schmiedebergs Archives of Pharmacology*, Vol. 369, No 1, pp. 23-37, 0028-1298.

Zhang, W., Z.P. Lin, F.T. Nan, P. Guo, H. Zhao, M.Q. Huang, K. Bertelsen&N.D. Weng, (2010), Simultaneous determination of tolbutamide, omeprazole, midazolam and dextromethorphan in human plasma by LC-MS/MS-A high throughput approach to evaluate drug-drug interactions. *Journal of Chromatography B-Analytical Technologies in the Biomedical and Life Sciences*, Vol. 878, No 15-16, pp. 1169-1177, 1570-0232.

Zhou, H.H., Z. Tong&J.F. McLeod, (2004), "Cocktail" approaches and strategies in drug development: Valuable tool or flawed science? *Journal of Clinical Pharmacology*, Vol. 44, No 2, pp. 120-134, 0091-2700.

Zhou, S.F., (2009), Polymorphism of Human Cytochrome P450 2D6 and Its Clinical Significance Part I. *Clinical Pharmacokinetics*, Vol. 48, No 11, pp. 689-723, 0312-5963.

Zhou, S.F., Z.W. Zhou, L.P. Yang&J.P. Cai, (2009), Substrates, Inducers, Inhibitors and Structure-Activity Relationships of Human Cytochrome P450 2C9 and Implications in Drug Development. *Current Medicinal Chemistry*, Vol. 16, No 27, pp. 3480-3675, 0929-8673.

Zlokarnik, G., P.D.J. Grootenhuis&J.B. Watson, (2005), High throughput P450 inhibition screens in early drug discovery. *Drug Discovery Today*, Vol. 10, No 21-24, pp. 1443-1450, 1359-6446.

Microdosing Assessment to Evaluate Pharmacokinetics and Drug Metabolism Using Liquid Chromatography-Tandem Mass Spectrometry Technology

Jinsong Ni and Josh Rowe
Department of Drug Safety Evaluation, Allergan, Inc., Irvine, CA,
USA

1. Introduction

Drug development is an expensive, complicated and time-consuming process. According to current estimates, a new drug approval, on average, takes about 10 years and costs around US$1.0 billion. For all approved drugs, an estimated 30% could make a return on the investment. In addition, large pharmaceutical companies will collectively lose about US$70 billion of revenue over the next five years because of patent expiration (Adams & Vu Brantner, 2010). As a result, there is tremendous sense of urgency for the pharmaceutical industry to develop new tools to accelerate the drug development process and to reduce attrition rate on drug candidates. Microdosing is one of these tools.

A "microdose" is defined as a dose less than 1/100 of the test substance calculated to yield a pharmacologic effect, with a maximum dose of 100 μg (Food and Drug Administration, 2006). The concept of microdosing to accelerate drug development was first introduced in 2004 by the Europe Medicines Agency in the position paper on non-clinical safety studies to support clinical trials with a single microdose (Europe Medicines Agency, 2004). The Food and Drug Administration in 2006 issued a guidance document on exploratory Investigative New Drug detailing the regulatory process for microdosing clinical studies (Food and Drug Administration, 2006). In 2008, the Ministry of Health, Labor and Welfare in Japan also issued a guidance on microdose clinical studies as the means to understand the bioavailability and pharmacokinetic profiles of test compounds in human, to evaluate the metabolic profiles of test compounds in human or to obtain the information on the tissue distribution of test compounds in human by using molecular imaging technology (Ministry of Health, Labor and Welfare, 2008). Since the dose is sub-pharmacological, the potential for adverse side effect to a human subject in the clinical study is considered to be minimal. As a result, only an abridged non-clinical package is required to support a microdosing clinical study. This makes the microdosing concept attractive when a speedy decision on drug candidate selection around pharmacokinetics and drug metabolism is critical, particularly when clear decisions cannot be made with in vivo animal and in vitro pre-clinical pharmacokinetic data.

2. Microdosing strategy on human pharmacokinetics, metabolism and drug development

There are many reasons drugs can fail in clinical trials. Although drug attrition due to unfavorable absorption, distribution, metabolism and excretion properties in humans has dropped from 40% in 1991 to 10% in 2000, while drug attrition for efficacy, toxicity and safety has increased to 20-30% during the same period (Frank & Hargreaves, 2003), one could argue that the reason for the insufficient pharmacological effect in vivo might be related to the low concentrations at the target tissues. In addition, accumulation of the drug or its metabolites in organ tissues might lead to unwanted adverse effects in humans (Sugiyama & Yamashita, 2011). Therefore, issues related to lack of efficacy or safety of drug candidates may be attributed not only to the pharmacodynamics, but also to the pharmacokinetics and metabolism of the compound.

Typically, during the pre-clinical stage, a number of *in vitro* models and *in vivo* pharmacokinetic and drug metabolism studies are conducted in experimental animals such as rats, dogs and monkeys. The allometric scaling approach, or physiologically based pharmacokinetic models, have often been used to predict human pharmacokinetics. However, large genetic and species differences in drug metabolism, particularly for drugs with high first-pass metabolism, extra-hepatic metabolism, significant polymorphic metabolism, or that are transporter substrates sometimes make prediction of human pharmacokinetics difficult. As a result, unfavorable pharmacokinetic and metabolism properties such as low oral bioavailability, high clearance, short half-life and extensive drug distribution could lead to unexpected adverse effects or lack of efficacy in clinic trials. Therefore, in these circumstances, and where there is conflicting animal data that make predicting human pharmacokinetics and metabolism difficult, microdosing in the clinic could be useful to quickly obtain such information.

Conceptually, microdosing clinical studies could help (1) choose a drug from a series of candidates with the best human pharmacokinetic and metabolism properties for further development; (2) evaluate if sufficient exposure could be achieved at proposed clinical doses to test pharmacological activity; (3) provide valuable information for formulation optimization; and (4) estimate the amount of active pharmaceutical ingredient to support clinical drug development (Ings, 2009; Garner, 2010). The underlying fundamental assumption, however, for the success of the microdosing concept is that pharmacokinetics are linear from microdose to therapeutic dose in the clinic. In order to accurately characterize microdosing pharmacokinetics and drug metabolism, a highly sensitive and selective bioanalytical method is vital.

3. Analytical challenges: Advantages and disadvantages of liquid chromatography-tandem mass spectrometry, accelerator mass spectrometry and positron emission tomography to support microdosing studies

Microdosing studies for pharmacokinetics and drug metabolism investigations rely on analytical techniques with adequate sensitivity. Liquid chromatography-tandem mass spectrometry (LC-MS/MS), accelerator mass spectrometry (AMS) and positron emission tomography (PET) are currently three major analytical tools to study microdosing pharmacokinetics and drug metabolism, and each technique has its advantages and disadvantages.

AMS employs an instrument for measuring long-lived radionuclides that occur naturally in our environment. It uses a particle accelerator in conjunction with ion sources, large magnets, and detectors to separate out interferences and count single radionucleotide atoms in the presence of 1×10^{15} stable atoms. Because of the powerful magnet employed, AMS typically displays excellent sensitivity with the lower limit of quantitation at femtogram or attogram per mL levels (Lappin et al., 2006). Despite its ultra-low sensitivity, AMS has many limitations. It requires the synthesis of ^{14}C-radiolabeled drug, which can be costly and time-consuming (Wilding & Bell, 2005) and necessitates extra precautions during sample handling and preparation to prevent contamination by extraneous sources of ^{14}C. In addition, AMS measures total ^{14}C radioactivity, that is, drug plus metabolites. In order to accurately measure parent drug concentrations, the parent drug in plasma or blood extracts must first be separated by high performance liquid chromatography (HPLC) with fraction-collection followed by subsequent analysis using AMS (Sandhu et al., 2004). At present, unlike LC-MS/MS, there is no direct interface between HPLC and AMS. Furthermore, AMS methodology requires biological samples to be graphitized prior to analysis, which involves a time-consuming process of sample oxidation followed by reduction. These procedures result in low throughput, large instrument space and high operating cost (Lappin & Garner, 2005).

PET is a relatively new imaging technique that, due to its high sensitivity, has the potential to support microdosing studies. In pharmacokinetic studies using PET imaging technology, a drug labeled with a positron-emitting radiotracer, such as ^{11}C, is administered. Three dimensional images showing the distribution of the radiolabel with spatial resolution of 2-5 mm are then produced. In dynamic PET, the images can be acquired rapidly and the time-course can be followed with temporal resolution of a few seconds. Typically, the radiotracers employed have very high specific activity, which allows for doses of 10 μg or less, consistent with the microdosing concept (Lappin et.al., 2009). However, the short half-life of positron emitting radionucleotides typically limits the duration of these studies and prevents accurate assessment of pharmacokinetics beyond the initial distribution phase. The main advantage of PET compared with other analytical techniques is the ability to quantitatively image drug distribution in the clinic under a microdosing paradigm, gaining insight into concentrations of drug in specific tissues of interest. Another advantage of PET is that it is non-invasive. Although PET is mainly used to study pharmacokinetics of compounds in the target tissues, it could also be used to analyze blood or plasma samples. In this practice, an HPLC with radiodetection is used to separate parent drug from the metabolites, thereby gaining information on the quantities of both parent drug and metabolites. This procedure, however, could add considerably to the complexity of the experiments and can be challenging due to the short half-life of the radionucleotides. Other disadvantages of PET are that the instrument is expensive and only available at certain locations that have the specialized hot chemistry facilities, an on-site cyclotron and a positron emission tomography camera.

LC-MS/MS is widely available in the pharmaceutical industry and academic institutions as a powerful analytical tool to measure drug concentrations. It is easy to use and highly automated. Mass Spectrometry can also be directly linked to a HPLC system to separate parent drug from the metabolites. In addition, LC-MS/MS has the functionality to characterize drug metabolites. LC-MS/MS is relatively inexpensive compared to AMS or PET, and occupies much smaller footprint in the laboratory setting. At present, however, LC-MS/MS can only achieve lower limits of quantitation at picogram or femtogram per mL level, an order of magnitude less sensitive compared to AMS technique. Nevertheless, LC-MS/MS has gained considerable attention in the recent years as an analytical technique to study microdosing pharmacokinetics and drug metabolism.

4. Brief description on liquid chromatography-tandem mass spectrometry and sample preparation techniques

Since its widespread introduction more than 20 years ago, LC-MS/MS has made an enormous impact on biomedical research, particularly on the study of drug metabolism and pharmacokinetics (Kamel & Prakash, 2006) in the pharmaceutical industry (Lee, 2005). It has been the preferred technique for bioanalysis of small molecules in biological fluids for more than 10 years (Marzo & Dal Bo, 2007). Although considered as a mature technology, rapid and exciting advances continue to occur that promise even greater performance. The inherent sensitivity, selectivity, robustness and speed of LC-MS/MS make it an attractive technique for supporting microdosing studies even though sensitivity is still somewhat of a challenge at the extremely low doses. Advances in mass spectrometry technology, chromatography and sample preparation have made bioanalytical assays with sensitivities at the low pg/mL range more common, if not yet routine. As the technology continues to advance, improvements in sensitivity are likely to continue.

Several excellent books are available that cover LC-MS/MS in general (Niessen, 2006) and application to analysis of small molecule pharmaceuticals in biological matrices (Korfermacher, 2004), and numerous review articles (Xu et al., 2007) cover recent developments for the reader interested in a comprehensive review of LC-MS/MS technology. An excellent review on sample preparation, which is a key factor in bioanalysis, is also available (Wells, 2003). The objective of this brief introduction to LC-MS/MS is to provide an understanding of the technology, as well as its promise and limitations, that would assist a researcher interested in microdosing, but not necessarily familiar with analytical chemistry, with emphasis on aspects and recent developments relevant to microdosing studies.

4.1 Overall liquid chromatography-mass spectrometry analysis

LC-MS/MS is a joining of two techniques: HPLC and mass spectrometry (MS). A schematic diagram of a LC-MS/MS system is shown in Figure 1. In an HPLC system, the components of the sample are separated on the basis of physical properties by distributing into two immiscible phases, the stationary phase (contained in a column) and the mobile phase (which flows through the column). The effluent from the HPLC column is directed to the ionization source of the mass spectrometer, where the analyte(s) is converted into gas phase ions. These ions are then introduced in several stages to the high vacuum region of the mass analyzer, where the ions are separated by mass to charge ratio and measured by the detector. In most applications related to bioanalysis, tandem mass spectrometers are utilized.

4.2 Sample pretreatment

Prior to analysis by LC-MS/MS, complex samples such as plasma are typically pretreated to remove proteins and other potentially interfering materials. Table 1 lists the most common sample preparation techniques along with the key advantages and disadvantages.

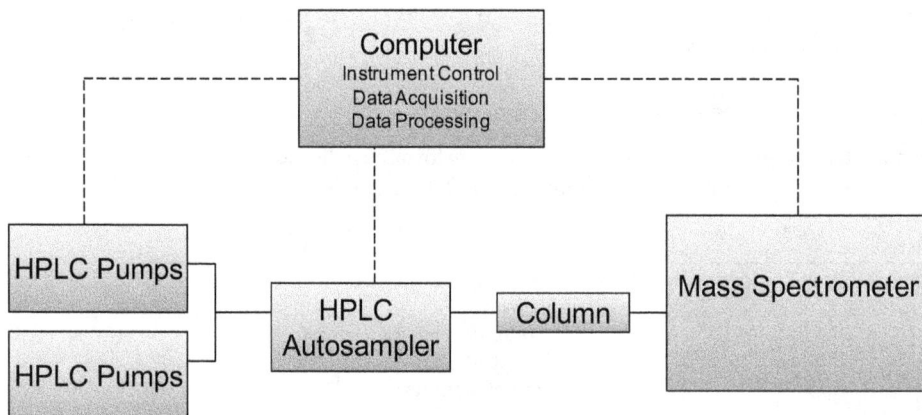

Fig. 1. Schematic diagram of a liquid chromatography-mass spectrometry system.

Typical bioanalytical assays involve preparing calibration standard and control samples, then pre-treating the samples prior to injection and analysis by LC-MS/MS. Thus, the technique can be divided into three parts: sample pretreatment, HPLC and MS/MS.

Technique	Pro	Con
Protein precipitation	• Little or no method development needed • Good recovery of wide variety of analytes (i.e. metabolites)	• Matrix ion suppression
Liquid-liquid extraction	• Provides clean extract • Concentrates sample to improve sensitivity	• Recovery of polar analytes (i.e. metabolites) may be poor • Less amenable to automation and high throughput
Solid phase extraction	• Provides clean extract • Concentrates sample to improve sensitivity • Amenable to high throughput • Large variety of SPE sorbents	• Extensive method development may be needed to optimize • Recovery of metabolites may be poor
Online sample preparation (turbulent flow, monolithic)	• No sample preparation needed • Amenable to automation and high throughput • High sensitivity can be achieved	• More complex valve switching system is needed • Extensive method development needed to achieve high sensitivity • Higher carry-over

Table 1. Summary of pros and cons of selected bioanalytical sample preparation techniques.

Solid phase extraction and liquid-liquid extraction are the two most common techniques applied to microdosing studies, since these techniques allow for concentration of the sample to help achieve high sensitivity. Adequate sample clean-up to remove background interferences and to reduce matrix ion suppression is critical for achieving highly sensitive and robust bioanalytical assays. Note that if analysis of metabolites is desired, a less specific sample preparation procedure (i.e. protein precipitation) may be necessary to ensure recovery of the metabolites.

4.3 High performance liquid chromatography

Selected techniques and advances in high performance liquid chromatography used in bioanalysis, along with key advantages and limitations, are shown in Table 2.

Technique	Pro	Con
Reverse phase liquid chromatography	• Most common mode to connect mass spectrometry • Predictable retention of metabolites • Larger variety of stationary phases available	• Difficult to retain highly polar analytes
Normal phase liquid chromatography	• Optimal mode for chiral separations	• Not amenable to electrospray • Unpredictable retention of metabolites
Ion pairing liquid chromatography	• Provides retention for very polar analytes	• Ion suppression
Very or ultra high pressure liquid chromatography	• Higher chromatographic efficiency improves sensitivity and speed	• Special columns and pumps needed
Fused core particle technology columns	• Higher chromatographic efficiency improves sensitivity and speed	• Ultra high pressure liquid chromatography - like performance without special pumps
Hydrophilic interaction liquid chromatography	• Provides retention and improves sensitivity for very polar analytes	• Unpredictable retention of metabolites
Two dimensional - high performance liquid chromatography	• Cleaner background improves sensitivity	• Special equipment and extensive method development needed

Table 2. Selected advances and techniques of HPLC along with a summary of the pros and cons of each.

Reverse-phase liquid chromatography, wherethe stationary phase is a non-polar material such as C8 or C18 and the mobile phase is a mixture of polar solvents, is by far the most common configuration. Normal phase, ion pairing (Gao *et al.*, 2005), ion exchange and chiral chromatography (Chen *et al.*, 2005) are less common modes used in bioanalysis. Key technology developments within reverse-phase HPLC that improve sensitivity include ultra-high-pressure liquid chromatography (Guillarme *et al.*, 2010) and fused-core particle columns (Song *et al.*, 2009), which improve the efficiency and speed of liquid

Microdosing Assessment to Evaluate Pharmacokinetics and Drug Metabolism
Using Liquid Chromatography-Tandem Mass Spectrometry Technology

227

chromatographic separations. Improving chromatographic efficiency increases sensitivity in two ways; by producing sharper, more concentrated peaks and by separating matrix components that could cause matrix ion suppression.

4.4 Mass spectrometry

4.4.1 Ionization source

The development of atmospheric pressure ionization, in particular electrospray and atmospheric pressure chemical ionization, was the key development that made the union of liquid chromatography and mass spectrometry successful. In electrospray (Figure 2), the mobile phase effluent is nebulized and a charge of 3-5 kV is applied to the spray needle. In the spray zone, small charged droplets are formed and as the solvent evaporates, the excess charge in the droplets becomes more concentrated and, at some point, the Coulomb repulsion overcomes the competing force of surface tension and causes the droplets to disintegrate and gas phase ions of the analyte(s) are produced. The exact mechanisms of how ions are produced from charged droplets are complex and still a matter of intense research and debate, and several reviews summarize practical implications of recent findings (Cech, 2002; Cole, 2000). Electrospray is capable of ionizing almost any polar analyte molecule, and works especially well with weakly basic or acidic compounds. For less polar or non-polar analytes, atmospheric pressure chemical ionization is often used.

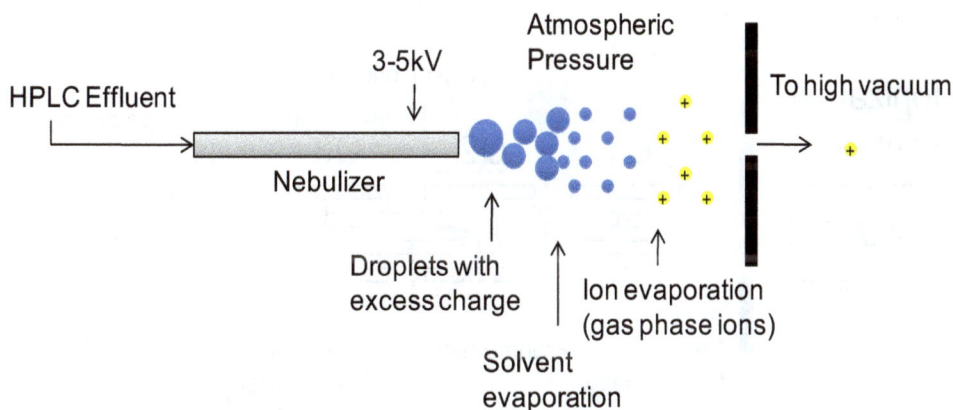

Fig. 2. Electrospray ionization.

In atmospheric pressure chemical ionization (APCI), the mobile phase effluent is almost completely evaporated in a heated quartz tube and a corona discharge reacts with gas molecules from evaporation of the various mobile phase components, which undergo a series of gas phase ion-molecule reactions, especially proton transfer reactions, that eventually result in the production of gas phase ions of the analyte(s). Unlike electrospray, in atmospheric APCI, ionization occurs in the gas phase, which could explain why atmospheric pressure chemical ionization is less susceptible to matrix ion suppression effects.

Both electrospray and atmospheric pressure chemical ionization are "soft" ionization methods, which typically result in protonated molecular ions, [MH]+, in positive mode or deprotonated molecular ions, [M-H]-, in negative mode. In either case, the composition of the mobile phase has a profound influence on ionization (Kostiainen *et al.*, 2009). The choice of composition of the mobile phase is therefore a compromise between its effects on the chromatography and the effects on ionization in the mass spectrometer. The ionization efficiency, and therefore assay sensitivity, is also highly compound dependent.

4.4.2 Mass analyzer types and configurations

There are many different types of mass spectrometers. In a tandem mass spectrometer, two mass analyzers are used to provide an additional dimension of selectivity, where the first mass analyzer selects ions of only the desired mass to charge ratio, which are fragmented and the resulting fragment ions analyzed by the second mass analyzer. Tandem mass spectrometers improve the selectivity and sensitivity for quantitative assays, and greatly expand the capabilities for gaining qualitative information of unknown metabolites.

4.4.2.1 Triple quadropole mass spectrometers for quantitative bioanalysis

LC-MS/MS utilizing a triple quadrupole mass spectrometer operated in multiple reaction monitoring mode is currently the method of choice for quantitative bioanalysis of small molecules. A schematic diagram of a triple quadrupole mass spectrometer is shown in Figure 3.

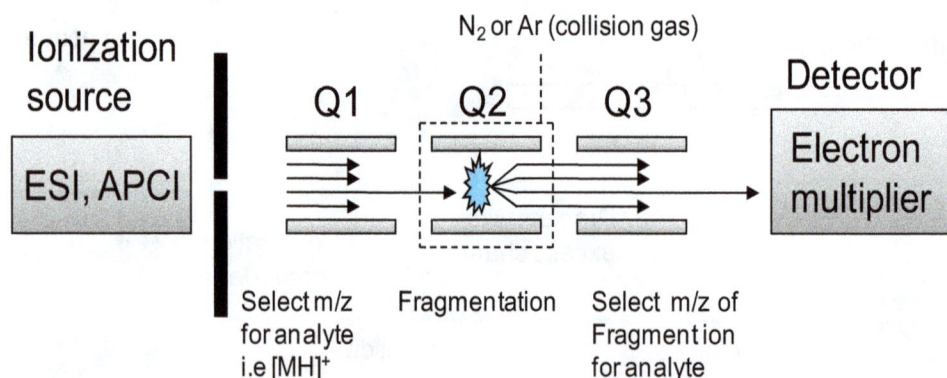

Fig. 3. Schematic diagram of a triple quadrupole mass spectrometer.

The first quadrupole acts as a mass filter to select only ions of a specific mass to charge ratio,typically of the [MH]+ or [M-H]- ions of the analyte, to enter into the second quadrupole. The second quadrupole is the collision cell, where collision with a gas (N_2 or Ar) causes the ions to fragment through a process known as collision activated dissociation. The resulting fragment ions are transmitted to third quadrupole, where only the fragment ions of the desired mass to charge ratio are allowed to pass and impinge on the detector (electron multiplier). The two levels of selectivity in the multiple reaction monitoring experiment, combined with the chromatographic separation, provided a very high level of selectivity and are critical to achieving high sensitivity.

4.4.2.2 Mass spectrometers for qualitative analysis

Despite the current predominance of triple quadrupole mass spectrometers in quantitative bioanalysis, other instrument types show promise and may prove to be powerful tools for use in microdosing studies. Several mass spectrometer configurations are available that, in addition to quantifying parent drug and known metabolites, offer the ability to gain information about metabolite pathways even without a priori knowledge of metabolism. These instruments vary widely in their configurations, principles of operation, but can provide structural information on metabolites. Several examples are briefly discussed below.

High resolution mass spectrometers, including time-of-flight (Williamson et al., 2007; Williamson et al., 2008), orbitrap instruments (Zhang et al., 2009; Bateman et al., 2009) and linear ion trap-fourier transform ion cyclotron mass spectrometers (Yamane et al., 2009) provide high selectivity and are able to characterize metabolites.

Ion trap and hybrid triple quadrupole-ion trap mass spectrometers are low resolution instruments that could provide the ability to simultaneously measure and characterize metabolites along with quantitative bioanalysis. The hybrid linear ion trap–triple quadrupole mass spectrometer, or Quadrupole-Trap, by configuring third quadrupole to function either as a quadrupole mass filter or a linear ion trap, combines the features of a triple quadrupole instrument with the features of an ion trap instrument (King & Fernandez-Metzler, 2006). The quadrupole-trap instruments can therefore provide the same sensitivity as a triple quadrupole mass spectrometer and also provide simultaneous qualitative metabolite characterization data, which has allowed these instruments to be used to support microdosing studies.

5. Application of liquid chromatography-tandem mass spectrometry to support microdosing pharmacokinetic studies

LC-MS/MS has been successfully used to investigate the pharmacokinetic linearity of drugs in animals as well as in clinical trials. Balani et al. first reported the evaluation of microdosing to assess pharmacokinetic linearity of fluconazole, tolbutamide and an investigational compound MLNX in rats using LC-MS/MS (Balani et al., 2006). In this study, fluconazole was orally administered at 0.001, 0.005, 0.05 and 5 mg/kg; tolbutamide at 0.001, 0.002, 0.01, 0.1 and 1 mg/kg; and MLNX at 0.01, 0.1, 1, 10 mg/kg to rats. Because of the low plasma clearance, low volume of distribution, and high oral bioavailability for these compounds, the plasma concentrations in rats declined slowly and were easily quantifiable in 24 hour postdose plasma samples. Thus, the LC-MS/MS sensitivity of 0.1 to 1 nM was adequate to support microdosing studies for these compounds in rats. Both fluconazole and tolbutamide showed linear pharmacokinetics throughout the entire dose range and MLNX showed linear pharmacokinetics between 0.1 and 1 mg/kg, but not to 10 mg/kg.

A more comprehensive study involving five drugs of antipyrine, metoprolol, carbamazepine, digoxin and atenolol from three different classes of the Biopharmaceutical Classifications Systems and with the diverse chemical structures were used as model compounds to evaluate the feasibility and sensitivity requirements of LC-MS/MS as an analytical tool to support microdosing studies (Ni *et al.*, 2008). These five drugs were individually administered orally to rats at 0.167, 1.67, 16.7, 167 or 1670 μg/kg doses, where 1.67 μg/kg was equivalent to the maximal microdose of 100 μg in 60 kg human. The 10,000 fold dose range from 0.167 μg/kg to 1670 μg/kg was designed to evaluate the linearity of pharmacokinetics. Using 100 μl plasma sample aliquots, the lower limits of quantitation for antipyrine (10 pg/ml), carbamazepine (1 pg/ml), metoprolol (5 pg/ml), atenolol (20 pg/ml) and digoxin (5 pg/ml) were achieved. Proportional pharmacokinetics were obtained from 0.167 to 1670 μg/kg for antipyrine and carbamazepine and from 1.67 to 1670 μg/kg for atenolol and digoxin, while metoprolol, which is known to undergo extensive metabolism in rats, exhibited non-proportional pharmacokinetics.

LC-MS/MS technology has also been successfully utilized in support of microdosing clinical studies. A validated assay using LC-MS/MS methodology was developed to support quantitative analysis of fexofenadine in human plasma for microdose and pharmacologic dose clinical trials (Yamane *et al.*, 2007). Calibration standards for microdosing study were prepared in the range from 10 to 1000 pg/ml while calibration standards for pharmacological dosing study were from 1 to 500 ng/ml. The results suggested that it was possible to obtain the plasma drug concentrations at all time points up to 12 hours after microdosing and the linear pharmacokinetic profiles were obtained for fexofenadine between microdose of 100 μg and therapeutic dose of 60 mg (Yamazaki *et.al.*, 2010). Similarly, a sample treatment procedure and LC-MS/MS method for quantitative determination of nicardipine in human plasma were developed for a microdose clinical trial with nicardipine (Yamane *et al.*, 2009). Bioanalytical methods were validated in the calibration ranges from 1 to 500 pg/ml and from 0.2 to 100 ng/ml to support microdosing and pharmacological dosing, respectively. Each method was successfully applied to measure drug concentrations in plasma using LC-MS/MS after administration of 100 μg microdose and 20 mg pharmacological dose to each of six healthy volunteers.

In order to obtain information on absolute oral bioavailability, a technique utilizing simultaneous intravenous microdosing of ^{14}C-labeled drug with oral dosing of non-labeled drug in dogs was exemplified using an investigational compound R-142086 (Miyaji *et al.*, 2009). Plasma concentrations of R-142086 were measured by LC-MS/MS and plasma concentrations of ^{14}C-R-142086 were measured by AMS following R-142086 oral dosing at 1 mg/kg and simultaneous ^{14}C-R-142086 intravenous dosing at 1.5 μg/kg (71.25 nCi/kg). Using this strategy, the oral bioavailability of R-142086 was calculated as 16.1% in dogs. In addition, the correlation between the plasma R-142086 concentration data obtained by AMS and LC-MS/MS was examined at an intravenous dose of 0.3 mg/kg (71.25 nCi/kg). The plasma concentration-time curves for ^{14}C-R-142086 determined by AMS and for R-142086 determined by LC-MS/MS in each dog are compared in Figure 4. Although plasma concentrations of R-142086 determined by LC-MS/MS were approximately 20% higher than those of ^{14}C-R-142086 as determined by AMS, there was excellent correlation (r=0.994) between both concentrations.

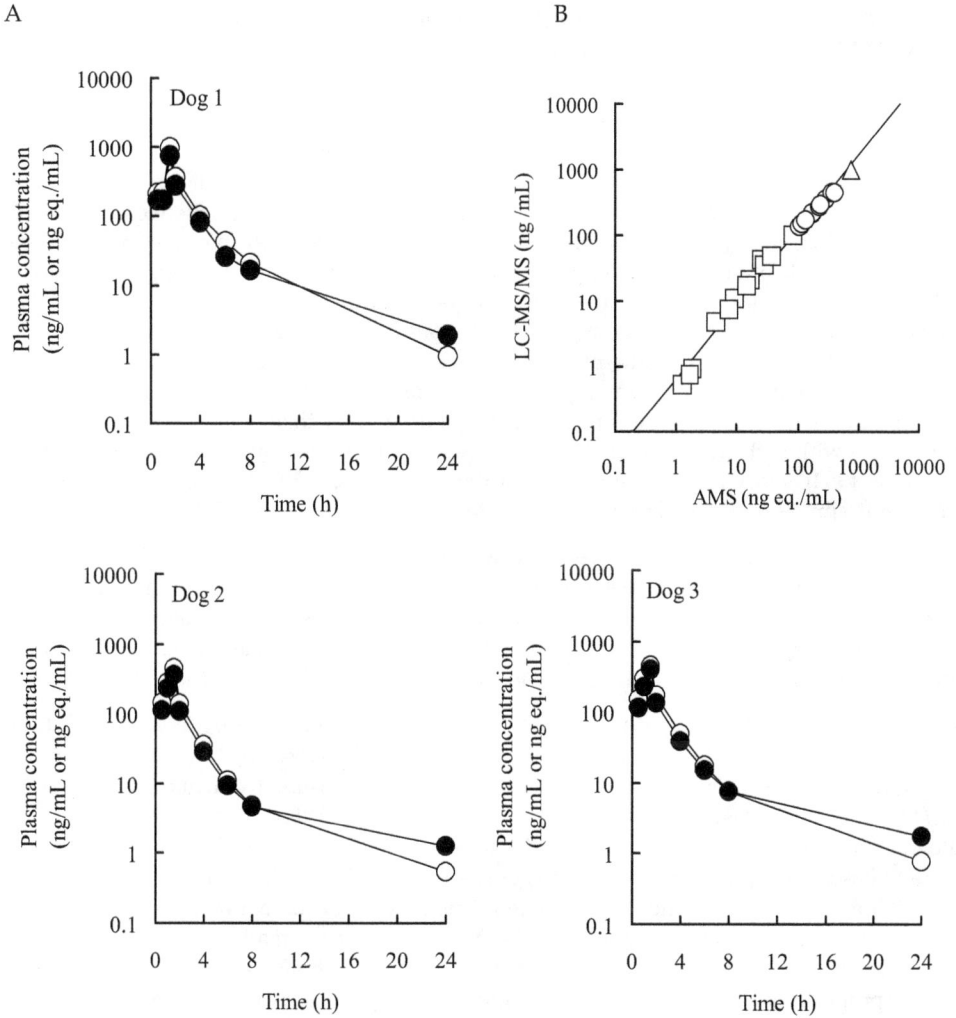

Fig. 4. Correlation between AMS and LC-MS/MS analyses. Panel A: Comparison of plasma concentrations of R-142086 determined by LC-MS/MS (o) versus those of ^{14}C-R-142086 determined by AMS (•) after intravenous administration of ^{14}C-R-142086 at a higher dose (0.3 mg/kg, 71.25 nCi/kg) in each of three dogs. Panel B: Relationship of concentration of R-142086 in all dogs determined by LC-MS/MS and those of ^{14}C-R-142086 determined by AMS after intravenous dosing of a higher dose (0.3 mg/kg, 71.25 nCi/kg). The coefficient of correlation (r) was 0.994. The regression line was y = 1.14 x -0.191.For AMS analysis, the plasma samples were diluted 5-fold (open square), 20-fold (open circle) or 50-fold (open triangle).
(Reprinted with permission from [Miyaji 2009],©2009, The Japanese Society for the Study of Xenobiotics)

6. Application of liquid chromatography-tandem mass spectrometry to support microdosing metabolism studies

LC-MS/MS technology has also been used to characterize and quantify metabolites in microdosing animal and clinical studies. Ni *et al.* (Ni *et al.*, 2008) reported the characterization of carbamazepine metabolites in both *in vitro* liver microsomes and *in vivo* rat at ultra-low concentrations or dose level. Concentrations of 100 nM or 3 nM carbamazepine were incubated in rat liver microsomes, and metabolites were characterized by LC-MS/MS. Incubation concentration at 3 nM was selected because of its close equivalency with plasma C_{max} of carbamazepine at the microdose of 1.67 μg/kg in rats. *In vitro* metabolism data showed the presence of oxidative and conjugated metabolites following incubations at 3 nM and 100 nM. Four metabolites of carbamazepine were detected and characterized in the plasma of rats dosed with 1.67 μg/kg of carbamazepine. The carbamazepine epoxide, among the four metabolites characterized, was the major human circulating metabolite of carbamazepine at the therapeutic doses. Through comparing with carbamazepine metabolism reported in the literature (Lertratanangkoon & Horning, 1982), study results suggested that the metabolic profile *in vivo* at a microdose is, in general, similar to that at therapeutic doses in rats for carbamazepine.

The metabolites of nicardipine were characterized using linear ion trap-fourier transform ion cyclotron resonance mass spectrometry for *in vitro* human liver microsomal incubation with 10 μM nicardipine, where the chemical structures and possible fragmentation patterns for nine metabolites were proposed. These nine metabolites were subsequently monitored and detected in human plasma in a microdosing clinical study (Yamane *et al.*, 2009).

Further evaluation took place on the sensitivity requirement for LC-MS/MS as an analytical tool to characterize metabolites in plasma and urine at microdose level in rats. In addition, the investigation of the proportionality of metabolite exposure from microdose of 1.67 μg/kg to a high dose of 5000 μg/kg was conducted for four model compounds of atorvastatin, ofloxacin, omeprazole and tamoxifen (Ni *et al.*, 2010). For all targeted metabolites based upon literature reports, only a few metabolites including the glucuronide metabolite of ofloxacin, the hydroxylation metabolite of omeprazole and hydration metabolite of tamoxifen were detected by LC-MS/MS in rat plasma following microdosing. The exposure of detected metabolites of omeprazole and tamoxifen appeared to increase in a non-proportional manner with increasing doses. For atorvastatin metabolites, the exposure of atorvastatin lactone increased non-proportionally with increasing doses while the exposure of ortho- and para-hydroxyatorvastatin did show proportional increase (Table 3). Following a single oral microdose or high dose to rats, the exposure of area under the curve of detected metabolites of atorvastatin, omeprazole or tamoxifen did not always display a proportional relationship from a microdose of 1.67 μg/kg to high dose of 5000 μg/kg. Therefore, it was concluded that the exposure of metabolites at the microdose level cannot simply be used to predict their exposure at higher doses.

7. Discussion

Microdosing could provide tremendous value to the drug development, particularly for the evaluation of pharmacokinetics and metabolism properties of compounds. In cases where human pharmacokinetic prediction becomes difficult due to conflicting animal

	Dose	C_{max} (ng/mL)		T_{max} (hour)		$AUC_{0-tlast}$ (ng*hours/ml)	
	µg/kg	Mean	SD	Mean	SD	Mean	SD
Atorvastatin	1.67	0.158	0.0508	0.556	0.193	0.208	0.0116
	25	0.508	0.193	0.444	0.193	0.426	0.0474
	350	2.68	1.32	0.333	0.00	2.54	0.806
	5000	34.8	17.7	0.555	0.385	36.5	21.0
ortho-Hydroxy atorvastatin	1.67	0.0985	0.124	0.777	0.507	0.0628	0.0485
	25	0.463	0.185	0.333	0.00	0.497	0.249
	350	5.12	2.76	0.665	0.576	6.63	2.89
	5000	50.9	35.5	0.777	0.507	67.4	47.6
para-Hydroxy atorvastatin	1.67	NC	NC	NC	NC	NC	NC
	25	0.0233	0.0133	0.665	0.576	0.0208	0.0111
	350	0.241	0.149	0.665	0.576	0.258	0.110
	5000	2.13	1.33	0.888	0.508	2.18	1.25
Lactone of atorvastatin	1.67	2.33	1.20	0.999	0.332	2.82	1.39
	25	4.08	0.427	0.444	0.193	5.33	0.648
	350	7.58	1.06	0.444	0.193	11.4	0.862
	5000	23.8	10.7	0.556	0.193	27.3	8.90

NC: not calculable

Table 3. The pharmacokinetic parameters of atorvastatin and its metabolites following a single oral dose to male Sprague-Dawley rats.

pharmacokinetic data, a microdose clinical study could help to determine if a drug has desirable pharmacokinetic properties that warrant further development. Highly sensitive and selective analytical tools such as LC-MS/MS and AMS have made it possible to characterize pharmacokinetics and metabolism of drug candidates at the microdose level. In the past several years, a lot of attention has been focusing on evaluating pharmacokinetic linearity of drug molecules from microdose to therapeutic doses in animals as well as in the clinic. It has been summarized that out of 26 drugs examined so far, 21 compounds, approximately 80%, have demonstrated linear pharmacokinetics between microdose to therapeutic doses (Lappin, 2010). For compounds which have failed to demonstrate pharmacokinetic linearity, there are a number of possible causes. For instance, drug candidates with saturable first-pass metabolism or saturable elimination at therapeutic doses would often result in under-prediction of exposure based upon microdose data. On the other hand, drug candidates with poor solubility would produce over-prediction of exposure based upon microdose data. Therefore, the understanding of physical and chemical properties of compounds and of enzyme kinetics *in vitro* could be very important prior to the commitment to a microdosing study. In practice, if there is a concern that compound would display nonlinear pharmacokinetics from a microdose to therapeutic doses in the clinic, a pharmacokinetic study could be performed to exam pharmacokinetic linearity in a relevant animal species.

Microdosing could also be very valuable to obtain an earlier understanding of metabolism of drug candidates in the clinic. This has become more important with the release of the recent guidance document "safety testing of drug metabolites" by the FDA (Food and Drug Administration, 2008). The guidance document stated that metabolites found only in human plasma or metabolites present at disproportionately higher levels in humans than in any of the animal test species should be considered for safety assessment. In particular, human metabolites that are formed at greater than 10% of parent drug systemic exposure at steady state can raise a safety concern. As a result, it has become very important to obtain human drug metabolism information as early as possible in the drug development stage, and to compare with preclinical metabolism data. Although microdosing studies in the clinic would be ideal to understand the metabolism of drug candidates early on, caution must be exercised to extrapolate the learning from microdose to therapeutic doses. This could be particularly true for compounds where metabolism enzymes have low substrate capacities and can be saturated at low substrate concentrations. For example, the P450 isoform CYP2D6 is a low capacity enzyme and if a novel drug candidate is metabolized primarily through the CYP2D6 pathway, the metabolic pathway of this drug candidate at microdose may be different from that at therapeutic doses. The levels of a particular metabolite relative to parent drug, as the means to identify major metabolites, may be different from microdose to therapeutic doses. In this case, a thorough understanding of metabolic pathways with animals and *in vitro* would be very useful to assess reliability of drug metabolism prediction from microdose to therapeutic doses. In addition, a microdose clinical study would help to identify if human-specific metabolites are present so that a thorough evaluation of these human unique metabolites could take place in the relevant toxicological species.

8. Conclusion

The highly selective and sensitive technology of LC-MS/MS has become a powerful analytical tool that provides the opportunity to understand clinical pharmacokinetics of compounds using the microdosing approach. Furthermore, LC-MS/MS has demonstrated its usefulness for detecting and characterizing metabolites in plasma and urine at microdose level. Although the extrapolation of parent drug exposure from a microdose to a therapeutic dose appears to be promising, such extrapolation for metabolites may be compound and/or metabolite dependent. Extrapolation of metabolite exposure would particularly be difficult if there is involvement of enzyme inhibition, induction or saturation.

9. References

Adams, C. & Vu Brantner.V. (2010). Spending on New Drug Development. *Health Economics*, Vol.19, No.2, pp. 130-141.

Balani, S. K., Nagaraja, N. V., Qian, M. G., Costa, A. O., Daniels, J. S., Yang, H., Shimoga, P. R., Wu, J. T., Gan, L. S., Lee, F. W. & Miwa, G. T. (2006). Evaluation of Microdosing to Assess Pharmacokinetic Linearity in Rats Using Liquid Chromatography – Tandem Mass Spectrometry. *Drug Metabolism and Disposition*, Vol.34, No.3, pp. 384-388.

Bateman, K. P., Kellman, M., Muenster, H., Papp, R. & Taylor, L. (2009). Quantitative-Qualitative Data Acquisition Using a Benchtop Orbitrap Mass Spectrometer. *Journal of American Society on Mass Spectrometry*, Vol. 20, No.8, pp. 1441-1450.

Cech, N. B. & Enke, C. J. (2002). Practical Implications of Some Recent Studies in Electrospray Ionization Fundamentals. *Mass Spectrometry Reviews*, Vol. 20, No.6, pp. 362-387.

Chen, J., Korfermacher, W. A. & Hsieh, Y. (2005). Chiral Liquid Chromatography-Tandem Mass Spectrometric Methods for Stereoisomeric Pharmaceutical Determinations. *Journal of Chromatography B* Vol. 820, No.1, pp. 1-8.

Cole, R. B. (2000). Some Tenets Pertaining to Electrospray Ionization Mass Spectrometry. *Journal of Mass Spectrometry*, Vol. 35, pp. 763–772.

European Medicines Evaluation Agency (2004). European Agency for Evaluation of Medicines for Human Use. A position paper on the nonclinical safety studies to support clinical trials with a single microdose. CPMP/SWP2599/02/Rev 1. http://www.emea.eu.int/pdfs/human/swp/259902en.pdf.

Food and Drug Administration. (2006). Guidance for Industry, Investigators, and Reviewers. Exploratory IND Studies. http://www.fda.gov/downloads/Drugs/GuidanceComplianceRegulatoryInform ation/Guidances/UCM078933.pdf.

Food and Drug Administration. (2008). Safety Testing of Drug Metabolites. http://www.fda.gov/downloads/Drugs/GuidanceComplianceRegulatoryInform ation/Guidances/UCM079266.pdf.

Frank, R. & Hargreaves, R. (2003). Clinical biomarkers in drug discovery and development, *Nature Reviews Drug Discovery*, No.2, pp. 566-580.

Gao, S., Zhang, Z. & Karnes, H. T. (2005). Sensitivity Enhancement in Liquid Chromatography/Atmospheric Pressure Ionization Mass Spectrometry Using Derivitization and Mobile Phase Additives. *Journal of Chromatography B*, Vol. 825, No.2, pp. 89-110.

Garner, R.C. (2010). Practical experience of using human microdosing with AMS analysis to obtain early human drug metabolism and PK data, *Bioanalysis*, Vol.2, No.3, pp. 429-440.

Guillarme, D., Schappler, J., Rudaz, S. & Veuthey, J. (2010). Coupling Ultra-High-Pressure Liquid Chromatography with Mass Spectrometry. *Trends in Analytical Chemistry* Vol.29, No.1, pp. 15-27.

Ings, R. (2009). Microdosing: a valuable tool for accelerating drug development and the role of bioanalytical methods in meeting the challenge, *Bioanalysis*, Vol.1, No.7, pp. 1293-1305.

Kamel, A. & Prakash, C. (2006). High Performance Liquid Chromatography/Atmospheric Pressure Ionization /Tandem Mass Spectrometry (HPLC/API/MS/MS) in Drug Metabolism and Toxicology. *Current Drug Metabolism*, Vol. 7, No.8, pp. 837-852.

King, R. & Fernandez-Metzler, C. (2006). The Use of Qtrap Technology in Drug Metabolism. *Current Drug Metabolism*, Vol. 7, No.5, pp. 541-545.

Korfermacher, W. A. (2004). Using Mass Spectrometry for Drug Metabolism Studies. CRC Press, Boco Raton.

Kostiainen, R. & Kauppila, T. J. (2009). Effect of Effluent on the Ionization Process in Chromatography-Mass Spectrometry. *Journal of Chromatography A*, Vol. 1216, No.4, pp. 685-699.

Lappin, G. (2010). Microdosing: Current and the Future. *Bioanalysis* Vol.2, No.3, pp. 509-517.

Lappin, G. & Garner, R. C. (2005). The Use of Accelerator Mass Spectrometry to Obtain Early Human ADME/PK Data. *Expert Opinion on Drug Metabolism & Toxicology*, Vol. 1, No.1, pp. 23-31.

Lappin, G., Kuhnz, W., Jochemsenm R., Kneer, J., Chaudhary, A., Oosterhuis, B., Drijfhout, W. J., Rowland, M. & Garner, R. C. (2006). Use of Microdosing to Predict Pharmacokinetics at the Therapeutic Dose: Experience with Five Drugs. *Clinical Pharmacology & Therapeutics*, Vol.80, No.3, pp. 203-215.

Lappin, G., Wagner, C. C. & Merbel, N. (2009). New Ultrasensitive Detection Technologies for Use in Microdosing Studies. *Bioanalysis*. Vol.1, No.2, pp. 357-366.

Lee, H. (2005). Pharmaceutical Applications of Liquid Chromatography Coupled with Mass Spectrometry (LC/MS). *Journal of Liquid Chromatography & Related Technologies*, Vol.28, No.7-8, pp. 1161-1202.

Lertratanangkoon, K., & Horning, M. G. (1982). Metabolism of Carbamazepine. *Drug Metabolism and Disposition*, Vol. 10, No.1, pp. 1-10.

Marzo, A. & Dal Bo, L. (2007). Tandem Mass Spectrometry (LC-MS-MS): a Predominant Role in Bioassays for Pharmacokinetic Studies. *Arzneimittel Forschung*, Vol.57, No.2, pp. 122-128.

Ministry of Health, Labor and Welfare. Guidance (2008). Microdose clinical studies, Ministry of Health, Labor and Welfare, Pharmaceutical and Medical Safety Bureau, Tokyo, Japan.

Miyaji, Y., Ishizuka, T., Kawai, K., Hamabe, Y., Miyaoka, T., OH-Hara, T., Ikeda, T. & Kurihara, A. (2009). Use of an Intravenous Microdose of ^{14}C-Labeled Drug and Accelerator Mass Spectrometry to Measure Absolute Oral Bioavailability in Dogs; Cross-Comparison of Assay Methods by Accelerator Mass Spectrometry and Liquid Chromatography-Tandem Mass Spectrometry. *Drug Metabolism and Pharmacokinetics*, Vol. 24, No.2, pp. 130-138.

Ni, J., Ouyang, H., Aiello, M., Seto, C., Borbridge, L., Sakuma, T., Ellis, R., Welty, D. & Acheampong, A. (2008). Microdosing Assessment to Evaluate Pharmacokinetics and Drug Metabolism in Rats Using Liquid Chromatography-Tandem Mass Spectrometry. *Pharmaceutical Research*, Vol. 25, No.7, pp. 1572-1582.

Ni, J., Ouyang, H., Seto, C., Sakuma, T., Ellis, R., Rowe, J., Acheampong, A., Welty, D. & Szekely-Klepser, G. (2010). Sensitivity and Proportionality Assessment of

Microdosing Assessment to Evaluate Pharmacokinetics and Drug Metabolism
Using Liquid Chromatography-Tandem Mass Spectrometry Technology

237

Metabolites from Microdose to High Dose in Rats Using LC-MS/MS. *Bioanalysis*, Vol.2, No.3, pp. 407-419.

Niessen, W. M. A. (2006). Liquid Chromatography-Mass Spectrometry, third ed., CRC Press, Boco Raton.

Sandhu, P., Vogel, J. S., Rose, M. J., Ubick, E. A., Brunner, J. E., Wallace, M. A., Adelsberger, J. K., Baker, M. P., Henderson, P. T., Pearson, P. G. & Baillie, T. A. (2004). Evaluation of Microdosing Strategies for Studies in Preclinical Drug Development: Demonstration of Linear Pharmacokinetics in Dogs of a Nucleoside Analog Over a 50-Fold Dose Range. *Drug Metabolism and Disposition*, Vol. 32, No.11, pp. 1254-1259.

Song, W., Pabbisetty, D., Groeber, E. A., Steenwyk, R. C. & Fast, D. M. (2009). Comparison of Fused-Core and Conventional Particle Size Columns by LC-MS/MS and UV: Application to Pharmacokinetic Study. *Journal of Pharmaceutical and Biomedical Analysis*, Vol. 50, No.3, pp. 491-500.

Sugiyama, Y. & Yamashita, S. (2011). Impact of microdosing clinical study – why necessary and how useful ? *Advanced Drug Delivery Reviews*, Vol.63, No.7, pp. 494-502.

Wells, D. A. (2003). High Throughput Bioanalytical Sample Preparation. Methods and Automation Strategies. Elsevier Science, Amsterdam, The Netherlands.

Wilding, I. R. & Bell, J. A. (2005). Improved Early Clinical Development Through Human Microdosing Studies. *Drug Discoveries & Therapeutics*, Vol. 10, No.13, pp. 890-894.

Williamson, L. N. & Bartlett, M. G. (2007). Quantitative Liquid Chromatography/Time-of-Flight Mass Spectrometry. *Biomedical Chromatography* Vol. 21, No.6, pp. 567-576.

Williamson, L. N., Zhang, G., Alvin, T. V. & Bartlett, M. G. (2008). Comparison of Time-of-Flight Mass Spectrometry to Triple Quadropole Tandem Mass Spectrometry for Quantitative Bioanalysis: Application to Antipsychotics. *Journal of Liquid Chromatography & Related Technologies*, Vol. 31, No.18, pp. 2737-2751.

Xu, R. N., Fan, L., Rieser, M. & El-Shourbagy, T. (2007). Recent Advances in High Throughput Quantitative Bioanalysis by LC-MS/MS. *Journal of Pharmaceutical and Biomedical Analysis*, Vol. 44, No.2, pp. 342-355.

Yamane, N., Takami, T., Tozuka, Z., Sugiyama, Y., Yamazaki, A. & Kumagai, Y. (2009). Microdose Clinical Trial: Quantitative Determination of Nicardipine and Prediction of Metabolites in Human Plasma. *Drug Metabolism and Pharmacokinetics*, Vol. 24, No.4, pp. 389-403.

Yamane, N., Tozuka. Z., Sugiyama, Y., Tanimoto, T., Yamazaki, A. & Kumagai, Y. (2007). Microdose Clinical Trial: Quantitative Determination of Fexofenadine in Human Plasma Using Liquid Chromatography/Electrospray Ionization Tandem Mass Spectrometry. *Journal of Chromatography B*, Vol. 858, No.1-2, pp. 118-128.

A. Yamazaki, Y. Kumagai, N. Yamane, Z. Tozuka, Y. Sugiyama, T. Fujita, S. Yokota & M. Maeda. (2010) "Microdose study of a P-glycoprotein substrate, fexofenadine, using a non-radioisotope-labelled drug and LC/MS/MS", *Journal of Clinical Pharmacy and Therapeutics*, Vol. 35, pp. 169-175.

Zhang, N. R., Yu, S., Tiller, P., Yeh, S., Mahan, E. & Emary, W. B. (2009). Quantitation of Small Molecules Using High-Resolution Accurate Mass Spectrometers-a Different Approach for Analysis of Biological Samples. *Rapid Communications in Mass Spectrometry* Vol.23, No.7, pp. 1085-1094.

Electrochemical Methods for the *In Vitro* Assessment of Drug Metabolism

Alejandro Álvarez-Lueje, Magdalena Pérez and Claudio Zapata
University of Chile,
Chile

1. Introduction

The development of new chemical compounds with promising pharmacological activities is a very time-consuming and costly process because it requires many studies and evaluations prior to obtaining final approval for use in humans. Thus, for the safe use of any new drug, it is necessary to first know its physical, chemical and biological properties, as well as its efficacy, stability, pharmacokinetic properties (i.e., absorption, distribution, metabolism and excretion) and toxicity.

Usually, the toxicity of a new drug or of its metabolites is the main reason most candidate drugs are removed from the development process and are not approved for human use. For this reason, it is very important to determine in the early development stages the tendency of a drug of interest to undergo bioactivation into toxic metabolites and, additionally, the reactivity of these metabolites toward biomolecules (Baumann & Karst, 2010). Therefore, an ideal drug metabolism study should include a complete identification of all metabolites generated and their bioactivation pathways, in addition to the reactions between the drug and its metabolites with endogenous molecules or xenobiotics. For this purpose, different *in vitro* and *in vivo* experimental models are commonly applied prior to clinical trials, which include the use of enzymes, liver cells, liver cell extracts and laboratory animals, among others (Brandon et al., 2003).

Rat and human liver microsomes (RLM and HLM) are the most widely used cell extracts for studying metabolic reactions because they contain high concentrations of the cytochrome P450 enzymatic complex (CYP), which catalyzes the majority of oxidative reactions in organisms (Brandon et al., 2003). However, the use of conventional *in vitro* and *in vivo* methods makes it very difficult to detect the formation of reactive metabolites or intermediates with short half-lives because these short-lived species tend to covalently bond to cellular macromolecules, such as proteins and DNA (Lohmann & Karst, 2007). For this reason, the early 1980s ushered in the development and application of new methods for studying drug metabolism. In this context, the use of electrochemistry, a purely instrumental technique, has emerged as an interesting alternative to generate and detect metabolites in the drug development process because it can mimic the predominant redox reactions that occur in the human body (Álvarez-Lueje & Bollo, 2010; Jurva et al., 2003).

Electrochemistry is useful for the study of metabolism, as it has certain advantages compared to conventional methods. Namely, it allows the generation and direct identification, in a rapid and clean manner, of both stable species and metabolites with short half-lives. Consequently, electrochemistry can be a powerful tool in interaction studies with specific cellular components, which is more difficult to realize with conventional *in vivo* or *in vitro* methods. Additionally, electrochemistry is a cost-effective, rapid and clean system that does not require the use of laboratory animals or organ extracts.

Different electrochemical methods have been applied to mimic drug metabolism and the reactivities of metabolites toward biomolecules, but the most frequently used system consists of an electrochemical cell coupled to a mass spectrometer (EC-MS). A modification of this system has involved the incorporation of a chromatographic separation between the cell and the detector, which permits on-line electrochemistry-liquid chromatography-mass detection (EC-LC–MS) (Lohmann et al., 2010). To improve this system and obtain more information about metabolic reactions, different modifications have also been utilized. For example, the incorporation of trapping agents (i.e., glutathione (GSH) or other thiols) that can form stable adducts with the reactive intermediates generated in the electrochemical cell is commonly used to detect the interactions of metabolites (Lohmann & Karst, 2006; van Leeuwen et al., 2005; Lohmann & Karst, 2009). Other electrochemical applications useful for metabolic studies include the development of enzyme-based biosensors, antibodies and DNA, among others (Joseph et al., 2003).

In the following sections, the most important electrochemical aspects that can help explain how metabolic reactions can be emulated using different electrochemical methods and the advantages of these over conventional methods are presented. Additionally, the main metabolic pathways that can be electrochemically emulated and comparisons with *in vivo* and *in vitro* assays are summarized and discussed. Finally, both the application of electrochemical tools for studying interactions between metabolites and biomolecules and the application of biosensors in this field are presented.

2. General aspects of electrochemistry

Electrochemistry involves the study of chemical phenomena associated with the separation and transfer of charge that occurs at the interface of an electrode and solution. Electrochemistry is applicable in areas ranging from basic studies to environmental and clinical applications (Speiser, 2007).

Electron transfer causes the reduction or oxidation of a substance when a sufficiently negative or positive potential is applied, respectively. As the potential values can be controlled externally, redox processes of interest can be carefully chosen, making electrochemistry useful for studying the redox behavior of any substance, inorganic or organic, including drugs, toxics, biomolecules and metabolites.

Commonly, measurements are realized in an electrochemical cell using a system of three electrodes, the working, reference and auxiliary electrodes, immersed in a solution containing the compound of interest and a supporting electrolyte. The working electrode is usually constructed from inert materials, such as allotrope derivatives of carbon (graphite or glassy carbon) or metals (mercury, platinum or gold). Reference electrodes provide a fixed potential against which the potential applied to the working electrode is measured and controlled, and they often consist of a saturated calomel electrode or $Ag/AgCl_{(sat)}$. A third electrode, the auxiliary electrode, is often included, which normally consists of a platinum wire. Because the reference electrode has a constant potential value, any change in the electrochemical cell is due to the working electrode and the redox process. The three electrodes are connected to a potentiostat, which controls the potential applied to the working electrode, and the results are recorded by a computer (Bard & Faulkner, 2001; Brett & Oliveira Brett, 1993). A schematic representation of this system is shown in figure 1A.

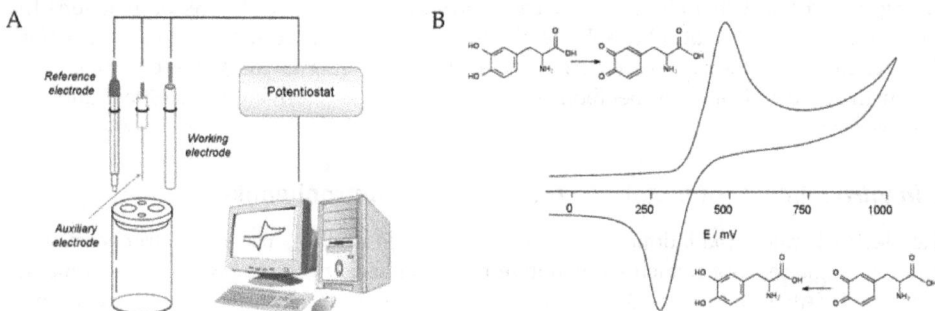

Fig. 1. A) Electrochemical cell with a three-electrode system. B) Typical redox couple obtained using cyclic voltammetry on levodopa and the respective oxidative and reductive reactions.

Different techniques are often employed in electrochemistry for the study of electroactive substances. These include linear sweep, differential pulse and cyclic voltammetry, chronoamperometry, chronocoulometry and bulk electrolysis, among others. All of these techniques can provide important information about substances of interest and the characteristics of their redox processes, but voltammetric and electrolytic methods are more relevant to the study of electroactive drugs, their metabolites and the metabolites' interactions with biomolecules.

Voltammetric methods are based on measuring changes in current by applying a fixed potential, or a potential sweep, onto the working electrode. According to the potential applied, the compound under study is oxidized or reduced at the electrode surface, while the bulk of the solution remains unchanged. Voltammetric measurements are two-dimensional, where the potential is related to the qualitative properties of the substance, and the current is related to its quantitative properties.

In linear sweep and pulse voltammetry, the potential sweep is applied in one direction only. However, the cyclic voltammetry technique makes successive potential sweeps in both directions, i.e., oxidation and reduction, between two potential values. A typical cyclic voltammogram is shown in figure 1B. Thus, cyclic voltammetry is useful for the study of both the redox properties of a substance and the behavior of the product generated during the electrochemical reaction. The applicability of this technique mainly depends on the number of compounds that are electroactive in the potential range applied, among other parameters. One highlight of cyclic voltammetry is that the rate of experiments can be regulated and, as a result, can be rapidly performed, allowing the study of species with short half-lives.

When the controlled potential electrolysis technique is used, a fixed potential is applied to the working electrodes, which have large surfaces so that the entire bulk solution can be oxidized or reduced. As a result, measurable amounts of compounds that are identifiable by other techniques, e.g., mass spectrometry, can be obtained. Thus, electrochemistry coupled to mass spectrometry (EC-MS) permits the reproduction of the redox reactions involved in drug metabolism, allowing the detection of final products or stable intermediaries (Lohmann et al., 2010).

Taking into account that electrochemistry allows investigations of the redox reactions that drugs undergo and that phase I metabolism in the liver occurs via redox reactions, electrochemical methods have emerged as a promising alternative and a complementary tool in the study of *in vitro* metabolism because they are relatively simple, fast and cost-effective systems.

3. *In vitro* mimicry of metabolic reactions by electrochemistry

The electrochemical oxidations of organic compounds and the use of electrochemistry to mimic biologic reactions, such as oxidative drug metabolism, have been well documented and revised (Álvarez-Lueje & Bollo, 2010; Jurva et al., 2000, 2003). Electrochemistry has been used to emulate different phase I reactions, such as aromatic hydroxylation, dehydrogenation and O- and N-dealkylation, by introducing the compound of interest into an electrochemical cell and applying a specific potential for a determined period of time. During this time, the entire sample is oxidized to generate one or more products, depending on the applied potential. Thus, from this method, the generated products can be identified, characterized and studied separately. Furthermore, the simulation of phase II reactions, including conjugation with GSH or other thiols from electrochemically generated phase I metabolites, has also been achieved. For example, the metabolism of clozapine, including both phase I and phase II reactions, has successfully been mimicked (van Leeuwen et al., 2005), as well as the detoxification of acetaminophen (Lohmann & Karst, 2006) and the conjugation of diclofenac (Madsen et al., 2008a) by the electrochemical oxidation of the parent drugs.

The replication of drug metabolism using electrochemistry is a faster, more cost-effective instrumental technique than the widely used *in vivo* and *in vitro* methods that utilize liver cells or isolated enzymes. On-line EC-MS has been introduced as an alternative for early-stage metabolite discovery, and its ability to mimic biological oxidation patterns is currently being explored because it allows both the oxidation of a drug and the identification of the oxidized species. In this on-line system, the sample flows through an electrochemical cell that normally contains a working electrode made of porous glassy carbon, which posses a great area. On the working electrode occurs the quantitative conversion of the tested compound, depending on the working conditions, such as the nature of the analyte, the potential applied, the flow rate and the pH. Especially in high-throughput screening, EC-MS is superior to the conventional methods, as it can be completely automated. Because of these features, on-line EC-MS is of particular importance to the pharmaceutical industry. Although the EC-MS results are not completely transferable to the conditions of the human liver, this methodology can provide primary data concerning the metabolism of drugs in the human body. Thus, the instrumental method EC-MS may have advantages or may be complementary to the existing methods of screening that involve *in vitro* studies or organ fractions, e.g., microsomes, hepatocytes and liver slices. Additionally, with an on-line EC-MS system, the complexity of a biological system is reduced, and the optimization of the electrochemical and MS parameters can be realized more rapidly. The ternary combination of EC-LC-MS is able to detect reaction products with lifetimes on the order of several minutes; therefore, short-lived intermediates are not detected, as they react to more stable products during the chromatographic run. Direct EC-MS allows the detection of less stable compounds with lifetimes of a few seconds (van Leeuwen et al., 2005). In figure 2, a schematic representation of both systems is shown.

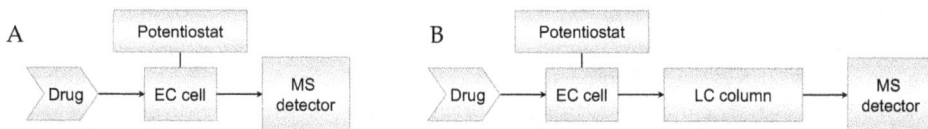

Fig. 2. Schematic representation of different on-line electrochemical set-ups used for the study of drug metabolism reactions. A) EC-MS system; B) EC-LC-MS system (adapted from Baumann & Karst, 2010).

The use of on-line EC-MS began in the early 1970s. Early studies included the development of a thin-layer electrochemical flow cell that was employed in combination with thermospray mass spectrometry for the study of the oxidation of uric acid and 6-thioxanthine (Volk et al., 1989, 1992). An analogous array in a flow injection experiment was used to study the formation of GSH and cysteine conjugates of acetaminophen. Later, the pattern of coupling an electrochemical flow cell to mass spectrometry was extended to other ionization techniques, e.g., fast-atom bombardment, particle beam, atmospheric-pressure chemical ionization and electrospray (Baumann & Karst, 2010; Jurva et al., 2000; Lohmann et al., 2008).

The first coupling of electrochemistry to particle-beam mass spectrometry was applied for the study of the oxidation pathway of dopamine (Regino & Brajter-Toth, 1997). Later, different electrochemical cells were coupled to an electrospray mass spectrometer to study the different products of biologically relevant redox reactions (Zhou & Van Berkel, 1995). In addition, an on-line electrochemistry-electrospray ionization mass spectrometry system using a microflow electrolytic cell was developed and applied to study the electrochemical oxidation of caffeic acid (Arakawa et al., 2004).

The first example of the application of EC-LC-MS for the study of drug metabolism was reported in 1989 for comparing the enzymatic and electrochemical oxidation pathways of uric acid. This study found that the enzymatic and chemical reactions yielded the same intermediates and products of those observed in the electrochemical oxidation. A similar array was used to oxidize 3-hydroxy-*dl*-kynurenine (a tryptophan metabolite) in an electrochemical cell, eventually separating the oxidation products by reversed-phase LC and identifying the products by UV and MS detection (Deng & Van Berkel, 1999).

Comparisons on the mechanistic level have been made for most reactions to explain why certain reactions can and other reactions cannot be mimicked by electrochemical oxidations. The EC system successfully mimics metabolic pathways in cases where the CYP-catalyzed reactions are supposed to proceed via a mechanism initiated by one-electron oxidation, such as N-dealkylation, S-oxidation, P-oxidation, alcohol oxidation, dehydrogenation and hydroxylation of aromatic rings that contain electron-donating groups. In contrast, the CYP-catalyzed reactions initiated via direct hydrogen abstraction, such as O-dealkylation, aliphatic hydroxylation and hydroxylation of aromatic rings without electron-donating groups, generally have a very high oxidation potential for electrochemical oxidation and cannot always be mimicked using EC (Johansson et al., 2007). However, even when the EC system is not able to mimic all oxidations performed by CYP, valuable information can be obtained regarding the sensitivity of the substrate toward oxidation and the molecular position where oxidation is likely to occur.

For the reason described above, to be able to mimic all CYP-catalyzed oxidations, electrochemistry must be complemented with other oxidative systems. This is the case for the electrochemically assisted Fenton reaction (EC-Fenton) that is able to mimic aliphatic hydroxylation, benzylic hydroxylation, aromatic hydroxylation, N-dealkylation, N-oxidation, O-dealkylation, S-oxidation and dehydrogenation (Johansson et al., 2007). In EC-Fenton, the regeneration of Fe^{+2} is achieved by the reduction of Fe^{+3} at the working electrode. The hydroxyl radical generated from this system is highly electrophilic and readily reacts with aromatic rings and double bonds. In addition, the hydroxyl radical can abstract a hydrogen atom from various organic compounds.

Studies on drug metabolism by electrochemical techniques will be presented, discussed and compared with conventional *in vitro* (e.g., microsomes, hepatocytes and porphine system) and *in vivo* assays and divided by each main representative chemical functional group, including aliphatic hydroxylation; aromatic hydroxylation; N-, S- and O-dealkylations; heteroatom (N, S and P) oxidation; dehydrogenation; and other oxidative reactions, such as the oxidations of alcohols, aldehydes and benzylic groups. In addition, examples of drug metabolism mimicked by EC are summarized in table 1.

Drug	Predicted metabolism	Products	Urine	Plasma	RLM	HLM	Rat Bile	EC	References
Acetaminophen	Phases I, II	N-acetyl-*p*-benzoquinoneimine *p*-benzoquinoneimine-GSH				√ √		√ √	Lohmann & Karst,2006; Madsen et al., 2007
Albendazole	Phase I	albendazole sulfoxide albendazole sulfone	√# √#	√ √	√ √			√ √	Galvão de Lima et al., 2003
Amodiaquine	Phases I, II	N-deethylated quinoneimine Quinoneimine Aldehyde GSH adducts N-deethylation			√ √ √ √ √	× √ × √ √		√ √ √ √ √	Johansson et al., 2007; Johansson et al., 2009; Lohmann & Karst,2007; Madsen et al., 2007
Boscalid	Phases I, II	hydroxylation, dehydrogenation GSH adducts	√* √*					√ √	Lohmann et al., 2009
Chlorpromazine	Phase I	N-demethylation S-oxidation N-oxidation aromatic hydroxylation				√ √ √ √		√ √ × ×	Nozaki et al., 2006

Drug	Predicted metabolism	Products	Urine	Plasma	RLM	HLM	Rat Bile	EC	References
Clozapine	Phases I, II	N-dealkylation			√	√		√	Dain et al., 1997; Schaber et al. 2001; van Leeuwen et al., 2005;
		N-oxide	√#	√#	√	√		×	
		aromatic	√#		×	×		√	
		hydroxylation	√#						
		GSH adducts			√	√		√	
Diclofenac	Phases I, II	4'-OH-diclofenac			√	√	√	√	Madsen et al., 2008a
		5-OH-diclofenac			√	√	√	√	
		GSH adducts			√	√	√	√	
Estradiol	Phases I, II	2-hydroxyestradiol			√	√		√	Gamache et al., 2003
		4-hydroxyestradiol			√	√		√	
		GSH adducts			√	√		√	
7-ethoxycoumarin	Phase I	O-dealkylation			√	√	√	√	Johansson et al., 2007; Jurva et al., 2000;
Lidocaine	Phase I	N-dealkylation			×	√	√	√	Baumann & Karst 2010; Johansson et al., 2007; Jurva et al., 2003;
		N-oxidation			√	√	×	√	
Mephenytoin	Phase I	dydroxylation			√	√		√	Johansson et al., 2007
S-methylthiopurine	Phase I	S-oxidation			√	√		√	Johansson et al., 2007
		S-demethylation			√	√		√	
Metoprolol	Phase I	benzylic hydroxylation			√	√		√	Baumann & Karst 2010; Johansson et al., 2007
		aromatic hydroxylation			√	×		√	
		N-dealkylation			√			√	
		O-dealkylation			√	√		√	
Mitoxantrone	Phase I	quinone			√			√	Lohmann & Karst, 2007
Parathion	Phase I	phosphine oxide	√*					√	Jurva et al., 2003
Procainamide	Phase I	N-monodealkyl procainamide			×	√		√	Odijk et al., 2010
		N-hydroxylamine procainamide			√	√		√	
		N-oxide derivative procainamide			√	×		√	
2-(N-propyl-N-2-thienylethyl amino)-5-hydroxitetralin	Phase I	N-dealkylation			√			√	Jurva et al., 2000
		hydroxylation			√			√	
Testosterone	Phase I	aliphatic hydroxylation			√	√		√	Johansson et al., 2007
Tetrazepam	Phase I	cyclohexenyl hydroxylations	√#		√			√	Baumann et al., 2009
		3-hydroxytetrazepam	×#		√			√	
		diazepam	√#		√			√	
		nortetrazepam	√#		√			√	
Toremifene	Phases I, II	N-demethylation			√	√		√	Lohmann & Karst, 2009
		N-oxide			√	√		×	
		quinone methide			√	√		√	
		GSH adducts			√	√		√	

Drug	Predicted metabolism	Products	Urine	Plasma	RLM	HLM	Rat Bile	EC	References
Triclocarban	Phase I	2'-hydroxytriclocarban	√#	√**	√	√	√	√	Baumann et al., 2010
		6-hydroxytriclocarban	√#	√**	√	√	√	√	
		3'-hydroxytriclocarban	√#		√	√	√	√	
		2',6-dihydroxytriclocarban	√*		×	×		√	
		3',6-dihydroxytriclocarban			×	×		√	
Troglitazone	Phases I, II	p-quinone derivative	√#		×	√		√	Madsen et al, 2008b; Tahara et al., 2007; Tahara et al., 2009
		o-quinone methide		×#	√	√		√	
		o-quinone methide conjugates			√	√		√	
Zotepine	Phase I	N-demethylation			√			√	Nozaki et al., 2006
		S-oxidation			√			√	
		N-oxidation			√			×	
		aromatic hydroxylation			√			×	

Table 1. Examples of drug metabolism mimicked by EC (√: generated; ×: not generated,*rat, #human).

Aliphatic hydroxylation

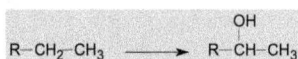

One limitation of the electrochemical method has been the difficulty in mimicking the metabolic hydroxylation of alkanes and alkenes due to the fact that electrochemical oxidation potentials for aliphatic hydrocarbons are generally very high (Jurva et al., 2003). Nevertheless, there have been some examples where this experimental limitation has been overcome, as in the oxidation of the muscle relaxant tetrazepam. In this case, a platinum working electrode was used, with an enhanced potential range of up to 2000 mV, instead of the typical porous glassy carbon working electrode, and the hydroxylation of the tetrazepam cyclohexenyl group at five different positions was successfully achieved (compounds 2, 3, 6, 8 and 10 in figure 3). In this study, an on-line EC-LC-MS system was used to analyze the metabolic pathway of the drug. Additionally, a comparison of the EC method with urine analyses and a conventional rat liver microsomal approach was performed, which found that eleven different metabolites were indentified in the urine samples, and only two of them were not found after microsomal incubation (table 2). These differences were explained as a result of different CYP isoforms with different catalytic activities in each organism; therefore, the metabolism in humans and in rat liver microsomes may result in different metabolites or a different distribution of them. As can be seen in this example, the comparison of both methods shows that electrochemistry combined with LC-MS is an adequate complementary tool to conventional *in vitro* methods in the prediction of metabolic processes of tetrazepam (Baumann et al., 2009).

A second example of aliphatic hydroxylation is testosterone, in which two different hydroxylation products were found in liver microsomes, one in RLM and the other in HLM. Both metabolites were generated using the EC-Fenton system and the porphine system (Johansson et al., 2007).

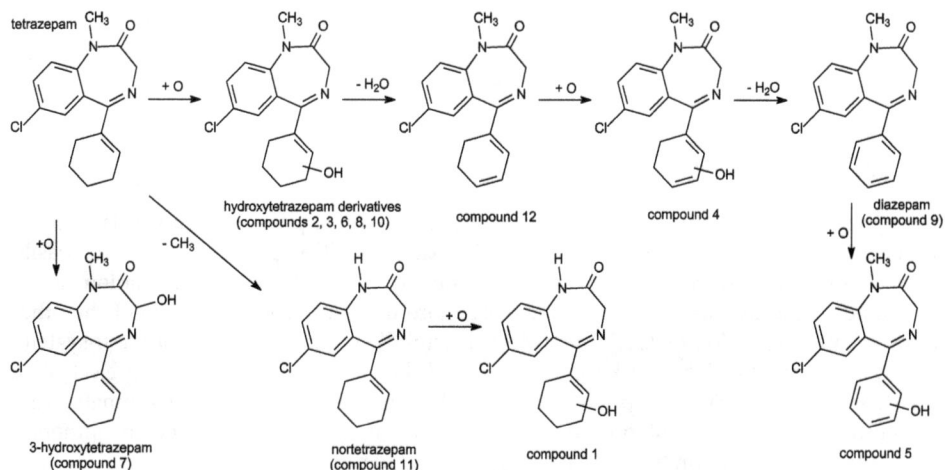

Fig. 3. Oxidative metabolism of tetrazepam (adapted from Baumann et al., 2009).

	Compound											
	1	2	3	4	5	6	7	8	9	10	11	12
Urine	x	x	x	x	x	x		x	x	x	x	x
RML	x	x	x	x			x	x	x	x	x	x
EC		x	x		x	x	x	x	x	x	x	x

Table 2. Tetrazepam metabolites produced in different systems. For compound identification, see figure 3 (adapted from Baumann et al., 2009).

Aromatic hydroxylation

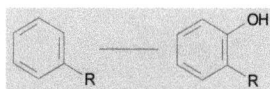

Contrary to aliphatic hydroxylation, a variety of drugs and compounds have been tested for aromatic hydroxylation using EC-MS, including coumarin, p-nitrophenol, diclofenac, xanthohumol, tyramine and N,N-dimethylaniline (Jurva et al., 2003).

In general, to be oxidized electrochemically within the potential limits of water, the aromatic ring must be activated by an electron-donating group (e.g., a hydroxyl or amino group). For an aromatic ring without an electron-donating group, the starting compound is more difficult to oxidize than the product. For example, benzene is oxidized at a potential approximately 1300 mV more anodic than phenol. Furthermore, the oxidation cannot be stopped at the phenol stage but instead proceeds immediately to benzoquinone (figure 4). The hydroxylation of aromatic compounds by CYP shows some mechanistic similarity to electrochemical oxidation. However, due to the lack of an active iron-oxygen species in the electrochemical system, the radical intermediate achieved after the initial oxidation and deprotonation steps will react further in different pathways, which are determined by the specific substituents (Jurva et al., 2003).

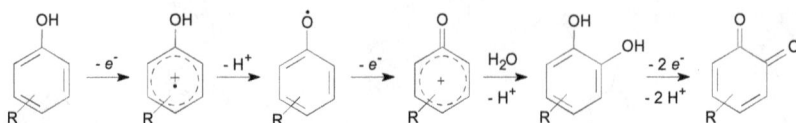

Fig. 4. Electrochemical oxidation mechanism of phenols.

The suggested mechanism for the electrochemical oxidation of phenols (figure 4) is initiated in the same way as the CYP-catalyzed oxidation. Compounds that are easily electrochemically oxidized likely follow this pathway for CYP-catalyzed oxidation, while compounds with high oxidation potentials are more likely to proceed via one of the other pathways after oxidation by CYP. In an electrochemical system, the nature of the π-system, the physical features of the working electrode and the nature of the supporting electrolyte will determine the final compound. Thus, different substituents on the aromatic ring frequently result in different products, e.g., phenols are generally oxidized to quinones, while other substituents on the aromatic ring will lead to different products.

The beta blocker metoprolol and the antiepileptic mephenytoin are good examples of compounds in which aromatic hydroxylation has been investigated. Metoprolol contains an aromatic ring with oxygen as an electron-donating group. In contrast, mephenytoin does not contain any strong electron-donating groups, and it represents an aromatic ring with lower electron density. The aromatic hydroxylation of metoprolol has been studied in RLM, and it was also simulated using a conventional EC system, the EC-Fenton system and the porphine system (figure 5). A different situation occurred with mephenytoin, whose aromatic hydroxylation has been investigated in both RLM and HLM but could only be mimicked using the EC-Fenton system and the porphine system (Johansson et al., 2007).

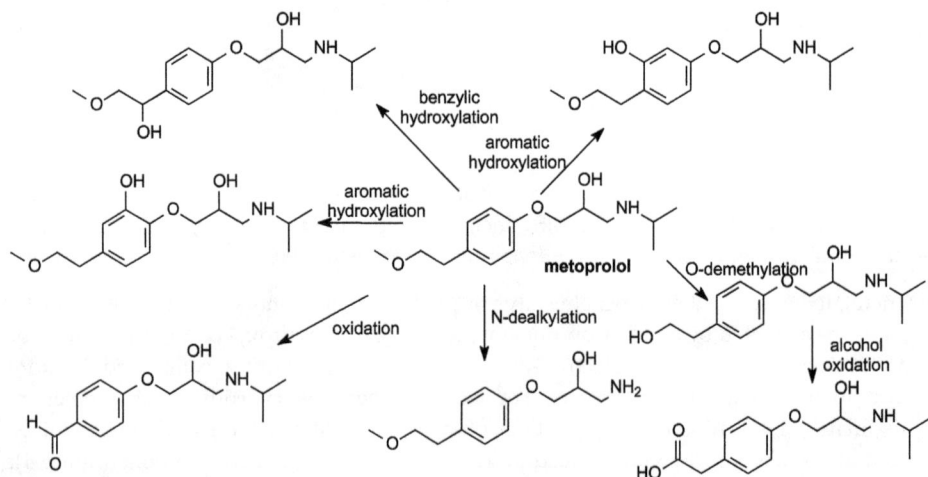

Fig. 5. Metabolism of metoprolol in HLM (Johansson et al., 2007).

The hydroxylation of estrogens has also been investigated in an EC system. Investigations with estradiol, which was subjected to EC oxidation, were interesting and produced two hydroxylated metabolites, 2-hydroxyestradiol and 4-hydroxyestradiol (figure 6) (Gamache et al., 2003). It has been shown that 2-hydroxylation of estradiol to its catechol derivative is a major metabolic pathway in rodent and human livers, whereas 4-hydroxylation to a different catechol represents a minor pathway in the liver. It has also been demonstrated that 2-hydroxylation is the major hydroxylation pathway in HLM, while the rate of 4-hydroxylation is 1/4 to 1/6 of that for the 2-hydroxylation of estradiol (Zhu & Lee, 2005).

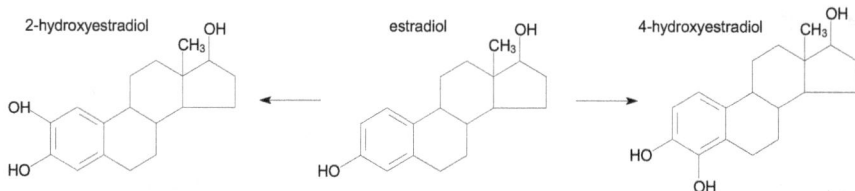

Fig. 6. Hydroxylation of estradiol produced by the EC system at 900 mV as well as in RLM and HLM.

N-, S- and O-Dealkylations

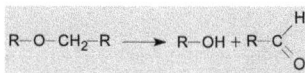

The dealkylation of amines and ethers can be replicated by EC systems. While the former can be readily mimicked, the dealkylation of ethers can only be obtained in low yields. However, the dealkylation of thioethers cannot yet be mimicked using EC.

The dealkylation of alkylamines is the main pathway in both EC and enzymatic oxidation. The parent compound undergoes one-electron oxidation to yield a heteroatom-centered cation radical. The cation radical is better stabilized by sulfur and phosphorus than by nitrogen. As a consequence, the main products from CYP-catalyzed oxidation and from EC oxidation are sulfoxides and phosphine oxides. If the heteroatom is oxygen, CYP is not able to complete a one-electron oxidation due to the poor ability of oxygen to carry the positive charge. Thus, the reaction proceeds via a direct hydrogen abstraction from the α-carbon. In the proposed mechanism for the EC oxidation of aliphatic amines (figure 7), the first two steps are the same for EC and CYP-catalyzed oxidation. One-electron oxidation gives an iminium cation radical, which produces the α-carbon-centered radical. In the CYP-catalyzed mechanism, the electron and the proton are transferred to the iron-oxygen of the enzyme, and the hydroxyl group is introduced to the α-carbon by reacting with the $[Fe–OH]^{3+}$ species. In the EC oxidation, the electron is transferred to the working electrode, and the proton is lost to any compound acting as a base in solution. Because there is no active iron-oxygen intermediary present in the EC system, the neutral radical is further oxidized at the working electrode to the iminium ion. Finally, hydrolysis of the iminium ion provides the dealkylated amine and the corresponding aldehyde (Jurva et al., 2003).

Many drugs contain substituted amine groups. For example, metoprolol undergoes N-dealkylation of the secondary amine and generates a product corresponding to a loss of its isopropyl group. This has been observed in both RLM and HLM, and the reaction has been successfully mimicked using conventional EC, EC-Fenton and porphine systems (figure 5). However, N-deethylation of the tertiary amine function of lidocaine has been observed in

HLM, and the same N-dealkylation was demonstrated for amodiaquine in RLM and HLM. Such N-dealkylation reactions were successfully mimicked in the EC system for lidocaine, while for amodiaquine, the reaction was mimicked in the EC and EC-Fenton systems (Johansson et al., 2009; Lohmann & Karst, 2007).

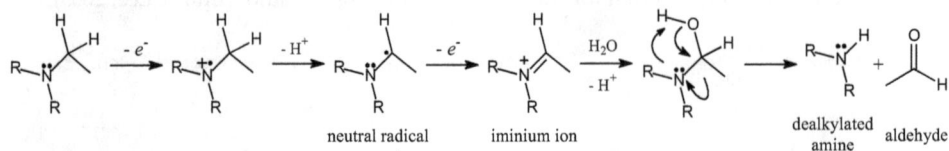

Fig. 7. Electrochemical oxidation mechanism of aliphatic amines.

More recently, an on-chip electrochemical cell was developed for routine use in drug metabolism studies. The chip was used for the metabolism study of the known antiarrhythmic drug procainamide, which found that the chip was able to generate all of the known metabolites produced in both RLM and HLM (figure 8). In the RLM incubation mixture, the metabolites N-hydroxylamine and N-oxide derivatives were identified. In contrast, in the HLM incubation mixture, the dealkylation product N-deethyl procainamide and the oxygenation product N-hydroxylamine derivative were detected. Using an on-line system consisting of the on-chip electrochemical cell, LC separation and subsequent MS detection, the metabolism of procainamide was achieved. In this case, on-chip oxidation actually demonstrated the ability to provide more information about the generated metabolites in a single experiment than the microsomal studies (Odijk et al., 2010).

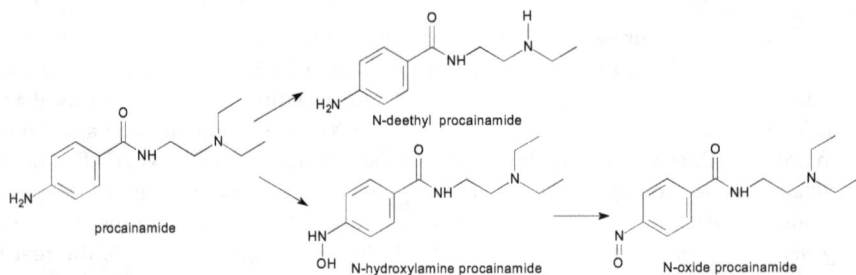

Fig. 8. Oxidative metabolism of procainamide (adapted from Odijk et al., 2010).

Finally, examples of O-dealkylations obtained from EC oxidation include metoprolol, which undergoes O-demethylation (figure 5), and 7-ethoxycoumarin, which generates its corresponding O-deethyl derivative. For both drugs, the same reactions have been found in RLM and HML (Johansson et al., 2007).

Heteroatom (N, S, P) oxidation

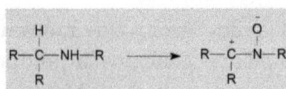

As a general rule, S-oxide and N-oxide formation can be successfully mimicked using EC, but unlike the formation of S-oxides, N-oxide formation can only be detected in low yields.

Thus, heteroatom (N, S and P) oxidation has successfully been proven for different drugs when compared with the typical *in vitro* systems. In all cases, the three types of oxidation were observed in both RLM and HLM, and the oxidation was mimicked in the EC, EC-Fenton and porphine systems. Typical examples of such reactions include lidocaine (N-oxidation) and S-methylthiopurine (S-oxidation). In figure 9, representative reactions of each type are presented. In heteroatom oxidation, the porphine system and the EC-Fenton system are preferable due to higher yields of the oxidation product than the EC-system (Jurva et al., 2003).

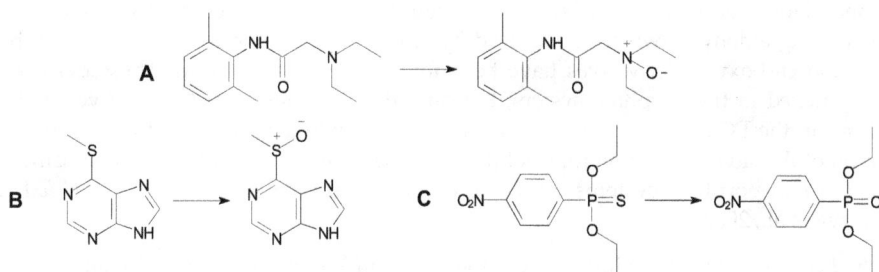

Fig. 9. Typical examples of heteroatom oxidations. A) lidocaine (N-oxidation), B) S-methylthiopurine (S-oxidation) and C) parathion (P-oxidation).

Compounds containing phosphorus generally have a lower oxidation potential than sulfur-containing compounds, and CYP-catalyzed oxidation and electrochemical oxidation of phosphorus-containing compounds almost exclusively result in phosphine oxides. An example of this kind of reaction is the CYP-catalyzed phosphothionate oxidation of the pesticide parathion (figure 9). Indeed, electrochemical oxidation of parathion yielded the same oxidation product at a potential of 600 mV in 0.1 M acetic acid (Jurva et al., 2003).

Dehydrogenation

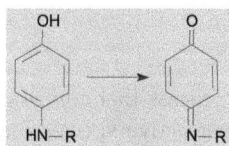

Dehydrogenation reactions can be readily mimicked using EC, especially when followed by quinone or quinone imine formation. Acetaminophen is oxidized by several human CYP enzymes to its toxic metabolite N-acetyl-p-benzoquinoneimine. The dehydrogenation of acetaminophen has been mimicked by the EC system as well. The proposed mechanism for its EC oxidation included the formation of a radical intermediary, likely via electron transfer followed by proton abstraction. Then, another one-electron oxidation followed by a second proton abstraction yields the final product. This mechanism for EC oxidation is nearly the same as the suggested enzymatic mechanism (Jurva et al., 2003).

A similar reaction occurs with the oxidation of the aminophenol moiety of the antimalarial agent amodiaquine to form the quinoneimine derivative (shown in figure 10). This has been observed in both RLM and HLM, and mimicry has been achieved with the EC-system, the

EC-Fenton system and the porphine system. The generated quinoneimine is an electrophilic species that reacts with nucleophiles present in the system. Therefore, cysteine is usually added to all of the systems, and the detection of amodiaquine cysteinyl conjugates is evidence of quinoneimine formation (Johansson et al., 2007; Lohmann & Karst, 2007).

Other oxidation reactions

Alcohol and aldehyde oxidation. Metoprolol has also been used to illustrate alcohol and aldehyde oxidation. Presumably, the formation of the final carboxylic metabolites from the O-demethylation of metoprolol, shown in figure 5, includes alcohol oxidation to the corresponding aldehyde, which is followed by aldehyde oxidation to carboxylic acid. Both alcohol and carboxylic derivatives have been found in RLM and HLM. These derivatives were mimicked in the porphine system, but only the O-demethylated derivative has been generated in the EC and EC-Fenton systems. The aldehyde derivative that comes from the oxidation of the side chain of metoprolol (figure 5) has been successfully obtained using EC, EC-Fenton and porphine systems but has only been observed in RLM (Baumann & Karst 2010; Jurva et al., 2003).

Benzylic hydroxylation. This kind of oxidative reaction has been mimicked using EC, EC-Fenton and the porphine systems for metoprolol. This metabolite (in figure 5), which is formed through benzylic hydroxylation, is the major hydroxylated metabolite of metoprolol in both RLM and HLM (Baumann & Karst 2010; Jurva et al., 2003).

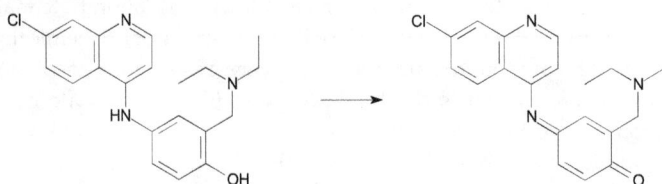

Fig. 10. Formation of the quinoneimine derivative from amodiaquine.

4. Interaction studies

Drug metabolism is regarded as a process that contributes to detoxification, but in some cases, the produced metabolites are reactive species that are more toxic than the parent drug. These reactive intermediates, which are classified as electrophiles and free radicals, can covalently bond to certain endogenous molecules, resulting in cell damage and toxicity.

The application of cyclic voltammetry can provide a first approach to study the reactivities of electrochemically generated species toward endogenous molecules, such as GSH, proteins and DNA. Usually, incubation with biomolecules in an electrochemical cell produces the appearance or disappearance of electrochemical signals in typical voltammograms of the drug of interest. These changes are due to adduct formations between the reactive species and the biomolecules, which could be part of the biological detoxification process. Furthermore, this technique allows an estimate of the electrochemical potential necessary to generate a desired product from the oxidation or reduction of its parent compound. Nevertheless, the small amount of electrolyzed product obtained from this technique does not allow the identification of the adducts formed. For this reason, the controlled potential electrolysis technique is useful for generating considerable amounts of reactive intermediaries, thereby facilitating the identification of adducts formed using other techniques, e.g., MS.

In this sense, EC-MS and EC-LC-MS systems allow the electrochemical generation and direct detection of reactive intermediaries that are short-lived and unstable, which are difficult to detect using the conventional methods of studying drug metabolism. The incorporation of biomolecules into the electrochemical cell or between EC and MS, as is presented in figure 11, is useful for determining the reactivity of metabolites and the respective adducts formed. This system has already been applied to study the interactions between endogenous molecules, especially with GSH, making it possible to establish relationships and obtain more information about phase II metabolism and drug detoxification mechanisms.

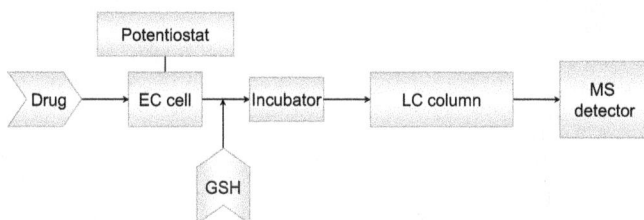

Fig. 11. Schematic representation of the on-line EC-LC-MS system to study adducts formation with GSH or other biomolecules (adapted from Baumann & Karst, 2010).

By using an on-line system, it has been possible to mimic metabolic reactions that involve phase I oxidation products and phase II conjugates of different drugs, such as clozapine, acetaminophen, toremifene, amodiaquine and mitoxantrone, among others (table 1). Some examples of interaction studies and the importance of the information obtained are described below.

The antipsychotic drug clozapine undergoes extensive hepatic metabolism, with the major metabolites found in humans being clozapine N-oxide and N-demethylclozapine. In addition, many other metabolites and adducts have been identified in humans and rats.

Cyclic voltammograms of clozapine have shown one signal in the oxidative scan direction (O1 at 450 mV) and two signals in the reverse scan (R1 at 390 mV and R2 at 75 mV) (figure 12). The potential difference between the O1 and R1 signals revealed a reversible redox process, which means that the oxidation product of clozapine (nitrenium ion) was reduced to the parent molecule. The second signal, R2, was attributed to a chemical reaction subsequent to the clozapine oxidation, with the formation of a new reduced species (hydroxylated). Upon repetitive scans, a new oxidation peak appeared (O2 at 300 mV), which was probably related to the oxidative process of the R2 product (quinone imine derivative). In the presence of GSH, the reduction peaks R1 and R2 disappeared completely in the presence of a ten-fold excess of GSH. These changes in the cyclic voltammetric profiles were due to adduct formations between GSH and the generated reactive intermediaries. Interestingly, upon increasing the GSH concentration, two new oxidation peaks appeared at potentials more positive than O1, which indicated that oxidation of the produced thioadducts occurred.

Using EC-MS and EC-LC-MS systems with a working electrode consisting of porous glassy carbon, different metabolites were obtained for clozapine, depending on the applied potential (figure 13). Upon oxidation to 400 mV, hydroxyl clozapine derivatives and nitrenium ions were the predominant products formed. Increasing the potential to 700 mV, the generation of an additional product, N-demethyl clozapine, was observed. No N-oxide derivative was detected by this system, probably because it was only generated to a small extent. When the oxidation of clozapine was performed in the presence of GSH, the formation of adducts between the metabolites that were generated and GSH were detected. These adducts were identified as hydroxy-GSH clozapine and GSH-demethyl clozapine. Additionally, a bis-GSH adduct and at least three isomers of a GSH-clozapine adduct were formed. Despite the fact that not all oxidative metabolic pathways of clozapine were mimicked by this system, the production of similar metabolites (phases I and II) confirmed the *in vitro* and *in vivo* reports concerning the metabolism of clozapine (van Leeuwen et al., 2005).

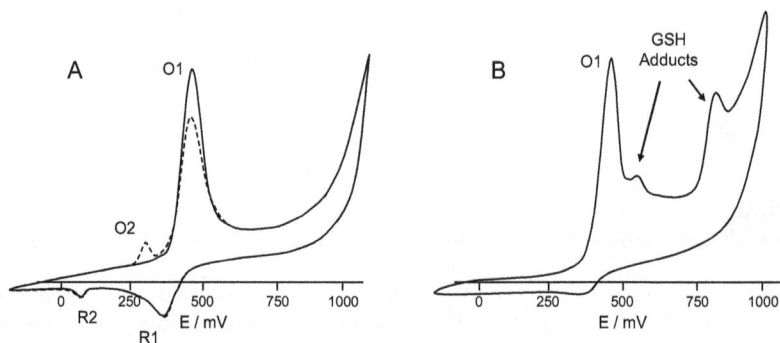

Fig. 12. Cyclic voltammograms of clozapine (A) without GSH and (B) with GSH (adapted from van Leeuwen et al., 2005).

The most studied drug in metabolite-biomolecule interactions is acetaminophen, and it is a classic example of the importance of these studies to measure the potential metabolic toxicity of a substance. Acetaminophen is a drug that is well known to cause liver toxicity in humans by its oxidative metabolic pathway in which the highly reactive electrophile intermediate N-acetyl-*p*-benzoquinoneimine (NAPQI) is generated. This species is normally detoxified by conjugation with reduced GSH, but in an acetaminophen overdose, the total liver GSH is depleted. EC-MS and EC-LC-MS experiments using either acetaminophen alone or in the presence of GSH or N-acetylcysteine (NAC) have been conducted to study the detoxification pathway of acetaminophen.

The electrochemical oxidation of acetaminophen leads to NAPQI, which is also observed *in vivo*. After applying a potential of 600 mV, at which acetaminophen shows an oxidation wave in cyclic voltammetry measurements, three major additional signals were observed in the presence of GSH or NAC, which indicated the formation of acetaminophen adducts. In the presence of these thiol-containing molecules, NAPQI was quenched by adduct formation (figure 14). This mechanism is the common detoxification pathway of NAPQI in the human liver. MS measurements showed only the formation of GSH and NAC monoadducts, but in each case, two different isomers were produced, which could correspond to 2- and 3-conjugated-acetaminophen. In general, NAPQI has two possible reaction sites, namely, the 2- and 3-substitution positions. Unlike in the human body, only conjugates at position 2 of acetaminophen are formed. This selectivity is a result of the CYP enzymatic system that is involved in *in vivo* adduct formation, which is not possible to achieve using only electrochemical methods and trapping agents. Despite this, the electrochemical oxidation of acetaminophen, alone and in the presence of GSH or NAC, allowed the successful replication of the metabolic detoxification pathway that occurs in the human liver (Lohmann et al., 2006).

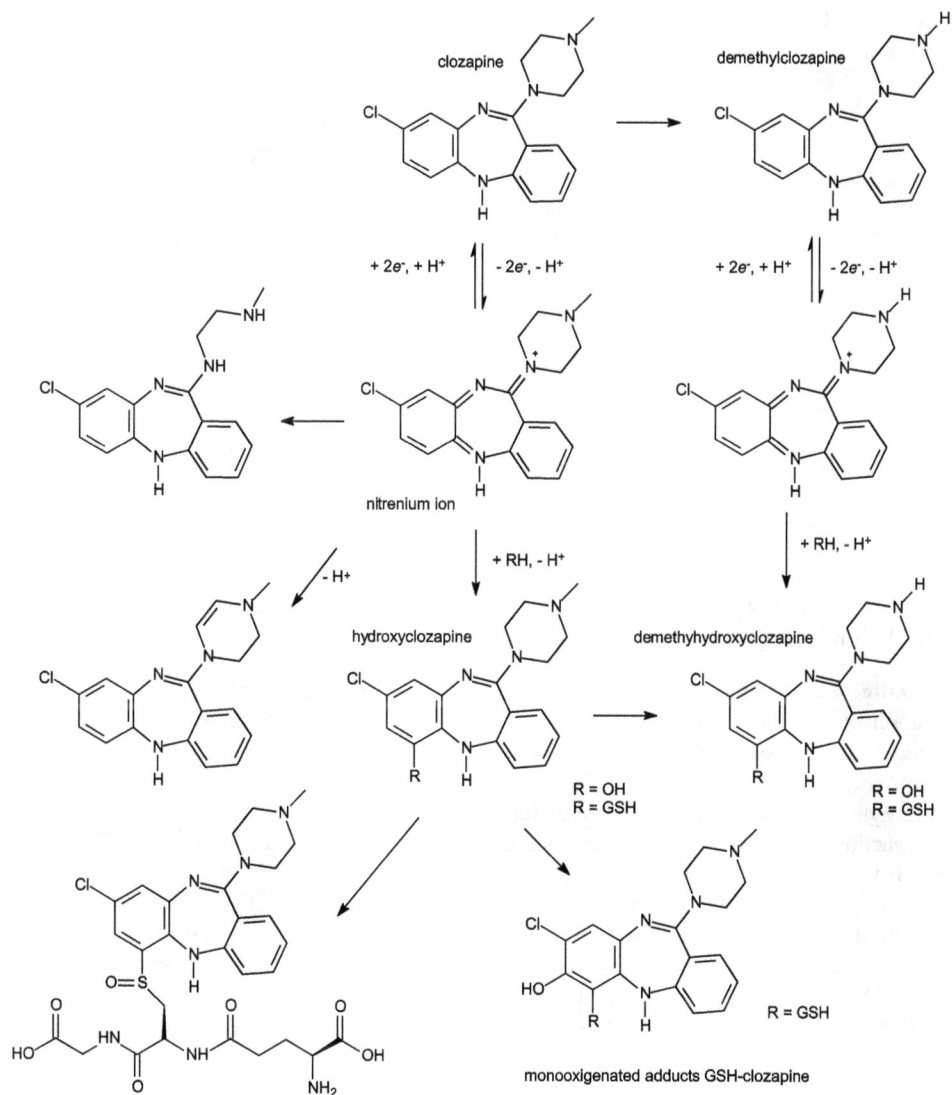

Fig. 13. Electrochemical oxidation of clozapine (van Leeuwen et al., 2005).

A modification of the conventional on-line system was introduced to simulate conjugative phase II reactions. This system consisted of the incorporation of an enzymatic reactor between the electrochemical cell and the separation system and was applied to investigate the phase II metabolism of toremifene, a selective estrogen receptor modulator.

It is well known that toremifene metabolism by CYP is comprised mainly of hydroxylation, O-dealkylation, N-dealkylation and N-oxide formation, which are observed in rat, mouse, and human liver microsomes. All are produced electrochemically, except for the N-oxide derivative (figure 15). Furthermore, the generation of reactive quinone methides may occur, which are detoxified by reacting with GSH, the reaction of which is catalyzed by glutathione-S-transferase (GST).

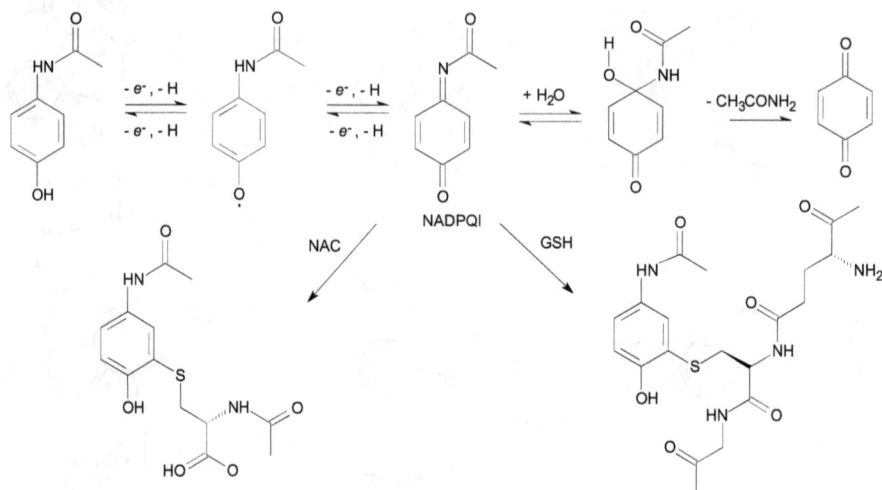

Fig. 14. Detoxification mechanism of acetaminophen by adduct formation with GSH and NAC (Lohmann et al., 2006).

Generally, the conjugation of quinoid compounds with GSH observed in phase II metabolism has been successfully mimicked by electrochemical methods because the conjugation proceeds spontaneously via a 1,4-Michael addition reaction. In the case of toremifene, the conjugation with GSH occurs by nucleophilic substitution of the chloride atom, which normally is not possible using electrochemical techniques, which suggests that this reaction requires enzymatic catalysis to proceed. However, using only an EC-LC-MS system with GSH incubation, it was possible to identify the adduct formed between GSH and the quinone methide derivative by chloride atom substitution. Furthermore, the incorporation of GST to the system made it possible to obtain an additional conjugate that is only generated by enzymatic catalysis. Thus, the use of metabolic enzymes in the on-line EC-LC-MS provided important information about metabolites that are not normally identified by conventional *in vitro* and *in vivo* assays or by simple electrochemical systems (Lohmann & Karst, 2009).

Other interesting approaches that involved this on-line system included interaction studies of metabolites with more complex biomolecules, such as plasma proteins and DNA. To perform and evaluate the covalent protein binding of reactive phase I metabolites, the oxidation products of acetaminophen, amodiaquine and clozapine have been evaluated with regard to adduct formation with beta-lactoglobulin A and human serum albumin. The experiments demonstrated that mainly covalent binding took place between the free thiol groups of these proteins and the reactive metabolites, which is analogous to endogenous detoxification pathways. Thus, this experimental system offered interesting features in the risk assessment of the covalent protein binding of drug metabolites due to the significance of the protein structure and its function (Lohmann et al., 2008).

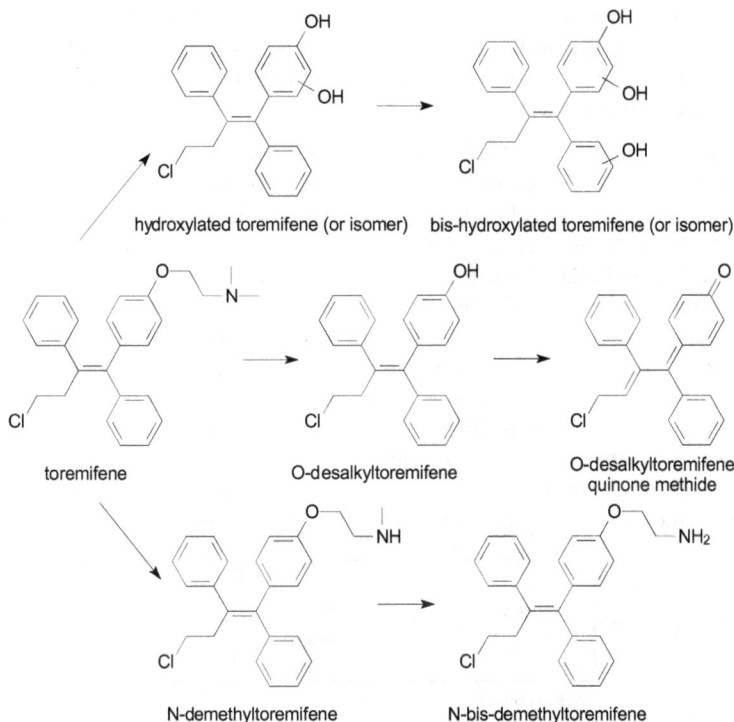

hydroxylated toremifene (or isomer)   bis-hydroxylated toremifene (or isomer)

toremifene   O-desalkyltoremifene   O-desalkyltoremifene
                                                       quinone methide

N-demethyltoremifene   N-bis-demethyltoremifene

Fig. 15. Electrochemical oxidation of toremifene (Lohmann & Karst, 2009).

In relation to reductive metabolism, the redox chemistry of different nitro compounds of biological significance have been studied to understand how the reduction of the nitro group can play an active role in free radical generation and free radical reactivity. Some drugs that were studied corresponded to calcium antagonists, antibacterial and antiprotozoan agents, among others (Squella et al., 2005). Cyclic voltammetric technique using mercury as the working electrode permitted the simulation of the enzymatic formation of the nitro radical anion, a product of the one-electron reduction of nitro compounds, and an evaluation of chemical and biological characteristics.

Using this electrochemical technique, it was also possible to detect and quantify the interaction between the nitro radical anion derivative and several targets of biological significance, such as oxygen, thiols and DNA. In fact, the addition of a target compound with which the nitro radical anion derivative could interact produced changes in the cyclic voltammetric response that could be used to quantitatively calculate the interaction constant value. One of the main advantages of cyclic voltammetry in the study of nitro radical anions is that they can be generated and studied *in situ* (Bollo et al., 2000).

5. Biosensors for metabolic reactions

A biosensor is a device capable of detecting, recording and transmitting information about the presence, activity or concentration of a specific compound in solution with a biological recognition element and a physicochemical transducer (figure 16). These devices have become very important due to the advantages they possess as rapid tools for the screening and detection of substances and the possibilities of miniaturization that would allow the development of portable devices.

As can be seen in figure 16, the biological recognition element can include enzymes, antibodies, cell receptors, tissues, or microorganisms, whereas the transducers that are often used are electrochemical, optical and piezoelectrical. The biorecognition process can either be a bio-affinity (affinity ligand-based biosensor) or bio-metabolism (enzyme-based biosensor) reaction, and this interaction results in biochemical and physicochemical changes that are converted to a quantifiable signal by the transducer. The biosensor selectivity for the target drug is mainly determined by the recognition element, while its sensitivity is greatly influenced by the transducer. In this sense, the most common biosensors are based on electrochemical transducers that confer high detection sensitivity (D'Orazio, 2003). In electrochemical biosensors, the main transducing elements include working electrodes of noble metals (e.g., platinum or gold) or carbon derivatives (e.g., glassy carbon or carbon paste). These electrodes can be modified to improve the connection to the recognizing agent, which would make them applicable to a large variety of samples.

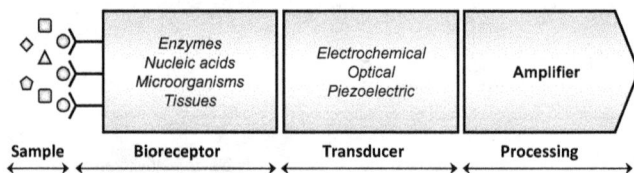

Fig. 16. Representation of a typical biosensor, including the different constituent parts.

Although biosensors have been successfully developed and used in different areas, with the glucose biosensor being the most common example, their application in metabolism is relatively new, and most of the works in this area have focused on optimizing the immobilization process of the biological element. Because most electrochemical biosensors are based on enzymatic reactions, they are a promising strategy for studying metabolic reactions, particularly by CYP-catalyzed oxidations. For example, modified electrodes with CYP enzyme films could be used as a screening tool to study drug metabolism, focusing mainly on drug interactions with the enzyme and on the toxicity of metabolites toward biomolecules, such as proteins and DNA (Bistolas et al., 2005).

A critical step in the construction of any biosensor is the immobilization of the biorecognition element onto the electroactive surface because an incorrect immobilization can lead to the loss of the native structure and therefore a loss of activity of the biological compound. In general, direct electrochemistry of CYP enzymes on unmodified electrodes has proven very difficult due to the deeply buried heme cofactor and instability of the biological matrix upon interaction with the electrode surface. To solve this problem, an immobilization material can be used, which is often a membrane or matrix that acts only as a biological component support or that participates in the signal transduction system. In addition to this problem, when the CYP is used as the biorecognition element, an extra component to provide external electrons (e.g., flavin, iron–sulfur proteins or NAD(P)H) is required, which makes biosensor development more complex. Despite these limitations, there are results that suggest that human enzyme CYP3A4 immobilized onto a gold electrode is electrically and catalytically active (Joseph et al., 2003). Additionally, some authors have studied the possibility of a direct electrochemical delivery of the required electrons using the CYP catalytic cycle, which would result in an interesting alternative that facilitates biosensor development without the need of redox transfer proteins and cofactors (Bistolas et al., 2004; Yang et al, 2009).

Yang et al. developed an electrochemical biosensor for the mimicry metabolism of warfarin, which is almost exclusively biotransformed by CYP2C9 to the primary inactive metabolite 7-hydroxy-warfarin and to 6-hydroxy-warfarin. The system consisted of the immobilization of CYP2C9 onto a gold electrode through an 11-mercaptoundecanoic acid and octanethiol self-assembled monolayer, without the presence of cofactors or other redox transfer proteins (figure 17). Using cyclic voltammetry, the reduction peak on the forward scan suggested the direct electron transfer from the electrode to the heme group of the enzyme and the consequent oxidation of the substrate, whereas the peak on the reverse scan indicated the re-oxidation of the reduced enzyme. The electrochemical behavior of this system demonstrated that warfarin was oxidized by CYP2C9. By controlled potential electrolysis and analysis of the electrolyzed solution using LC, the metabolite 7-hydroxywarfarin was identified, which was also obtained in an *in vitro* enzymatic assay (Yang et al, 2009). Thus, the developed system was efficient in the generation of the main metabolite of warfarin and therefore could be used to mimic oxidative drug metabolism in a more accurate form, without the necessity of enzymatic cofactors.

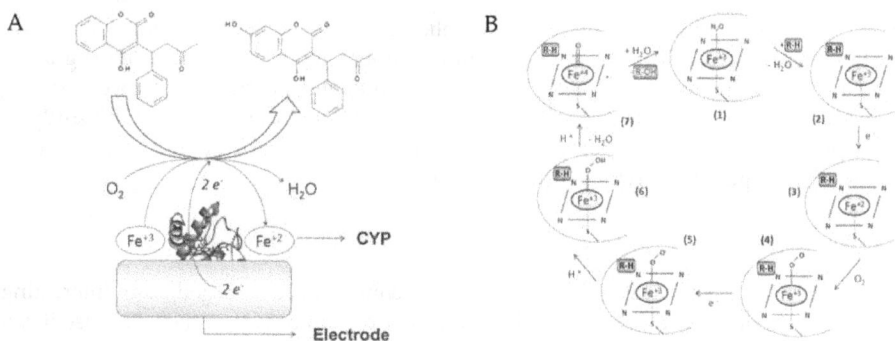

Fig. 17. A) Schematic representation of the CYP2C9 biosensor and the electrochemical oxidation of warfarin catalyzed enzymatically (adapted from Bistolas et al., 2005). B) Catalytic cycle of the CYP heme group and the reactions of the oxidation process (adapted from Lohmann & Karst, 2008).

A similar metabolic biosensor using the more predominant isoform of cytochrome P450 CYP3A4 was developed based on the redox properties and electronic transfer of the heme protein. In this case, the alternate adsorption of a CYP3A4 layer on top of a polycation layer was assembled onto gold electrodes. Under anaerobic conditions, a reversible electron transfer between the electrode and CYP3A4 was observed using cyclic voltammetry. However, in the presence of oxygen, the reduction peak increased 2- to 3-fold, and the oxidation peak of the hemoprotein disappeared. The addition of CYP3A4 substrates, such as verapamil, midazolam, quinidine and progesterone, to the oxygenated solution caused a concentration-dependent increase in the reduction current in cyclic voltammetric and amperometric experiments, which indicated an interaction between the enzyme and substrate. Controlled potential electrolysis of verapamil and midazolam and analysis by LC-MS revealed that the metabolites generated by this system were comparable to those produced by the microsomal incubation of human CYP3A4 with an NADPH-generating system. In addition, the presence of ketoconazole or catalase in the medium inhibited the catalytic activity of the enzyme and consequently led to a reduction in the amount of metabolites generated. Thus, important information was obtained from this system in the evaluation of new drugs as potential substrates or inhibitors of CYP3A4 (Joseph et al., 2003).

Inhibition and induction studies of metabolic enzymes are important in drug development processes because they can modulate or change the toxicity related to a drug. In this sense, Hull et al. developed an electrochemical biosensor to screen the metabolic inhibition of xenobiotics. This device consisted of films of bacterial cytochrome P450cam and DNA on a pyrolytic graphite electrode using a $Ru(bpy)_3^{2+}$ complex as a mediator of DNA voltammetric oxidation. For this study, styrene was chosen as the enzymatic substrate because its metabolite is genotoxic toward guanine in DNA. Styrene metabolism initiated by hydrogen peroxide was evaluated with and without the following inhibitors: imidazole, imidazole-4-acetic acid and sulconazole. The initial rates of DNA damage decreased with increasing inhibitor concentrations, and the calculated inhibition constants were directly related to the changes in styrene metabolism and DNA adduct formation in the presence of the inhibitor, which confirmed the usefulness of this enzyme/DNA biosensor as a rapid screening tool for metabolic inhibition studies of pharmaceutical candidates (Hull et al., 2009).

Therefore, modified electrodes with metabolic enzymes could provide significant information about metabolism, drug-drug metabolic interactions and whether a drug is the substrate of a specific enzymatic isoform. Furthermore, the possibility of incorporating different biomolecules into this system may provide additional advantages to the study of drug toxicity. In this sense, DNA biosensors that have been developed could be used in the future to assess the genotoxicity of drug metabolites.

6. Conclusions

The use of electrochemistry, a purely instrumental technique, has emerged as an interesting alternative to generate and detect metabolites in drug development processes because it can mimic the main oxidative reactions that occur in the human body, providing a good approximation of what occurs *in vivo*. However, it is important to take into account that not all compounds can be electrochemically oxidized; therefore, a complementary approach to this system is necessary, such as the incorporation of enzymes useful for studying metabolism.

Electrochemistry exhibits certain advantages compared to conventional methods because it allows the generation and direct identification, in a rapid and clean manner, of both stable species and metabolites with short half-lives without the need to use laboratory animals or organ extracts. Additionally, it can be a powerful tool in the interaction studies with specific cellular components, which is more difficult to realize with *in vivo* or *in vitro* methods.

In the future, this technique will most likely be supplemented with different enzymes or cofactors to expand its coverage to all metabolic reactions. It appears that biosensors could follow that trajectory to an increase in coverage and specificity. Additionally, the development of biosensors based on the use of metabolic enzymes and a biomolecular target that is susceptible to damage by the generated metabolites is a promising strategy to investigate enzyme inhibition in future metabolism studies.

7. References

Álvarez-Lueje, A. & Bollo, S. (2010). Stability and Drug Metabolism Assessed by Electrochemical Methods. *Combinatorial Chemistry & High Throughput Screening*, Vol.13, No.8, (January 2010), pp.712-727, ISSN 1386-2073

Arakawa, R., Yamaguchi. M., Hotta, H., Toshiyuki Osakai, T. & Kimoto, T. (2004).Product Analysis of Caffeic Acid Oxidation by On-Line Electrochemistry/Electrospray Ionization Mass Spectrometry, *Journal of The American Society for Mass Spectrometry*, Vol.15 , No.8 , (May 5, 2004), pp. 1228–1236, ISSN 1044-0305

Bard, A. & Faulkner, L. (2001). Introduction and overview of electrode process, In: *Electrochemical methods: fundamentals and applications*, J. Lipkowski & P. Ross, (Eds.), pp. 1-39, John Wiley & Sons Australia, Limited, ISBN 978-0-471-04372-0, United Kingdom

Baumann, A., Lohmann, W., Schubert, B., Oberacher, H. & Karst, U. (2009). Metabolic studies of tetrazepam based on electrochemical simulation in comparison to *in vivo* and *in vitro* methods. *Journal of Chromatography A*, Vol.1216, No.15, (February 2009), pp. 3192–3198, ISSN 0021-9673

Baumann, A. & Karst, U. (2010). Online electrochemistry/mass spectrometry in drug metabolism studies: principles and applications. *Expert Opinion on Drug Metabolism and Toxicology*, Vol.6, No.6, (October 2010), pp. 715-731, ISSN 1742-5255

Baumann, A., Lohmann, W., Rose, T., Ahn, K.C., Hammock, B.D., Karst, U. & Schebb, N.H. (2010). Electrochemistry-Mass Spectrometry Unveils the Formation of Reactive Triclocarban Metabolites *Drug Metabolism and Disposition*, Vol. 38, No. 12, (September 2010), pp. 2130–2138, ISSN 0090-9556

Bistolas, N., Christenson, A., Ruzgas, T., Jung, C., Scheller, F.W. & Wollenberger, U. (2004). Spectroelectrochemistry of cytochrome P450cam. *Biochemical and Biophysical Research Communications*, Vol.314, No.3, (December 2003), pp. 810-816, ISSN 0006-291X

Bistolas, N., Wollenberger, U., Jung, C. & Scheller, F.W. (2005). Cytochrome P450 biosensors—a review. *Biosensors and Bioelectronics*, Vol.20, No.12, (November 2004), pp. 2408-2423, ISSN 0956-5663

Bollo, S., Núñez-Vergara, L.J., Carbajo, J. & Squella, J.A. (2000). Electroreduction of Nitroaryl-1,4-dihydropyridines on a Mercury Pool Electrode in Mixed Media Analysis of the Reaction Products and Their Reactivity with Biomolecules. *Journal of The Electrochemical Society,* Vol.147, No.9, (December 1999) 3406-3413, ISSN 0013-4651

Brandon, E., Raap, C., Meijerman, I., Beijnen, J. & Schellens, J. (2003). An update on in vitro test methods in human hepatic drug biotransformation research: pros and cons. *Toxicology and Applied Pharmacology,* Vol. 189, No.3, (March 2003), pp. 233-246, ISSN 0041-008X

Brett, C. & Oliveira Brett, A.M. (1993). *Electrochemistry: Principles, Methods, and Applications* (First edition), Oxford University Press, ISBN 0198553889, New York, USA

D'Orazio, P. (2003). Biosensors in clinical chemistry. *Clinica Chimica Acta,* Vol.334, No.1-2, (May 2003), pp. 41–69, ISSN 0009-8981

Dain, J.G., Nicoletti, J. & Ballard, F. (1997). Biotransformation of Clozapine in Humans. *Drug Metabolism and Disposition,* Vol. 25, No. 5, (February 1997), pp. 603-609, ISSN 0090-9556

Deng, H. & Van Berkel. G.J. (1999). AThin-Layer Electrochemical Flow Cell Coupled On-Line with Electrospray-Mass Spectrometry for the Study of Biological Redox Reactions. *Electroanalysis,* Vol.11, No.12, (April 1999), pp. 857-865, ISSN 1040-0397

Galvão de Lima, R., Sueli Bonato, P. & Santana da Silva, R. (2003). Analysis of albendazole metabolites by electrospray LC_/MS/MS as a probe to elucidate electro-oxidation mechanism of albendazole. *Journal of Pharmaceutical and Biomedical Analysis,* Vol.32, No.2, (March 2003), pp. 337-343, ISSN 0731-7085

Gamache, P., Smith, R., McCarthy, R., Waraska, J. & Acworth, I. (2003). ADME/Tox Profiling Using Coulometric Electrochemistry and Electrospray Ionization Mass Spectrometry. *Spectroscopy,* Vol.18, No.6, (June 2003), pp. 14-21, Available from http://spectroscopyonline.findanalytichem.com/spectroscopy/data/articlestandard/spectroscopy/222003/58236/article.pdf

Hull, D.O., Bajrami, B., Jansson, I., Schenkman, J.B. & Rusling, J.F. (2009). Characterizing Metabolic Inhibition Using Electrochemical Enzyme/DNA Biosensors. *Analytical Chemistry,* Vol.81, No.2, (November 2008), pp. 716- 724, ISSN 0003-2700

Johansson, T., Weidolf, L. and Jurva, U. (2007). Mimicry of phase I drug metabolism – novel methods for metabolite characterization and synthesis. *Rapid Communications in Mass Spectrometry,* Vol.21, No.14, (May 2007), pp. 2323-2331, ISSN 0951-4198

Johansson, T., Jurva, U., Grönberg, G., Weidolf, L. & Masimirembwa, C. (2009). Novel Metabolites of Amodiaquine Formed by CYP1A1 and CYP1B1: Structure Elucidation Using Electrochemistry, Mass Spectrometry, and NMR. *Drug Metabolism and Disposition,* Vol. 37, No. 3, (December 2008), pp. 571–579, ISSN 0090-9556

Joseph, S., Rusling, J.F., Lvov, Y.M., Friedberg, T. & Fuhr, U. (2003). An amperometric biosensor with human CYP3A4 as a novel drug screening tool. *Biochemical Pharmacology,* Vol.65, No.11, (February 2003), pp. 1817–1826, ISSN 0006-2952

Jurva, U., Wikström, H.V. & Bruins, A.P. (2000). In vitro mimicry of metabolic oxidation reactions by electrochemistry/mass spectrometry. *Rapid Communications in Mass Spectrometry,* Vol.14, No.6, (January 2000), pp. 529–533, ISSN 0951-4198

Jurva, U., Wikström, H., Weidolf, L. & Bruins, A.P. (2003). Comparison between electrochemistry/mass spectrometry and cytochrome P450 catalyzed oxidation reactions. *Rapid Communications in Mass Spectrometry,* Vol.17, No.8, (February 2003), pp. 800–810, ISSN 0951-4198

Jurva, U., Holmén, A., Grönberg, G., Masimirembwa, C. & Weidolf, L. (2008). Electrochemical Generation of Electrophilic Drug Metabolites: Characterization of Amodiaquine Quinoneimine and Cysteinyl Conjugates by MS, IR, and NMR. *Chemical Research in Toxicology*, Vol.21, No.4, (November 2007), pp. 928–935, ISSN 0893-228X

Lohmann, W. & Karst, U. (2006). Simulation of the detoxification of paracetamol using on-line electrochemistry/liquid chromatography/mass spectrometry. *Analytical and Bioanalytical Chemistry*, Vol.386, No.6, (August 2006), pp. 1701–1708, ISSN 1618-2642

Lohmann, W. & Karst, U. (2007). Generation and Identification of Reactive Metabolites by Electrochemistry and Immobilized Enzymes Coupled On-Line to Liquid Chromatography/Mass Spectrometry. *Analytical Chemistry*, Vol.79, No.17, (July 2007), pp. 6831-6839, ISSN 0003-2700

Lohmann, W., Hayen, H. & Karst, U. (2008). Covalent Protein Modification by Reactive Drug Metabolites Using Online Electrochemistry/Liquid Chromatography/Mass Spectrometry. *Analytical Chemistry*, Vol.80, No.24, (October 2008) pp. 9714–9719, ISSN 0003-2700

Lohmann, W. & Karst, U. (2008). Biomimetic modeling of oxidative drug metabolism Strategies, advantages and limitations. *Analytical and Bioanalytical Chemistry*, Vol.391, No. , (December 2007), pp. 79–96, ISSN 1618-2642

Lohmann, W., Dötzer, R., Gütter, G., Van Leeuwen, S.M. & Karst, U. (2009). On-Line Electrochemistry/Liquid Chromatography/Mass Spectrometry for the Simulation of Pesticide Metabolism. *Journal of The American Society for Mass Spectrometry*, Vol.20, No.1, (September 2008), pp. 138–145, ISSN 1044-0305

Lohmann, W. & Karst, U. (2009). Electrochemistry meets enzymes: instrumental on-line simulation of oxidative and conjugative metabolism reactions of toremifene. *Analytical and Bioanalytical Chemistry*, Vol.394, No.5, (December 2008), pp.1341–1348, ISSN 1618-2642

Lohmann, W., Baumann, A. & Karst, U. (2010). Electrochemistry and LC–MS for Metabolite Generation and Identification: Tools, Technologies and Trends. *LC GC Europe*, Vol.28, No.6, (January 2010), pp. 1-7, ISSN 1471-6577

Madsen, K.G., Olsen, J., Skonberg, C., Hansen, S.H. & Jurva, U. (2007). Development and Evaluation of an Electrochemical Method for Studying Reactive Phase-I Metabolites: Correlation to *in Vitro* Drug Metabolism. *Chemical Research in Toxicology*, Vol.20, No.5, (January 2007), pp. 821-831, ISSN 0893-228X

Madsen, K.G., Skonberg, C., Jurva, U., Cornett, C., Hansen, S.H., Johansen, T.N. & Olsen, J. (2008a). Bioactivation of Diclofenac *in Vitro* and *in Vivo*: Correlation to Electrochemical Studies. *Chemical Research in Toxicology*, Vol.21, No.5, (November 2007), pp. 1107–1119, ISSN 0893-228X

Madsen, K.G., Grönberg, G., Skonberg, C., Jurva, U., Hansen, S.H. & Olsen, J. (2008b). Electrochemical Oxidation of Troglitazone: Identification and Characterization of the Major Reactive Metabolite in Liver Microsomes. *Chemical Research in Toxicology*, Vol.21, No.10, (), pp. 2035–2041, ISSN 0893-228X

Nozaki, K., Kitagawa, H., Kimura, S., Kagayama, A. & Arakawa, R. (2006). Investigation of the electrochemical oxidation products of zotepine and their fragmentation using on-line electrochemistry/electrospray ionization mass spectrometry. *Journal of Mass Spectrometry*, Vol.41, No.5, (January 2006), pp. 606–612, ISSN 1076-5174

Odijk, M., A. Baumann, A., Olthuis, W., van den Berg, A. & Karst, U. (2010). Electrochemistry-on-chip for on-line conversions in drug metabolism studies. *Biosensors and Bioelectronics*, Vol.26, No.4, (July 2010), pp. 1521–1527, ISSN 0956-5663

Regino, M.C.S. & Brajter-Toth, A. (1997). An Electrochemical Cell for On-Line Electrochemistry/Mass Spectrometry. *Analytical Chemistry*, Vol.69, No.24, (October 1997) pp. 5067-5072, ISSN 0003-2700

Schaber, G., Wiatr, G., Wachsmuth, H., Dachtler, M., Albert, K., Gaertner, I. & Breyer-Pfaff, U. (2001). Isolation and Identification of Clozapine Metabolites in Patient Urine. *Drug Metabolism and Disposition*, Vol. 29, No. 6, (February 2001), pp. 923–931, ISSN 0090-9556

Speiser, B. (2007). Methods to Investigate Mechanisms of Electroorganic Reactions, In: *Encyclopedia of Electrochemistry*, Hans-J. Schäfer, pp. 1-23, Wiley-VCH, Available from http://media.wiley.com/product_data/excerpt/02/35273040/3527304002-2.pdf

Squella, J.A., Bollo, S. & Núñez-Vergara, L.J. (2005). Recent Developments in the Electrochemistry of Some Nitro Compounds of Biological Significance. *Current Organic Chemistry*, Vol.9, N.6, (April 2005), pp. 565-581, ISSN 1385-2728

Tahara, K., Yano, Y., Kanagawa, K., Abe, Y., Yamada, J., Iijima, S., Mochizuki, M. & Nishikawa, T. (2007). Successful Preparation of Metabolite of Troglitazone by In-Flow Electrochemical Reaction on Coulometric Electrode. *Chemical & Pharmaceutical Bulletin*, Vol.55, No.8, (May 2007), pp. 1207-1212, ISSN 0009-2363

Tahara, K., Nishikawa, T., Hattori, Y., Iijima, S., Kouno, Y. & Abe, Y. (2009). Production of a reactive metabolite of troglitazone by electrochemical oxidation performed in nonaqueous medium. *Journal of Pharmaceutical and Biomedical Analysis*, Vol.50, No.5, (June 2009), pp. 1030–1036, ISSN 0731-7085

van Leeuwen, S.M., Blankert, B., Jean-Michel Kauffmann, J.M & Karst, U. (2005). Prediction of clozapine metabolism by on-line electrochemistry/liquid chromatography/mass spectrometry. *Analytical and Bioanalytical Chemistry*, Vol.382, No.3, (December 2004), pp. 742–750, ISSN 1618-2642

Volk, K.J., Yost, R.A. & Brajter-Toth, A. (1989). On-Line Electrochemistry/Thermospray/ Tandem Mass Spectrometry as a New Approach to the Study of Redox Reactions: The Oxidation of Uric Acid. *Analytical Chemistry*, Vol.61, No.15, (April 1989) pp. 1709-1717, ISSN 0003-2700

Volk, K.J., Yost, R.A. & Brajter-Toth, A. (1992). Electrochemistry On Line with Mass Slsectrometrv Insight into Biologital Redox Reactions. *Analytical Chemistry*, Vol.64, No.1, (November 1991) pp. 21-33, ISSN 0003-2700

Yang, M., Kabulski, J.L., Wollenberg, L., Chen, X., Subramanian, M., Tracy, T.S., Lederman, D., Gannett, P.M. & Wu, N. (2009). Electrocatalytic Drug Metabolism by CYP2C9 Bonded to A Self-Assembled Monolayer-Modified Electrode. *Drug metabolism and disposition*, Vol.37, No.4, (January 2009), pp. 892- 899, ISSN 0090-9556

Zhou, F. & Van Berkel, G.J. (1995). Electrochemistry Combined On-Line with Electrospray Mass Spectrometry. *Analytical Chemistry*, Vol.67, No.20, (August 1995) pp. 3643-3649, ISSN 0003-2700

Zhu, B.T. & Lee, A.J. (2005). NADPH-dependent metabolism of 17β-estradiol and estrone to polar and nonpolar metabolites by human tissues and cytochrome P450 isoforms. *Steroids*, Vol.70, No.4, (January 2005), pp. 225–244, ISSN 0039-128X

11

Label-Free Quantitative Analysis Using LC/MS

Atsumu Hirabayashi
Hitachi, Ltd.,
Japan

1. Introduction

Quantitative analysis using liquid chromatography/mass spectrometry (LC/MS) is widespread, especially in drug metabolism and pharmacokinetics studies, and in many laboratories label-free LC/MS analyses are carried out, i.e., without using isotope labeling techniques. However, even if the analytical method is well validated, an unexpected change in matrix concentrations in biological samples may cause matrix effects such as ion suppression or ion enhancement. When ion suppression occurs, for example, the ionization efficiency of an analyte molecule decreases, and the ion intensity of the analyte decreases from the expected intensity (Tang et al., 2004; Buhrman et al., 1996). Then the linear relationship between the sample amount and the ion intensity is lost, as shown in Figure 1.

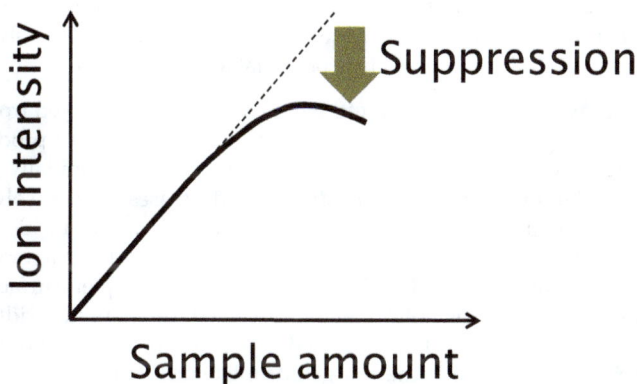

Fig. 1. When ion suppression occurs, the linear relationship between the ion intensity and the sample amount is lost, as shown by an arrow, and thus, label-free quantitative analysis becomes difficult.

The effects of ion suppression can be overcome by using stable-isotope labeling techniques such as $^{12}C/^{13}C$ and $^{14}N/^{15}N$ labeling, since an isotope-labeled molecule, used as an internal standard, exhibits chemical properties or effects of ion suppression almost identical to those of the unlabeled one. Eventually, though, label-free LC/MS analyses have to be carried out when we cannot employ isotope labeling techniques, which are rather laborious and expensive.

Ion suppression occurs in LC/MS interfaces such as electrospray ionization (ESI) and atmospheric pressure chemical ionization (APCI), which are used to analyze less volatile and volatile molecules, respectively. Because ESI is the more widely used technique, ion suppression in ESI is mainly described here, although that in APCI is also discussed later.

Because the effect of ion suppression depends on the chemical properties of the analyte molecule in ESI, it is difficult to correct for decreased intensity, so quantitative analysis becomes difficult. The potential occurrence of ion suppression can be reduced by desalting and fractionating the sample, reducing the sample volume, and the effect of ion suppression can be reduced by using a structural analog. Nevertheless, ion suppression may occur, and correcting for the decreased intensity remains difficult. Several sample preparation protocols for specific analytes have been proposed to reduce the effect of ion suppression by using internal standards (Matuszewski et al., 1998; Bonfiglio et al., 1999), but they are not widely used in label-free LC/MS.

We have developed a simple technique for detecting potential ion suppression in ESI (Hirabayashi et al., 2007, 2009). In this technique, a specific concentration of a probe molecule, which is sensitive to the occurrence of ion suppression, is added to an LC mobile phase, and the intensity of the protonated probe molecule is monitored. When ion suppression occurs, the intensity of the protonated probe is expected to decrease more than those of other protonated molecules, $[M+H]^+$.

2. Ion formation from a charged droplet in ESI

In this section, a brief explanation for why ion suppression occurs in ESI is presented, based on ion formation mechanisms of less volatile analyte molecules than solvent molecules, before explaining the technique for detecting potential ion suppression.

In ESI and other spray ionizations, an LC effluent in a capillary is sprayed from the capillary tip. Then, charged droplets are formed, from which gaseous ions are produced. Figure 2 shows a schematic view of a positively charged droplet. The droplet initially produced has a diameter of the order of 1 μm, and the diameter decreases as the solvent molecules evaporate. In the droplet, positive ions are concentrated near the inside of the droplet surface because of a Coulomb repulsive force. As solvent molecules evaporate, the gaseous ions are produced from the liquid-phase ions inside the droplet surface through ion evaporation (Iribarne & Thomson, 1976; de la Mora, 2000) or charged residue mechanisms (Dole et al., 1968). Therefore, most ions analyzed in a mass spectrometer originate from the liquid-phase ones near the inside of the charged droplet surface. In the charged droplet, the liquid-phase chemistry, ignoring the effect of the surface, is not necessarily valid but is a good approximation (Hirabayashi 1993).

Ion suppression occurs in the ionization processes when a component eluted from an LC column affects the ionization of coeluted analytes. In the droplet surface, the analyte molecules are charged in accordance with their chemical properties when the number of charges is much higher than that of analyte molecules. Then the ionization efficiency for each analyte molecule remains constant. Under these conditions, label-free quantitative analysis is readily performed. On the contrary, when the number of charges in the droplet is comparable to, or less than, that of analyte molecules, charge competition occurs among the analyte molecules. Because the decrease in the number of charges can be regarded as an increase in pH, the protonation for acidic molecules, for example, is likely to be reduced to a greater extent than that for neutral and basic ones. Of these molecules, those weakly dissociated near the surface tend to lose their charge in the competition, and their ionization efficiencies decrease, leading to ion suppression. Thus, in molecules with low ionization efficiencies, the ionization efficiencies tend to decrease further when ion suppression occurs. In contrast, when the number of charges in the droplet increases, the ionization efficiencies of some molecules increase. This leads to ion enhancement. The ionization efficiencies of molecules with low ionization efficiencies are expected to increase when ion enhancement occurs.

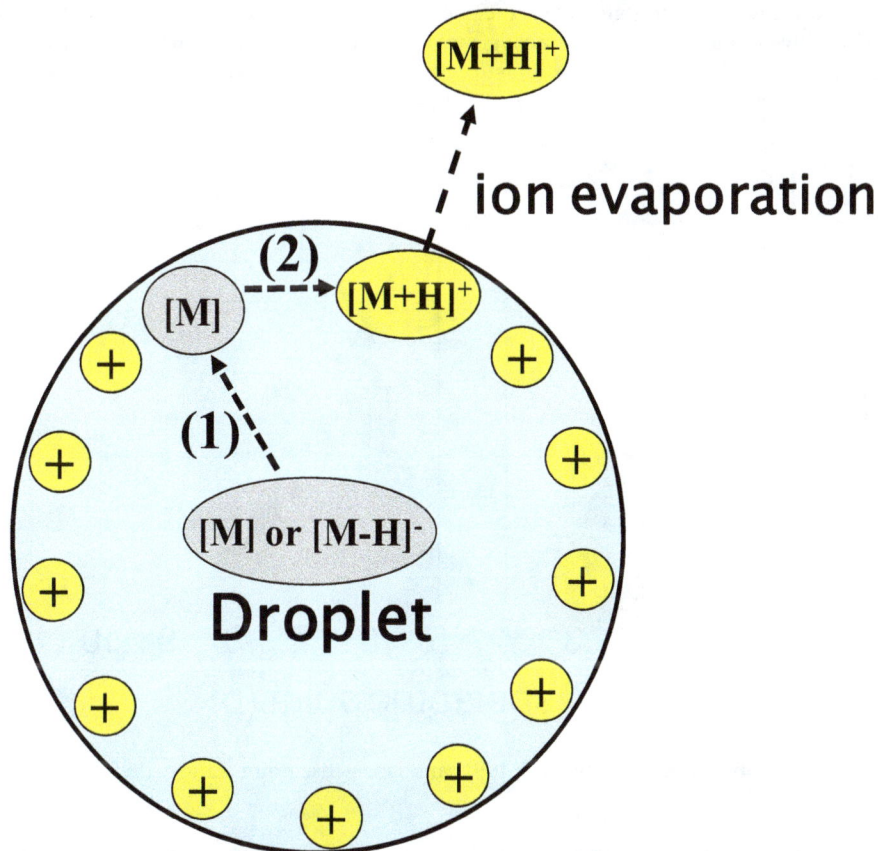

Fig. 2. Cross-sectional view of a positively charged droplet. The ionization processes of acidic molecules with low ionization efficiencies are shown: most of the molecules are deprotonated and concentrated in the central region of the droplet, but some do not undergo deprotonation because of their dissociation equilibrium. These neutral molecules with a low surface accessibility mostly remain in the droplet, but only a small part of the molecules can reach the droplet surface (1). Then, the protonated molecules may form near the surface (2). Gaseous ions are formed from the liquid-phase ions inside the droplet surface by ion evaporation or charge residue mechanisms.

3. Concept for ion suppression detection

In the following we consider the ionization processes of molecules with low ionization efficiencies in a charge droplet. In the droplet, the neutral or negatively charged molecules remain deep, as shown in Fig. 2. To be protonated, these molecules have to access the surface. Then, near the inside of the droplet surface, they are protonated in accordance with their isoelectric point, or dissociation constant. Therefore, the major factors determining the ionization efficiency are (1) surface accessibility (or hydrophobicity) and (2) isoelectric point (or dissociation constant) of the analyte molecule. Hydrophobic and basic molecules are expected to be insensitive to ion suppression, and their ionization efficiencies are rather high. On the contrary, the ionization efficiencies of quite hydrophilic and acidic molecules are much lower than those of the above molecules. However, these molecules would be quite sensitive to the occurrence of ion suppression and can potentially be used as probes for detecting ion suppression in the analysis of positive ions (protonated molecules).

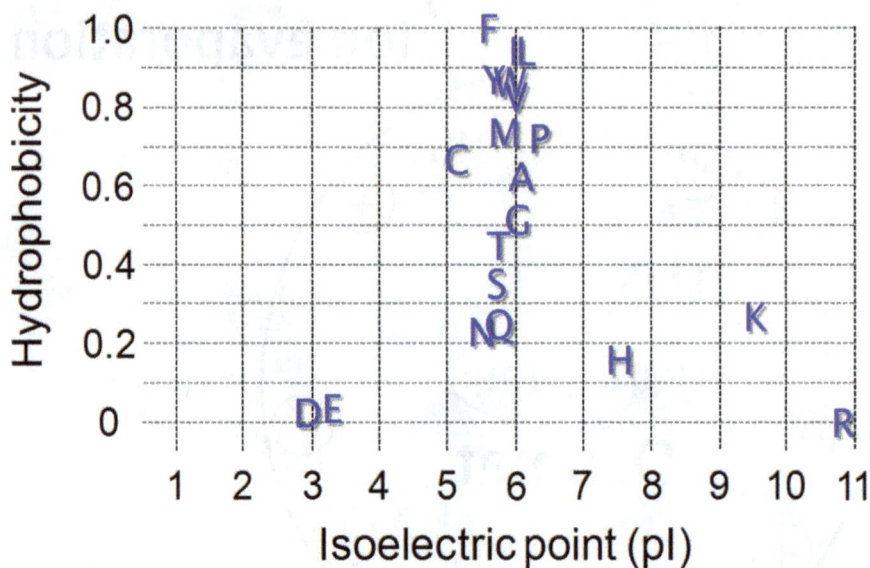

Fig. 3. Hydrophobicity (Black & Mould, 1991) and isoelectric point (Linde, 1995) for 20 amino acids.

In developing the probe, a convenient technique is to synthesize a quite hydrophilic and acidic peptide, which has an amino-acid sequence including a hydrophilic and neutral amino acid as well as an acidic one, as the probe for detecting ion suppression. Figure 3 compares 20 amino acids in terms of their hydrophobicity and isoelectric points (pI). Among the amino acids, serine (S), asparagine (N), and glutamine (Q) are very hydrophilic and neutral. On the other hand, aspartic acid (D) and glutamic acid (E) are very acidic, with a pK$_R$ of 3.65 and 4.25, respectively (Linde, 1995a), where pK$_R$ is the pK for the side chain of the amino acid. Then, as a probe for ion-suppression detection, we synthesized a peptide, DSSSSS, the isoelectric point of which is calculated to be 3.80 (Gasteiger et al., 2005). This probe is so acidic that no multiply protonated molecule of the probe is detected; only singly protonated ones can be detected at m/z 569.3 in a mass spectrometer. The molecular weight of the probe can be modified by altering the number of hydrophilic and neutral amino acids such as S. As mentioned above, the ionization efficiency of the probe is relatively low, whereas the probe concentration in the LC mobile phase should preferably be low, so as not to cause ion suppression. More acidic molecules than DSSSSS, for example, DDSSSS or DDDSSS with respective isoelectric points of 3.56 and 3.42, would be more sensitive to the occurrence of ion suppression, and could also be used as the probes. However, because of their higher acidities, their concentration should be higher than that of DSSSSS to be detected clearly in a mass spectrometer. Since the probe is rather insensitive to the occurrence of ion suppression of more acidic molecules than the probe, it is difficult to detect potential ion suppression for such acidic molecules if they are there. Note that the probe should be used to detect potential ion suppression for protonated molecules, not for cations and cationized molecules such as $[M]^+$ and $[M+Na]^+$.

For a probe used in negative-ion analysis, on the other hand, quite hydrophilic and basic peptides should be synthesized by using a very basic amino acid of R or K with a pK_R of 12.48 and 10.53, respectively (Linde, 1995) and the very hydrophilic ones. Then ion suppression of ions with the form of $[M-H]^-$ can be detected by monitoring the intensity of the deprotonated molecule of the probe.

In the following, the usability of the probe is examined. In most LC/MS analyses, the pH of the mobile phase ranges from 2 to 6, and the concentration of the organic solvent such as acetonitrile and methanol is below 90%. Figure 4 (a) plots the intensity of the protonated probe as a function of the acetonitrile concentration of the mobile phase under several pH conditions. The intensity appears to be almost independent of the mobile-phase pH. On the other hand, the intensity increases with an increase in the acetonitrile concentration. The increase in the ion intensity (or the ion formation efficiency of the probe) can be ascribed to the enhanced solvent evaporation of the charged droplets, since the surface accessibility (or hydrophobicity) of the probe has been confirmed to be almost independent of the organic solvent concentration by comparing the probe with a much more hydrophobic peptide of FDFSF (Hirabayashi, 2009). Furthermore, the number of charges in the droplet is likely to be almost independent of the organic solvent concentration. This is because the ion current, which is the current for all of the ions and charged droplets produced by ESI, is almost unchanged, as shown in Fig. 4 (b), and this trend is independent of the organic solvent such as acetonitrile and methanol. Thus, the probe is expected to be much less surface-accessible and quite acidic under the conditions used in LC/MS analyses.

4. Detection of ion suppression

As mentioned earlier, the effect of ion suppression depends on the sample amount. Therefore, different sample amounts of fractionated human plasma, as a typically crude sample, were analyzed with a nanoLC/TOF-MS system to detect the occurrence of ion suppression. An aqueous solution of the probe is added to the LC mobile phase at a gradient mixer-pump unit of the nanoLC system just before being introduced into a separation column. Then, a linear gradient of acetonitrile concentration from 7 to 50% is run at a flow rate of 50nL/min. Since the probe is very hydrophilic, it can pass through the reverse-phase separation column without adsorption when the organic solvent concentration of the LC mobile phase is above 4%. Then the protonated probe is detected in the mass spectrometer during the LC/MS analysis.

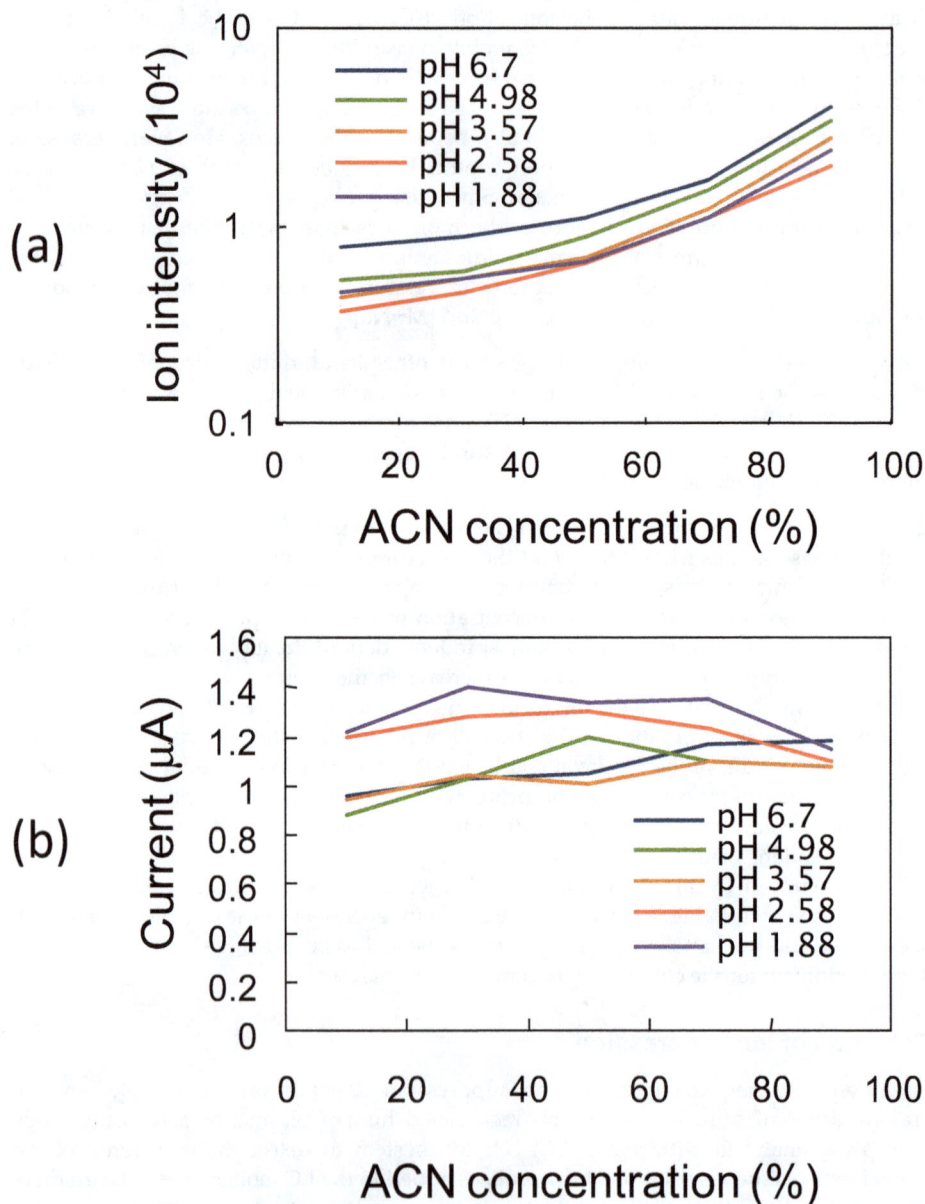

(a)

(b)

Fig. 4. (a) Intensity of the protonated probe molecule and (b) current for all the ions and charged droplets produced by ESI as a function of the acetonitrile (ACN) concentration of the mobile phase under several pH conditions.

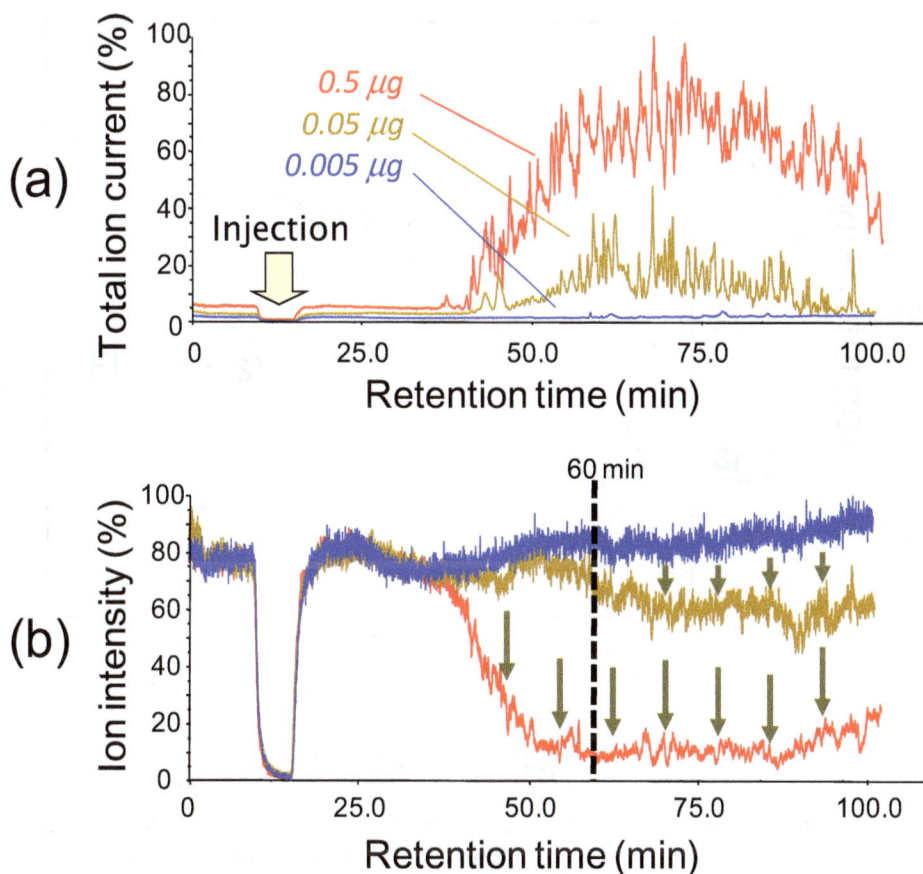

Fig. 5. (a) Total ion current chromatograms obtained from human plasma with injection amounts of 0.005, 0.05, and 0.5 µg, and (b) corresponding mass chromatograms of the protonated probe.

Figure 5 compares (a) chromatograms of the total ion current and (b) mass chromatograms of the protonated probe. For an injected amount of 0.005 µg, the mass chromatogram, shown in blue, is rather flat, except for the moment of sample injection using a manual injector. Thus, no ion suppression is likely to occur. However, for 0.05-µg injection, the intensity for the protonated probe, shown in yellow, decreases appreciably at a retention time above 50 min. For 0.5-µg injection, shown in red, a significant decrease in intensity is detected at a retention time above 40 min. For example, at 60 min (indicated by the vertical dashed line) the ion intensity for the 0.05-µg injection decreases by about 20%, and the decrease is above our experimental error of 10%. This means that potential ion suppression occurs and its maximum effect on ion intensity is 20%. Therefore, if an uncertainty of 20% is accepted, quantitative analysis is readily performed at the retention time. On the other hand, for the 0.5-µg injection, the effect of ion suppression is serious, and quantitative analysis would be difficult.

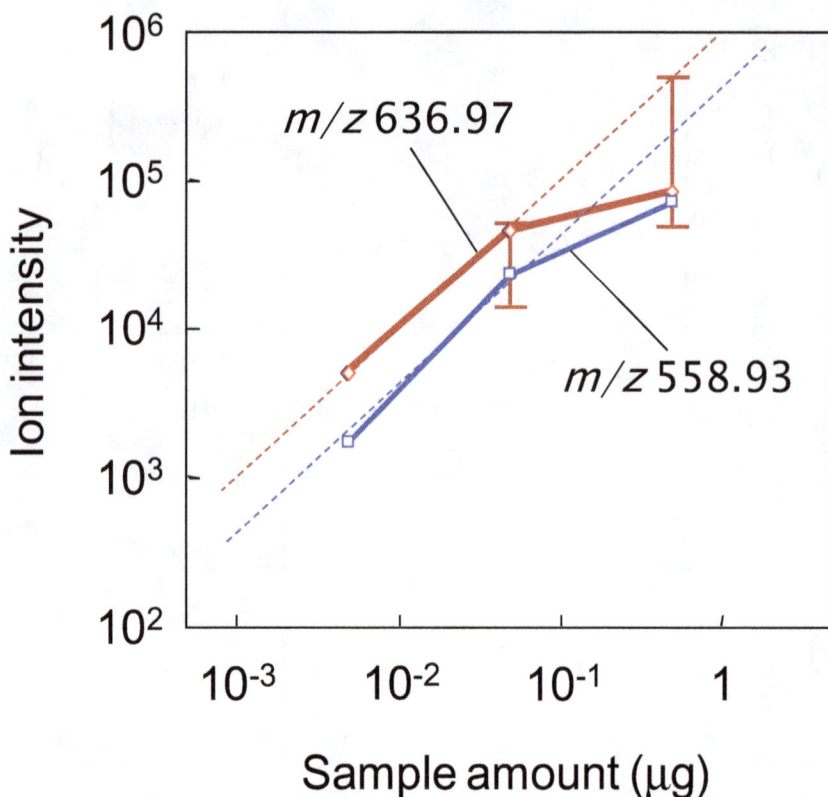

Fig. 6. Peak areas for the m/z 639.91 and 558.93 ions as a function of the injected sample amount. Broken lines with a slope of 1 are shown as a visual aid. Error bars show the decrease in intensity of the protonated probe.

The probe is expected to be so sensitive to the occurrence of ion suppression that the decrease in intensity for the protonated probe is stronger than those for other protonated molecules. Figure 6 shows the experimental results for protonated molecules chosen randomly. The red line shows the intensity or the peak area for a protonated molecule with m/z 636.97 detected at a retention time of about 60 min, as a function of the sample injection amount. As the injection amount increases, the difference between the observed intensity and the expected one, shown as a dashed line, increases, and this shows the effect of ion suppression. Another protonated molecule detected at m/z 558.93 is also shown in blue. Ion suppression for this ion is detected for the 0.5-μg injection, but the decrease in intensity of this ion is weaker than that for the protonated molecule with m/z 636.97. Furthermore, the error bars in the figure show the decrease in intensity for the protonated probe at 60 min. The decrease is actually stronger than those for the ion with m/z 636.97. Therefore, the results are consistent with the above expectation. For the 0.05-μg injection, ion suppression may occur for some ions but the intensities of the two ions with m/z 636.97 and 558.93 are not decreased.

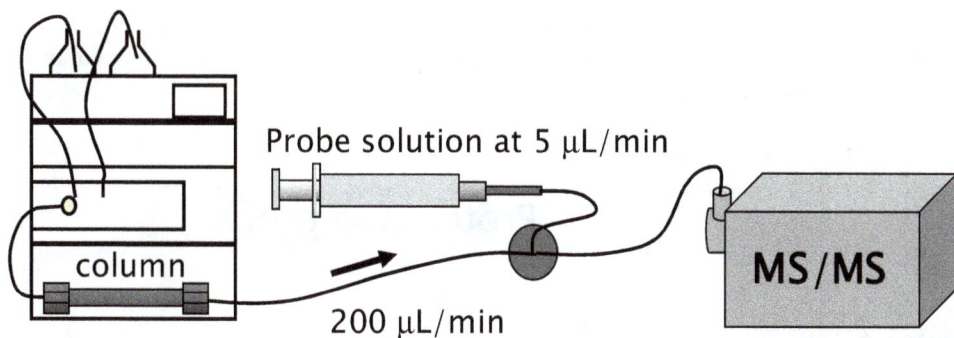

Fig. 7. Experimental setup for LC/MS/MS. An aqueous solution of the probe, pumped by a syringe pump, is mixed with the LC effluent at post-column with a tee.

For semi-micro or conventional LC/MS, the liquid flow rate is so high that the probe solution can be added to the LC mobile phase at post-column through a tee, since the band width of a component separated by the LC column is not expected to be degraded by using a tee with a small dead volume. A typical experimental setup is shown in Figure 7. An aqueous solution of the probe pumped at 5 µL/min is mixed with the LC mobile phase $(0.01M\text{-}CH_3COONH_4/CH_3CN/CH_3COOH, 600/400/0.15$; isocratic) in the tee, and the mixed solution is introduced into a triple-quadrupole mass spectrometer operated in selected reaction monitoring (SRM) mode.

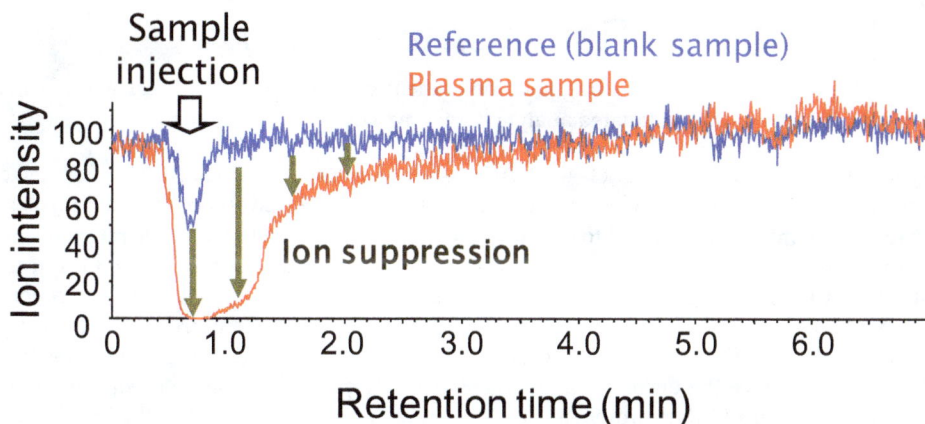

Fig. 8. Mass chromatograms of a fragment ion of the protonated probe for blank and plasma samples.

Before analyzing plasma samples, reference data are obtained using a blank sample such as water. In Figure 8, the mass chromatogram for a fragment (m/z 359.0) of the protonated probe obtained from the blank sample is shown in blue, and that from a plasma sample is shown in red, where the injection amount is about an order of magnitude higher than usual. It is clear that ion suppression is detected just after the sample injection until the retention time of 4 min. In particular, at a retention time of 0.6 min corresponding to the sample injection, the decrease in intensity for the plasma sample is much more significant than that for the reference data. This can be ascribed to an elution of very hydrophilic compounds in the plasma sample.

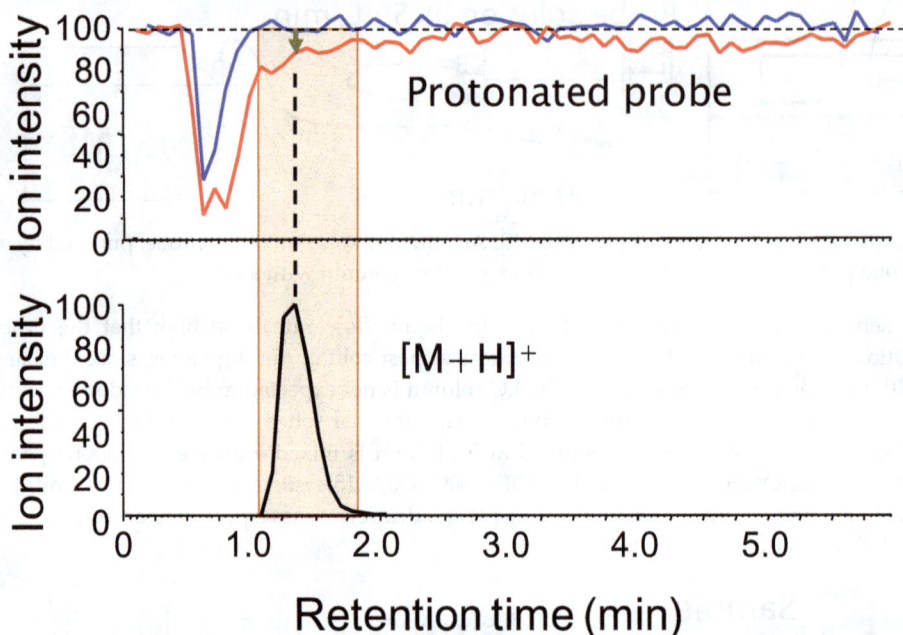

Fig. 9. Mass chromatograms of a fragment ion of the protonated probe for blank and plasma samples, and that of the protonated analyte (Omeprazole).

Figure 9 shows an example of ion-suppression detection obtained under our usual experimental conditions, in which no ion suppression is expected to occur. Omeprazole, a proton-pump inhibitor, is added to human plasma (4.5 µL). At a retention time ranging from 1.1 to 1.8 min, the fragment of the protonated Omeprazole is detected at m/z 198.1, but the intensity of the protonated probe (fragment) at 1.4 min decreases by 11%, which is beyond our experimental error of about 2%. This means that potential ion suppression occurs, and the intensity of the fragment of the protonated Omeprazole may be suppressed by less than 11% at 1.4 min since the decrease in the intensity of the protonated probe is expected to be stronger than that of other protonated molecules, as described earlier. On the other hand, the dependence of the peak area (intensity) of the fragment of the protonated Omeprazole on the amount of plasma is shown in Figure 10. The results are obtained under the condition that the injected amount of Omeprazole is constant. The figure shows that the peak area at 4.5 µL was 12% lower than those at 0 and 0.45 µL. This 12% decrease in peak area can be ascribed to the decrease in intensity of the protonated probe ranging from 8 to 22%, as shown in Fig. 9 (b). Thus, the decrease in peak area shown in Fig. 10 is almost consistent with the decrease (11%) in intensity of the protonated probe (fragment) at the retention time corresponding to the peak intensity for the protonated Omeprazole. Then, if the error of 11% obtained from the decrease in intensity of the protonated probe at the chromatogram peak is acceptable, the data can be readily analyzed quantitatively. If not, we may have to desalt the sample, reduce the injection amount, enhance the fractionation, or modify our LC separation conditions.

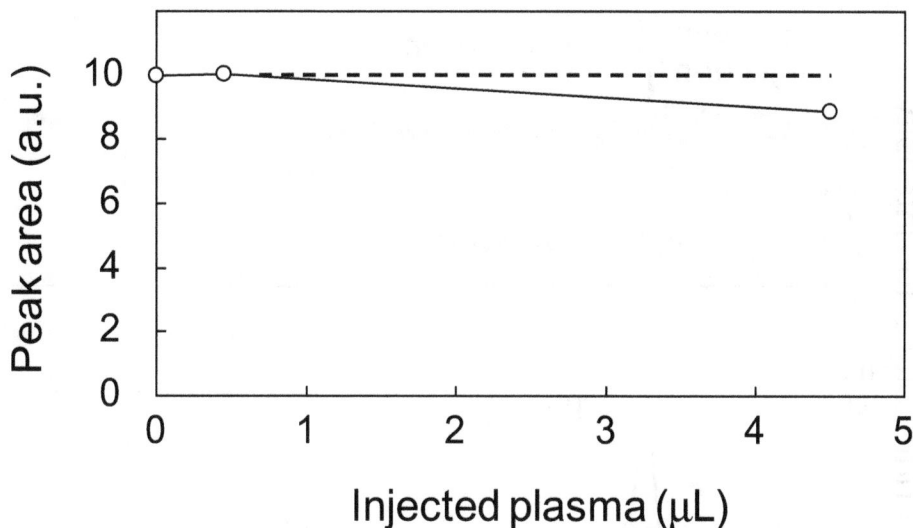

Fig. 10. Peak area (intensity) of the fragment of the protonated Omeprazole as a function of the injected plasma amount.

The detection of ion suppression has been described. As mentioned earlier, ion suppression occurs when the number of charges in the droplet is comparable to, or less than, those of analyte molecules. However, when the number of charges in the droplet increases, ion enhancement occurs. Then, intensities of the protonated molecules increase in accordance with the molecules' chemical properties. Since the increase in charge number can be regarded as a decrease in liquid pH, the protonation for acidic molecules is likely to be enhanced to greater degree than those for neutral and basic ones. This means that intensities of the protonated acidic molecules would increase more than those of other analyte molecules. Thus, when ion enhancement occurs, the intensity of the protonated probe is expected to increase more than those of other analyte molecules. An example of ion enhancement detection is shown in Figure 11. The reference mass chromatogram for the protonated probe, shown in blue, is compared with the mass chromatogram obtained from the plasma sample, shown in red. Ion enhancement is detected at a retention time of about 1.5 min. Furthermore, at 0.5-1.3 min ion suppression is also detected. Because complex matrix effects occur in this case, quantitative analysis of the data is difficult.

The probe can be used for optimizing the sample preparation protocol and analytical conditions as well as for analyzing label-free samples in LC/MS. Furthermore, by monitoring the intensity of the protonated probe, we can detect degradation or pollution of the LC/MS component clearly. Figure 12 compares the mass chromatograms of the protonated probe for the reference data obtained on different days. At about 0.6 min a decrease in intensity is observed in the green result. This decrease can be ascribed to ion suppression caused by contamination at the injection valve. Thus, when the decrease becomes serious, cleaning the valve is recommended.

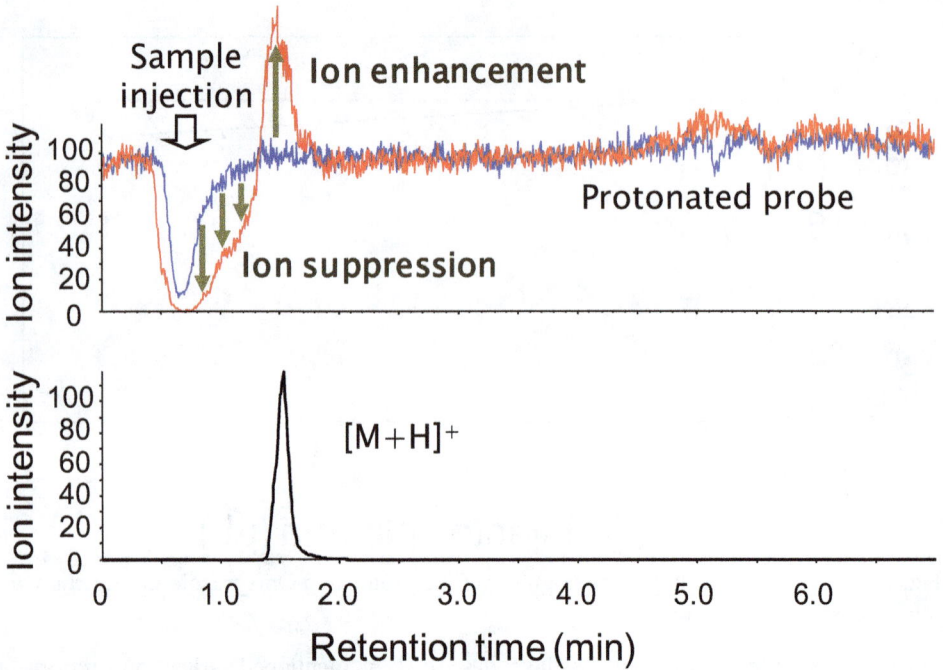

Fig. 11. Typical example of detection of ion enhancement as well as ion suppression. Also, mass chromatogram for a fragment (*m/z* 294.2) of the protonated analyte (Aminopterin) is shown in a lower figure.

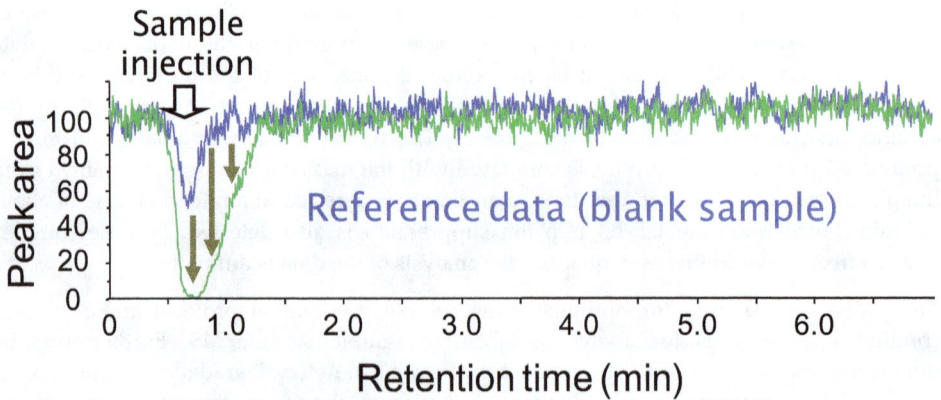

Fig. 12. Comparison of mass chromatograms for a fragment ion of the protonated probe. They were obtained from the blank sample on different days.

As described above, the potential occurrence of ion suppression and ion enhancement is detected with the probe when the intensity of the protonated probe molecule changes. However, there are some cases where the probe is not always useful for quantitative analysis. Even when neither ion suppression nor ion enhancement is detected with the probe, the intensity of the protonated analyte molecule may possibly have increased. The increase in intensity of the protonated analyte molecule can be ascribed to proton-transfer reactions in the gas-phase with other protonated molecules produced by ESI, not to the matrix effects. Such an increase in intensity occurs only when 1) the analyte such as Aminopterin has a proton affinity much higher than that of the probe and 2) molecules with proton affinities between those of the analyte and the probe are co-eluted with the analyte from LC with high concentrations.

5. Ion suppression in APCI (Atmospheric Pressure Chemical Ionization)

In APCI, volatile analyte molecules vaporized from an LC effluent by a nebulizer are introduced into a corona discharge plasma, which is generated under atmosphere. In the plasma, protonated solvent molecules such as H_3O^+ and their hydrated clusters are produced as major reagent ions for chemical ionization in positive ion analysis. In negative ion analysis, on the other hand, anions such as O_2^- and OH^- and their hydrated clusters are major reagent ions. In the plasma, positive and negative charges are balanced. Then, the analyte molecules are ionized by gas-phase ion/molecule reactions such as a proton-transfer reaction and an electron-transfer reaction with the reagent ions in the plasma, as shown below.

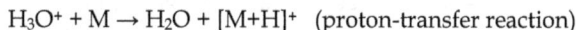

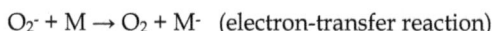

$$H_3O^+ + M \rightarrow H_2O + [M+H]^+ \quad \text{(proton-transfer reaction)}$$

$$O_2^- + M \rightarrow O_2 + M^- \quad \text{(electron-transfer reaction)}$$

Here, M is an analyte, and hydrated clusters are omitted for simplicity. The protonated analyte molecule $[M+H]^+$ is produced by the proton-transfer reaction when the analyte has a proton affinity higher than that of H_2O. Thus, the major factor determining the ionization efficiency for the protonated analyte molecule is the proton affinity of the analyte (Hunter& Lias, 1998). The negatively charged analyte molecule M^-, on the other hand, is produced by an electron-transfer reaction when the analyte has an electron affinity higher than that of O_2. Thus, the major factor determining the ionization efficiency for the negatively charged analyte molecule is the electron affinity of the analyte (Linde, 1995b). Although the ion/molecule reactions at atmospheric pressure are expected to be almost in equilibrium state, the density of the ion produced by APCI is proportional to that of the reagent ion for the ion/molecule reaction. That means that ion suppression occurs when the density of the reagent ions decreases appreciably. This situation is caused, for example, when the density of co-eluted molecules with proton affinities higher than that of the reagent molecule becomes significant.

In APCI, several kinds of ion/molecule reactions in the gas phase occur such as a proton-transfer reaction, electron-transfer reaction, anion-transfer reaction, and anion-attachment reaction (Moini, 2007). Therefore, it is important to identify the reagent ion for the ion/molecule reaction of the analyte molecule before the analysis. Then, the occurrence of ion suppression can be detected by monitoring the intensity of the reagent ion for the analyte molecule. Before analyzing biological samples, reference data should be obtained using a blank sample. Potential ion suppression is detected when the intensity of the reagent ion for a biological sample becomes lower than that for the reference sample. In the analysis of protonated analyte molecules, for example, ion suppression can be detected by monitoring the intensity of the protonated solvent molecule such as H_3O^+ or its hydrated cluster. In the analysis of negatively charged analyte molecules, it can be detected by monitoring the intensity of the anions such as O_2^- and OH^-. In APCI, however, ion suppression occurs less frequently than in ESI probably because charges or the current for the reagent ions, produced in the corona discharge plasma, are much higher than the charges produced by ESI.

6. Conclusion

In ESI as an interface in LC/MS, a technique to detect ion suppression or enhancement using a probe has been developed. In positive-ion analysis, the probe should be more hydrophilic and acidic than analyte molecules. In negative-ion analysis, it should be more hydrophilic and basic than analyte molecules. When ion suppression occurs in positive-ion analysis, for example, the intensity of the protonated molecule of the probe is expected to decrease more than those of other analytes. Furthermore, potential error for the intensity of the protonated analyte can be estimated from the decrease in the intensity of the protonated probe.

In preparing a stock solution of the probe, the probe powder is readily dissolved in pure water by adding a small amount of ammonia or trifluoroacetic acid (TFA) to adjust the solution's pH. In an organic-solvent/water solution, however, the very hydrophilic probe might be aggregated in several ten minutes. Thus, the aqueous solution of the probe should be mixed with the LC mobile phase just before the analysis, as shown in Fig. 7.

Directions for the use of the probe are summarized as follows:

1.   Add the probe in the LC mobile phase.
2.   Obtain reference LC/MS data with a blank sample.
3.   Obtain LC/MS data with a biological sample.
4.   Compare mass chromatogram for the protonated probe with that in the reference data.
5.   Measure potential error from the decrease in intensity for the protonated probe.

The probe can also be used to detect the occurrence of ion enhancement. When ion enhancement occurs, the intensity of the protonated molecule of the probe is expected to increase more than those of other analytes. When neither ion suppression nor ion enhancement occurs, the probe can be used as an internal standard in quantitative LC/MS analysis. Unlike isotope labeling techniques, however, it cannot be used as an internal standard in sample preparation.

In contrast, in APCI the occurrence of ion suppression can be detected by monitoring the intensity of the reagent ion for the analyte.

7. Acknowledgement

The author is grateful to M. Furukawa, M. Umeda, T. Bando, Y. Orii, and T. Mori of Hitachi High-Technologies for their help in the experiments and their contribution to our fruitful discussions. He also thanks M. Ishimaru, N. Manri, T. Yokosuka, and H. Hanzawa of Hitachi for their invaluable assistance.

8. References

Tang, K.; Page, J. & Smith, R. (2004). Charge Competition and the Linear Dynamic Range of Detection in Electrospray Ionization Mass Spectrometry, *Journal of the American Society for Mass Spectrometry*, Vol. 15, Issue 10, (April 2004), pp. 1416-1423, ISSN 1044-0305

Buhrman, D.; Price, P. & Rudewicz, P. (1996). Quantitation of SR 27417 in Human Plasma using Electrospray Liquid Chromatography-Tandem Mass Spectrometry: A Study of Ion Suppression, *Journal of the American Society for Mass Spectrometry*, Vol. 7, Issue 11, (June 1996), pp. 1099-1105, ISSN 1044-0305

Matuszewski, B.; Constanzer, M. & Chevez-Eng, C. (1998). Matrix Effect in Quantitative LC/MS/MS Analyses of Biological Fluids: A Method for Determination of Finasteride in Human Plasma at Picogram Per Milliliter Concentrations. *Analytical Chemistry*, Vol. 70, Issue 5, (December 1997), pp. 882-889, ISSN 1520-6882

Bonfiglio, R.; King, R.; Olah, T. & Merkle, K. (1999). The Effects of Sample Preparation Method on the Variability of the Electrospray Ionization Response for Model Drug Compounds. *Rapid Communications in Mass Spectrometry*, Vol. 13, Issue 12, (April 1999), pp. 1175-1185, ISSN 1097-0231

Hirabayashi, A.; Ishimaru, M.; Manri, N.; Yokosuka, T. & Hanzawa, H. (2007). Detection of Potential Ion Suppression for Peptide Analysis in Nanoflow Liquid Chromatography/Mass Spectrometry, *Rapid Communications in Mass Spectrometry*, Vol. 21, Issue 17, (June 2007), pp. 2860-2866, ISSN 1097-0231

Hirabayashi, A.; Furukawa, M.; Umeda, M.; Bando, T. & Orii, Y. (2009). Probe for Label-free Quantitative Analysis in Liquid Chromatography/Mass Spectrometry, *Analytical Sciences*, Vol. 25, Number 1, (January 2009), pp. 67-71, ISSN 0910-6340

Iribarne, J. & Thomson, B. (1976). On the Evaporation of Small Ions from Charged Droplets, *Journal of Chemical Physics*, Vol. 64, Number 6, (July 1975), pp. 2287-2294, ISSN 0021-9606

de la Mora, J. (2000). Electrospray Ionization of Large Multiply Charged Species Proceeds via Dole's Charged Residue Mechanism, *Analytica Chimica Acta*, Vol. 406, Issue 1, (February 1999), pp. 93-104, ISSN 0003-2670

Dole, M.; Mack, L.; Hines, R.; Mobley, R.; Ferguson, L. & Alice, M. (1968). Molecular Beams of Macroions, *Journal of Chemical Physics*, Vol. 49, Number 5, (April 1968), pp. 2240-2249, ISSN 0021-9606

Hirabayashi, A.; Takada, Y.; Kambara, H.; Umemura, Y.; Ito, H. & Kuchitsu, K. (1993). Mass Spectroscopic Studies of Protonation to Amino-acid Molecules in Atmospheric Pressure Spray, *Chemical Physics Letters*, Vol. 204, Number 1,2, (December 1992), pp. 152-156, ISSN 0009-2614

Black, S. & Mould, D. (1991). Development of Hydrophobicity Parameters to Analyze Proteins Which Bear Post- or Cotranslational Modifications, *Analytical Biochemistry*, Vol. 193, Issue 1, (July 1990), pp. 72-82, ISSN 0003-2697

Linde, D. (1995a). Section 7, Biochemistry, In: *CRC Handbook of Chemistry and Physics*, pp. 1, CRC Press, ISBN 0-8493-0476-8, Boca Raton

Gasteiger, E.; Hoogland, C.; Gattiker, A.; Duvaud, S.; Wilkins, M.; Appel, R. & Bairoch, A. (2005). *Protein Identification and Analysis Tools on the ExPASy Server*, In: *The Proteomics Protocols Handbook*, J.M. Walker (Ed), pp. 571-607, Humana Press, ISBN 798-1-58829-383-5, Available from
http://au.expasy.org/tools/pi_tool.html

Moini, M. (2007). Atmospheric Pressure Chemical Ionization: Principles, Instrumentation, and Applications, In: *The Encyclopedia of Mass Spectrometry Volume 6; Ionization Methods*, M. Gross & R. Caprioli, (Ed.), pp. 345-354, ISBN 978-0-08-0438016, Elsevier, Amsterdam

Hunter, E. & Lias, S. (1998). Evaluated Gas Phase Basicities and Proton Affinities of Molecules: An Update. *Journal of Physical and Chemical Reference Data*, Vol. 27, Issue 3, (August 1997), pp. 413-656, ISSN 0047-2689

Linde, D. (1995b). Section 10, Atomic, Molecular, and Optical Physics, In: *CRC Handbook of Chemistry and Physics*, pp. 180-188, CRC Press, ISBN 0-8493-0476-8, Boca Raton

12

Recent Advances in Pharmacogenomic Technology for Personalized Medicine

Toshihisa Ishikawa and Yoshihide Hayashizaki
Omics Science Canter, RIKEN Yokohama Institute,
Japan

1. Introduction

Genetic polymorphisms and mutations in drug metabolizing enzymes, transporters, receptors, and other drug targets (*e.g.*, toxicity targets) are linked to inter-individual differences in the efficacy and toxicity of many medications as well as risk of genetic diseases. Validation of clinically important genetic polymorphisms and the development of new technologies to rapidly detect clinically important variants are critical issues for advancing personalized medicine.

Pharmacogenomics, which deals with heredity and response to drugs, is the scientific field that attempts to explain individual variability of drug responses and to search for the genetic basis of such variations or differences (Evans et al., 2001). The inter-individual variation in the rate of drug metabolism has been known for many years. Initially, the study of pharmacogenetics was only of academic interest, but today it is of major concern to the pharmaceutical industry as a means for documenting the metabolism of a new drug in development before registration. The knowledge of how a drug is metabolized and which enzymes are involved may help to predict drug-drug interactions and the rate at which individual patients may metabolize a specific drug. Such information is now required for registration by the U.S. Food and Drug Administration (FDA) and similar authorities (Salerno & Lesko, 2004a, 2004b). To improve drug safety, the FDA has started to update the labels and package inserts of previously approved drugs as new clinical and genetic evidence accrues (Frueh et al., 2008; Lesko, 2008).

The current important step is to incorporate pharmacogenomics data into routine clinical practice. As a means of implementing personalized medicine, it is critically important to understand the molecular mechanisms underlying inter-individual differences in the drug response, namely, pharmacological effect vs. side effect. The occurrence of personal variations in the response to a drug may result from many different causes, for example, genetic variations and expression levels of drug-targeted molecules, including membrane receptors, nuclear receptors, signal transduction components, and enzymes, as well as those of drug-metabolizing enzymes and drug transporters (Evans et al., 2001). Recently, tools such as next-generation sequencing technologies and genome-wide association studies (GWAS) have been used to uncover a number of variants that affect drug toxicity and efficacy as well as potential risk of diseases. The costs involved in carrying out GWAS and sequencing have been dropping dramatically, while providing data at an unprecedented rate. The GWAS approach has been applied for identifying genetic contributions to variations in drug response (The SEARCH Collaborative Group, 2008; Kamatani et al., 2010; Cooper et al., 2008; Schuldiner et al., 2009; Ge et al., 2009; Daly et al., 2009). As a result, there have been dramatic increases in our understanding of the mechanisms of drug action and of the genetic determinants responsible for variable responses to both rarely and widely used drugs, such as warfarin, tomoxifen, and clopidogrel.

Technologies are evolving to transform diagnostic devices for rapid genetic testing. Portable devices are being engineered for use in a range of settings to perform robust assays for the diagnosis of disease that will improve patient management, and result in greater convenience and speed to answer.The genetic diagnostics is a growing field that is gradually becoming more user-friendly with the introduction of portable devices and quicker nucleic acid detection. Successful genetic diagnostics require 4 major elements, such as rapid reaction, low cost, low energy consumption, and simple analysis (with minimal technical training and inclusion of controls but no off-instrument processing or reagent preparation). In this context, we decided to develop a point-of-care "POC" technology and to apply it to medical advances.

Development of personalized medicine including POC technology requires integration of various segments of biotechnology, clinical medicine, and pharmacology. A key requirement for advancing personalized medicine is the ability to rapidly and conveniently test for patients' genetic polymorphisms and/or mutations. To address this urgent need, we have recently developed a rapid and cost-effective method, named Smart Amplification Process (SmartAmp), which enables us to detect genetic polymorphisms or mutations in target genes within 30 to 45 minutes under isothermal conditions that do not require DNA isolation and PCR amplification (Mitani et al., 2007; Mitani et al., 2009; Ishikawa et al., 2010; Aw et al., 2011; Ota et al., 2010; Lezhava et al., 2010; Toyoda et al., 2009; Aomori et al., 2009; Watanabe et al., 2007; Okada et al., 2010; Azuma et al., 2011). In this book chapter, we will present the technological development and clinical applications of the SmartAmp method.

2. SmartAmp method

The SmartAmp method was developed based on the principal concept that DNA amplification itself is the signal for detection of a genetic mutation or SNP. Differing from the widely-used PCR, the SmartAmp method is an isothermal DNA amplification reaction (Mitani et al., 2007; Mitani et al., 2009). In the SmartAmp method, the entire DNA amplification process requires five primers: turnback primer (TP), boost primer (BP), folding primer (FP), and two outer primers (OP1 and OP2) (Fig. 1). Primers are selected based on those algorithms considering the free energy, probability of base-pairing, product size range, optimal melting temperature, and product size range. The design of these primers contributes to the specificity of SmartAmp. In particular two primers (TP and FP) are critically important for the amplification process. The genomic sequence between the annealing sites of the TP and FP primers is the target region that will be amplified by the SmartAmp reaction. The other primers (BP, OP1, and OP2) are additionally employed to accelerate the process and enhance specificity.

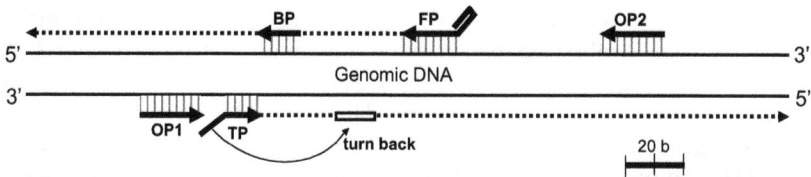

Fig. 1. Schematic illustration of five primers used for the SmartAmp method: turn-back primer (TP), boost primer (BP), folding primer (FP), and two outer primers (OP1 and OP2)

2.1 Molecular mechanism underlying isothermal DNA amplification

In isothermal DNA amplification by the SmartAmp method, the initial step of copying a target sequence from the genomic DNA is a prerequisite. FP and TP hybridize the template genomic DNA. Next, both products primed for the FP and TP are detached from template genomic DNA by strand-displacing DNA polymerase, whose extensions are primed by OP1 and OP2. Single-stranded DNA products, thus displaced, become templates in the second step for the opposing FP and TP. These single stranded DNA products are generated by the strand-displacement activity of the DNA polymerase, being primed from the flanking region of OP primers adjacent to the target sequence. The resulting DNA products are referred to as "intermediate products", IM1 and IM2, which play key roles in the subsequent amplification steps (Fig. 2).

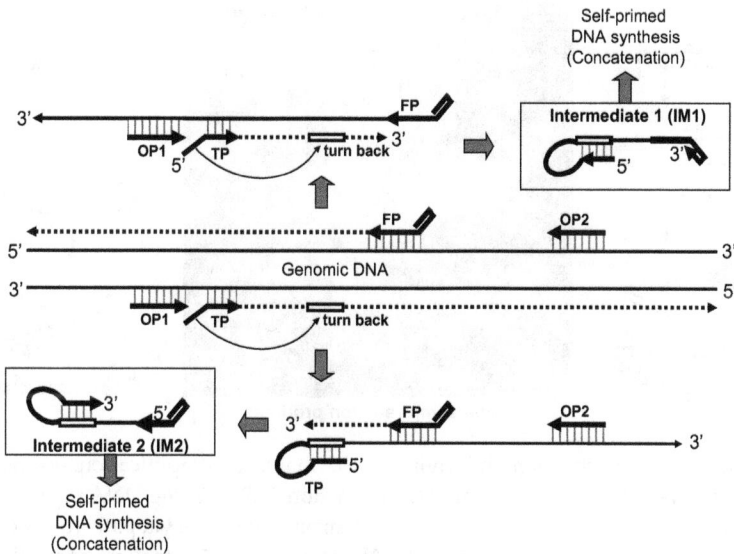

Fig. 2. Formation of intermediate products in the initial step of the SmartAmp reaction. The priming events of the SmartAmp reaction generate two intermediates (i.e., IM1 and IM2).

The formation of those intermediate products (IM1 ad IM2) is the rate-limiting step in SmartAmp-based isothermal DNA amplification. IM1 has the TP sequence at the 5′ end and the FP complementary sequence at the 3′ end; and IM2 is complementary to IM1 (Fig. 3).

The initial self-priming site on IM1 is the 3'-end of the FP sequence of IM1. Concatenated products of IM1 are synthesized by an elongation process termed pathway A. The characteristic feature of the products of pathway A is that the free 5' and 3' ends carry TP and its complementary sequence, forming long double stranded hairpin DNA. The initial self-priming elongation site on IM2 is located at the 3' end of the TP sequence of IM2. Long concatenated DNA products are synthesized as in pathway A, but end products in pathway B are different. The long-hairpin DNA products of pathway B carry FP and its complementary sequence at the free 5' and 3' ends respectively. There is another elongation pathway which starts from the 3' end of a free TP-primer that hybridizes to the looping structure of the TP complementary sequence, which is located at the intermediate region of the long products of pathway A. Thus, concatenated DNA products are formed in the SmartAmp reaction. The resulting DNA products could be detected by conventional agarose gel electrophoresis, where DNA ladder patterns represented the formation of concatenated DNA products (Mitani et al., 2007) (Fig. 3).

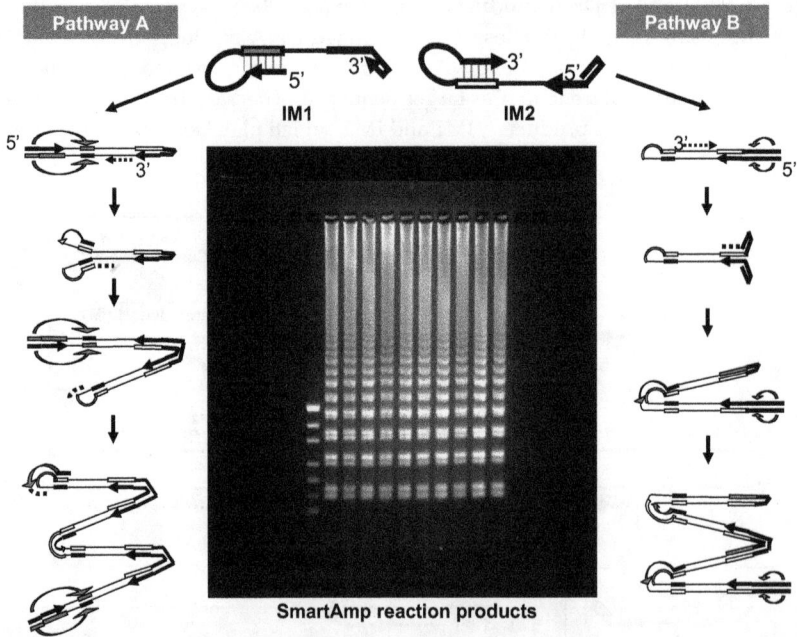

Fig. 3. The molecular mechanism underlying isothermal DNA amplification. Formation of concatenated DNA products in the SmartAmp reaction. Self-priming DNA synthesis from each of the intermediates, IM1 and IM2, creates hairpin molecules via pathway A or B. These structures lead to further self-primed DNA synthesis to create dimeric amplicons and then subsequently concatenated DNA products.

2.2 Molecular mechanism underlying SNP detection

To ensure the high fidelity of SNP detection by the SmartAmp method, exponential amplification of mis-primed DNA must be suppressed. In the original SmartAmp method, this was achieved by adding either the mismatch binding protein (MutS) *Thermus aquaticus* (Mitani et al., 2009) or a competitive probe (Toyoda et al., 2009) to the reaction mixture. MutS inhibits background DNA from entering the amplification cycle by specifically binding to mis-primed amplification products (Fig. 4). In addition, a combination of the asymmetrical primers, *i.e.*, TP and FP is used to minimize alternative mis-amplification pathways (Mitani et al., 2007).

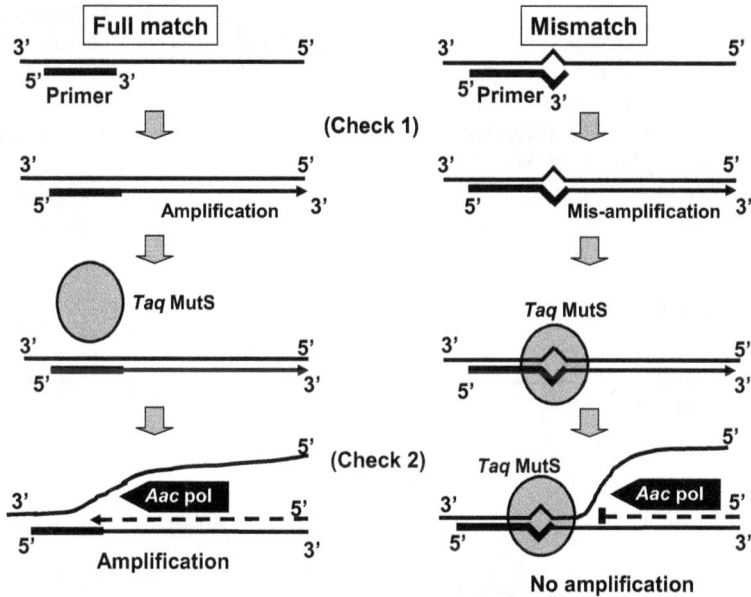

Fig. 4. The mechanism of allele discrimination as exercised by *Taq* MutS. SNP typing with a wild-type allele detection primer, using the wild-type allele (left) and the mutant-type allele (right) as templates. The wild-type allele detection primer is designed to encompass the SNP nucleotide site at each 3'-position. Amplification is not allowed when the primer mismatches with the mutant-type allele (Check 1). If check 1 fails, *Taq* MutS strongly binds to mismatched nucleotides and *Aac* DNA polymerase can not strand-displace or extend the newly synthesized strand (Check 2).

The SmartAmp method utilizes *Aac* polymerase as a DNA polymerase with strand-displacement activity. This DNA polymerase is highly resistant to cellular contaminants and hence works directly on blood samples, just after a simple heat treatment (98°C, 3 min) to degrade RNA and denature proteins. This is a great advantage of the SmartAmp method over the commonly used PCR-based techniques that require careful DNA extraction. In the conventional method, the enzymatic activity of *Taq* DNA polymerase is easily inhibited by impurities.

2.3 Example of SNP detection by SmartAmp method

Clinical application of SmartAmp to practical SNP detection should be evaluated with clinical samples (either blood or genomic DNA) according to the principle of amplification versus non-amplification as compared to threshold values. The amount of DNA-intercalating SYBR Green I dye during the reaction can be monitored in a real-time PCR system (e.g., Mx3000P), and thereby SNP typing can be determined by referring to the intensity of fluorescence.

Each SmartAmp2 reaction is performed in a 25 μl-volume tube at 60°C. The standard reaction mixture contains 3.2 μM each of TP and FP, 0.4 μM each of OP1 and OP2, 1.6 μM BP, 1.4 mM dNTPs, 5% dimethyl sulfoxide (DMSO), 20 mM Tris-HCl (pH 8.8), 10 mM KCl, 10 mM $(NH_4)_2SO_4$, 8 mM $MgSO_4$, 0.1% Tween 20, SYBR Green I (1/100,000-diluted), 40 units of *Aac* DNA polymerase, 1.5-2.4 μg of *Taq* MutS (optional) and 1 μl of blood or genomic DNA sample. Each reaction mixture should be incubated at 60°C for 40 - 60 minutes under isothermal conditions in a real-time PCR model Mx3000P system (Stratagene, La Jolla, CA, USA) where changes in the fluorescence intensity of SYBR Green I dye is monitored to detect the DNA amplification. Fig. 5 presents the results of the SmartAmp method when applied to detection of a clinically important SNP 460G>A in exon 7 of the human thiopurine S-methyltransferase (*TPMT*) gene. Clinical importance of this SNP will be discussed in the following section.

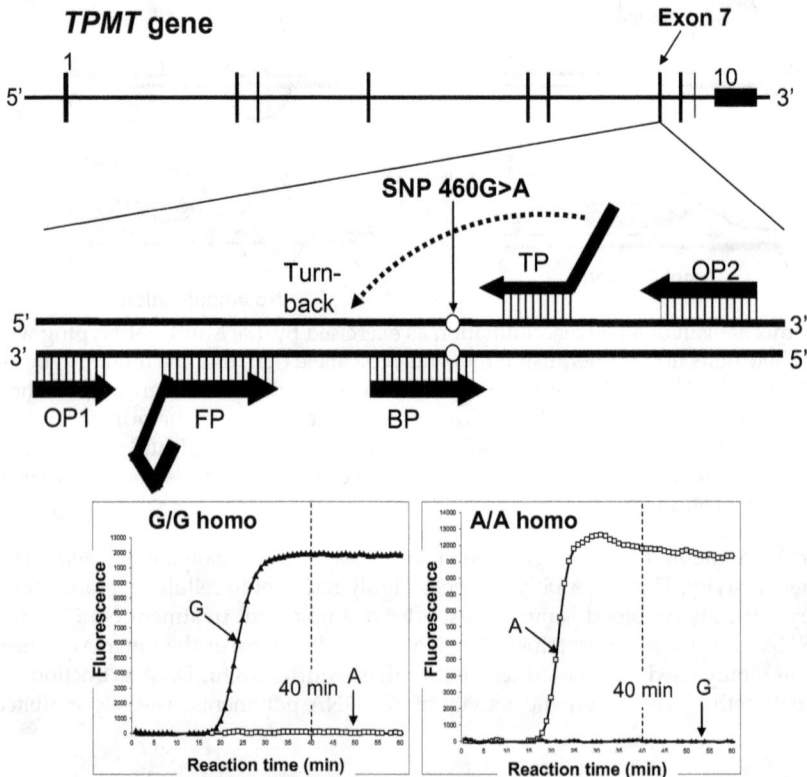

Fig. 5. Schematic illustration of the human *TPMT* gene and detection of the SNP 460G>A by the SmartAmp method. Two panels depict the time-courses of the SmartAmp assay reactions with *TPMT*-specific primers carrying WT (460G) or SNP (460A) alleles; namely, G/G homozygote and A/A homozygote.

3. Clinical applications of SmartAmp method

Hitherto, we have proven that the SmartAmp method is capable of detecting SNPs in drug transporter genes (*e.g.*, *ABCB1*, *ABCG2*, and *ABCC11*) (Ishikawa et al., 2010; Aw et al., 2011; Ota et al., 2010; Toyoda et al., 2009) as well as in drug metabolizing enzyme genes, including those of cytochrome P450s, vitamin K epoxide reductase (*VKORC1*), and UDP-glucuronosyltransferase *UGT1A1* (Aomori et al., 2009; Watanabe et al., 2007). Here we present other examples of SNP detection by the SmartAmp method, namely detection of genetic polymorphisms in human *TPMT* and *ABCC4* genes to predict thiopurine-induced adverse reactions in certain sub-populations of patients.

3.1 Thioprine toxicity and genetic polymorphisms in *TPMT* gene

Thiopurines are effective immunosuppressants and anticancer agents used for treating childhood acute lymphoblastic leukemia, acute myeloblastic leukemia, autoimmune disease, rheumatoid arthritis, and inflammatory bowel diseases. The intracellular accumulation of such active metabolites as 6-thioguanine nucleotides (6-TGN), however, causes dose-limiting hematopoietic toxicity (Weinshilboum & Sladek, 1980). TPMT deficiency has been reported to exacerbate thiopurine toxicity (Fig. 6).

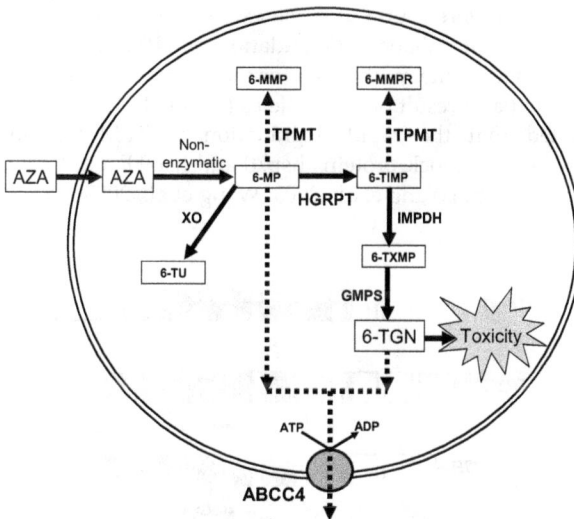

Fig. 6. Cellular metabolism of azathioprine (AZA) and transport. HGRPT, hypoxanthine-guanine phosphoribosyl transferase; IMPDH, inosine monophosphate dehydrogenase; XO, xanthine oxidase. 6-MMP, 6-methylmercaptopurine; 6-MMPR, 6-methylmercaptopurine ribonucleosides; 6-MP, 6-mercaptopurine; 6-TGN, 6-thioguanine nucleotide; 6-TIMP, 6-thiosine 5′-monophosphate; 6-TU; 6-thiouric acid; 6-TXMP, 6-thioxanthosine monophosphate; GMPS, guanosine monophosphate synthetase; 6-TGN, 6-thioguanine nucleotides. AZA is non-enzymatically converted to 6-MP in the cell. HGRPT is responsible for conversion of 6-MP to 6-TIMP. Thiopurine toxicity is caused by cellular accumulation of 6-TGN. Human ABC transporter ABCC4 plays a role of extruding the cytotoxic 6-TGN from the cells.

The enzyme TPMT operates in the main inactivation pathway for thiopurine drugs. The *TPMT* gene comprising 10 exons is located on chromosome 6p22.3 (Fig. 7). TPMT activity has been proven by numerous studies to be inversely correlated to 6-TGN levels in erythrocytes and other hematopoietic tissues (Krynetski et al., 1995; Evans, 2004; Anstey et al., 1992; Stolk et al., 1998; Yates et al., 1997; Black et al., 1998; Clunie et al., 2004). Polymorphisms in the *TPMT* gene can lead to intermediate, low, or no TPMT activity in certain patients, who are thus at an increased risk of developing thiopurine-induced life-threatening hematologic toxicity. Therefore, the thiopurine dose should be reduced by 50% for intermediate and by 80 to 90% for poor metabolizers to reduce the toxicity risk. There are a total of 24 functionally related alleles that have been reported to date, i.e., *TPMT*1* to *18* and *20* to *23* (Schütz et al., 2000; Schaeffeler et al., 2008; Lee et al., 2008). *TPMT*1* is the wild-type allele with high enzymatic activity. The *TPMT*2* allele has one non-synonymous SNP of 238G>C (Ala80Pro). The *TPMT*3A* allele carries two non-synonymous SNPs of both 460G>A (Ala154Thr) and 719A>G (Tyr240Lys), while the *TPMT*3B* and *TPMT*3C* alleles each carry one non-synonymous SNP of 460G>A (Ala154Thr) and 719A>G (Tyr240Lys), respectively. While *TPMT*2* is the first variant allele described, this allele is much less common than *TPMT*3A*. Population studies have shown that approximately 10% of Caucasians and African Americans inherit one non-functional *TPMT*3A* allele. This non-functional allele is not commonly seen in Asians. In Korean populations, *TPMT*3C* (0.88-2.54%) and *6* (0.25-1.27%) were found to some extents (Schaeffeler et al., 2008; Lee et al., 2008). Tai *et al.* reported that enhanced degradation of TPMT allozymes encoded by the *TPMT*2* and *TPMT*3* alleles is the mechanism for the decreased levels of TPMT protein and enzyme activity inherited as a result of these alleles (Tai et al., 1997). Subsequently, Wang *et al.* have demonstrated that the rapid degradation of TPMT*3A involves molecular chaperones, such as the heat shock proteins hsp70 and hsp90, and that TPMT*3A can also form intracellular aggresomes (Wang et al., 2003; Wang et al., 2005; Wang & Weinshilboum, 2006).

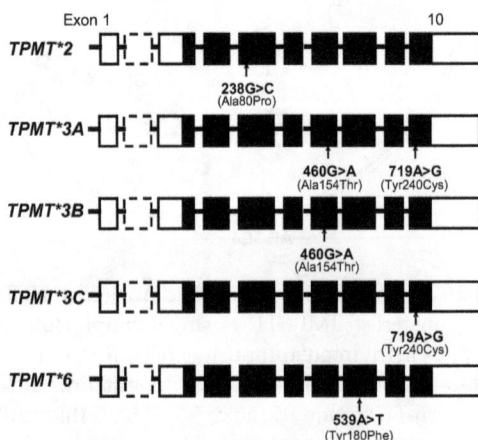

Fig. 7. The genomic organization of the human *TPMT* gene and five different alleles, *i.e.*, *TPMT*2, TPMT*3A, TPMT*3B, TPMT*3C, and TPMT*6*. Non-synonymous SNPs of 238G>C (Ala80Pro), 460G>A (Ala154Thr), 539A>T (tyr180Phe), and 719A>G (tyr240Cys) are indicated by arrows.

3.2 SNP 2269G>A (Glu757Lys) in *ABCC4* gene and thiopurine toxicity

For largely unknown reasons, there are subsets of Japanese patients who suffer from dose-limiting hematopoietic toxicity, but are not *TPMT* deficient (Takatsu et al., 2009). Recent studies have revealed that ABCC4 protects against thiopurine-induced hematopoietic toxicity by actively exporting thiopurine nucleotides (Krishnamurthy et al., 2008; Ban et al., 2010). ABCC4 is reportedly involved in the transport of antiviral agents, such as azidothymidine, adefovir, tenofovir, lamivudine, and ganciclovir (Shuetz et al., 1999; Adachi et al., 2002; Anderson et al., 2006; Imaoka et al., 2007), as well as anticancer drugs including 6-MP, 6-TG, methotrexate, and the camptothecins (Lee at al., 2000; Chen et al., 2002; Wielinga et al., 2002; Tian et al., 2005).

ABCC4 is a highly polymorphic gene with more than 20 missense genetic variants identified in the National Centre for Biotechnology Information (NCBI) database and the Pharmacogenetics Research Network (PGRN). Despite this situation, few data are available regarding the functions of these variants. Krishnamurthy *et al.* have recently shown that patients carrying SNP 2269G>A (Glu757Lys) in the human *ABCC4* gene have severely reduced ABCC4 function resulting from an impairment of its cell membrane localization (Krishnamurthy et al., 2008). ABCC4 protects against thiopurine-induced hematologic toxicity by actively exporting 6-TGN, a toxic metabolite in the thiopurine drug metabolic pathway. Interestingly, the *ABCC4* 2269G>A SNP is common in the Japanese population (15 to 18% frequency), which suggests that this non-synonymous SNP could provide an explanation for the unsolved thiopurine toxicity that is not associated with genetic polymorphisms of *TPMT* (Takatsu et al., 2009; Ban et al., 2010; Ando et al., 2001).

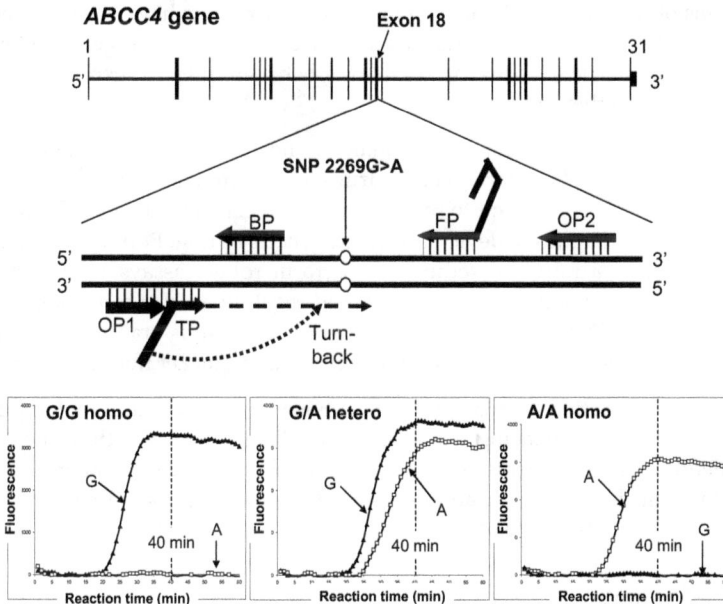

Fig. 8. Schematic illustration of the human *ABCC4* gene located on chromosome 13q32.1. The SNP 2269G>A that resides in exon 18 was detected by the SmartAmp method.

Unlike the situation for *TPMT*, the effects of the 2269G>A polymorphism in the *ABCC4* gene have been relatively unexplored. Most recently, Ban *et al.* have investigated an association between the 2269G>A polymorphism in the *ABCC4* gene and thiopurine sensitivity in Japanese patients with inflammatory bowel disease (IBD) (Ban et al., 2010). A total of 235 samples from IBD patients were analyzed in their clinical study. They showed that the 6-TGN levels in red blood cells were significantly higher in patients with the allele of *ABCC4* SNP 2269G>A than in patients with the wild-type allele ($P = 0.049$). The white blood cell count was significantly lower in patients with the SNP 2269G>A allele than in patients with the wild-type allele. Among 15 patients with leucopenia ($< 3 \times 10^9/l$), seven carried the SNP 2269G>A allele (Ban et al., 2010). The odds ratio of carrying the SNP allele and having leucopenia was 3.33 (95% confidence interval 1.03-10.57, $P = 0.036$) (Ban et al., 2010). As compared with the azathioprine (AZA) dose of 2 to 3 mg/kg recommended in Western countries (Lichtenstein et al., 2006), lower doses of AZA (0.6 to 1.2 mg/kg) are used in Japan because of the relatively higher sensitivity to AZA (Hibi et al., 2003). Those results strongly suggest that the *ABCC4* SNP 2269G>A is a new diagnostic marker indicative of thioprine toxicity/sensitivity in Japanese patients with IBD. In this context, the SmartAmp method for rapid detection of the *ABCC4* SNP 2269G>A (Fig. 8) provides a practical tool for prediction of thioprine toxicity/sensitivity in Japanese patients with IBD.

4. Conclusion

Accumulating evidence strongly suggests that genetic polymorphisms in drug metabolizing enzymes, transporters, receptors, and other drug targets (e.g., toxicity targets) are linked to inter-individual differences in the efficacy and toxicity of many medications. The genetic polymorphisms of drug metabolizing enzymes and transporters have been studied in many laboratories worldwide. In fact, efforts to discover and characterize gene polymorphisms resulted in new diagnostic tests for discriminating between different gene alleles and better strategies for pharmacotherapy.

To realize the promise of individualized medicine, however, genetic diagnosis should be further integrated with therapy for selecting drugs and treatments as well as for monitoring results. It is also critically important to reduce the cost of genetic diagnosis. Technologies are evolving to transform diagnostic devices for rapid genetic testing. Portable devices are being engineered for use in a range of settings to perform robust assays for the diagnosis of disease that will improve patient management, and result in greater convenience and speed to answer. Indeed, the POC diagnostics is a growing field that is gradually becoming more user-friendly with the introduction of portable devices and quicker nucleic acid detection.

The isothermal amplification technologies have a potential to cover different applications. A key requirement for the advancing personalized medicine resides in the ability of rapidly and conveniently testing patients' genetic polymorphisms and/or mutations. With this respect, isothermal nucleic acid amplification technologies, including the SmartAmp method, are expected to translate into less complex and less expensive instrumentation.

5. Acknowledgment

The authors thank Prof. John D. Schuetz (St. Jude Children's Hospital, Memphis, TN, USA) and Prof. Akira Andoh (Shiga University of Medical Science, Otsu, Japan) for their fruitful discussion about genetic polymorphisms of human *ABCC4* gene. Our thanks go to Drs. Alexander Lezhava and Wanping Aw (Omics Science Center, RIKEN) for their generous support in SmartAmp-based genotyping experiments. The authors' study was supported by a Japan Science and Technology Agency (JST) research project named "Development of the world's fastest SNP detection system" (to TI) and Research Grant for RIKEN Omics Science Center from the Ministry of Education, Culture, Sports, Science and Technology (to YH).

6. References

Adachi, M.; Sampath, J.; Lan, L.B.; Sun, D.; Hargrove, P.; Flatley, R.; Tatum, A.; Edwards, M.Z.; Wezeman, M.; Matherly, L.; Drake, R. & Schuetz, J. (2002) Expression of MRP4 confers resistance to ganciclovir and compromises bystander cell killing. *J. Biol. Chem.*, vol. 277, pp. 38998-39004

Anderson, P.L.; Lamba, J.; Aquilante, C.L.; Schuetz, E. & Fletcher, C.V. (2006) Pharmacogenetic characteristics of indinavir, zidovudine, and lamivudine therapy in HIV-infected adults: a pilot study. *J. Acquir. Immune Defic. Syndr.*, vol. 42, pp. 441-449

Ando, M.; Ando, Y.; Hasegawa, Y.; Sekido, Y.; Shimokata, K. & Horibe, K. (2001) Genetic polymorphisms of thiopurine S-methyltransferase and 6-mercaptopurine toxicity in Japanese children with acute lymphoblastic leukaemia. *Pharmacogenetics*, vol. 11, pp. 269-273

Anstey, A.; Lennard, L.; Mayou, S.C. & Kirby, J.D. (1992) Pancytopenia related to azathioprine–an enzyme deficiency caused by a common genetic polymorphism: a review. *J. Royal Soc. Med.*,vol. 85, pp. 752-756

Aomori, T.; Yamamoto, K.; Oguchi-Katayama, A.; Kawai, Y.; Ishidao, T.; Mitani, Y.; Kogo, Y.; Lezhava, A.; Fujita, Y.; Obayashi, K.; Nakamura, K.; Kohnke, H.; Wadelius, M.; Ekström, L.; Skogastierna, C.; Rane, A.; Kurabayashi, M.; Murakami, M.; Cizdziel, P.E.; Hayashizaki, Y. & Horiuchi, R. (2009) Rapid SNP detection of the cytochrome P-450 (CYP) 2C9 and the vitamin K oxide reductase (VKORC1) gene for the warfarin dose adjustment by Smart-Amplification prosess vesion 2. *Clin. Chem.*, vol. 55, pp. 804-812

Aw, W.; Lezhava, A.; Hayashizaki, Y. & Ishikawa, T. (2011) A new trend in personalized medicine: rapid detection of SNPs in drug transporter genes by SmartAmp method. *Clin. Pharmacol. Ther.*, vol. 89, pp. 617-620

Azuma, K.; Lezhava, A.; Shimizu, M.; Kimura, Y.; Ishizu, Y.; Ishikawa, T.; Kamataki, T,; Hayashizaki, Y. & Yamazaki, H. (2011) Direct genotyping of *cytochrome P450 2A6* whole gene deletion from human blood samples by SmartAmp method. *Clin Chim Actat*, vol. 412, pp. 1249-1251

Ban, H.; Andoh, A.; Imaeda, H.; Kobori, A.; Bamba, S.; Tsujikawa, T.; Sasaki, M.; Saito, Y. & Fujiyama, Y. (2010) The multidrug-resistance protein 4 polymorphism is a new factor accounting for thiopurine sensitivity in Japanese patients with inflammatory bowel disease. *J. Gastroenterol.*, vol. 45, pp. 1014-1021

Black, A.J.; McLeod, H.L.; Capell, H.A.; Powrie, R.H.; Matowe, L.K.; Pritchard, S.C.; Collie-Duguid, E.S. & Reid, D.M. (1998) Thiopurine methyltransferase genotype predicts therapy-limiting severe toxicity from azathioprine. *Ann. Internal Med.*, vol. 129, pp. 716-718

Chen, Z.S.; Lee, K.; Walther, S.; Raftogianis, R.B.; Kuwano, M.; Zeng, H. & Kruh, G.D. (2002) Analysis of methotrexate and folate transport by multidrug resistance protein 4 (ABCC4): MRP4 is a component of the methotrexate efflux system. *Cancer Res.*, vol. 62, pp. 3144-3150

Clunie, G.P. & Lennard, L. (2004) Relevance of thiopurine methyltransferase status in rheumatology patients receiving azathioprine. *Rheumatology*, vol.43, pp.13-18

Cooper, G.M.; Johnson, J.A.; Langaee, T.Y.; Feng, H.; Stanaway, I.B.; Schwarz, U.I.; Ritchie, M.D.; Stein, C.M.; Roden, D.M.;, Smith, J.D.; Veenstra, D.L.; Rettie, A.E. & Rieder, M.J. (2008) A genome-wide scan for common genetic variants with a large influence on warfarin maintenance dose. *Blood*, vol. 112, pp. 1022-1027

Daly, A.K.; Donaldson, P.T.; Bhatnagar, P.; Shen, Y.; Pe'er, I.; Floratos, A.; Daly, M.J.; Goldstein, D.B.; John, S.; Nelson, M.R.; Graham, J.; Park, B.K.; Dillon, J.F.; Bernal, W.; Cordell, H.J.; Pirmohamed, M.; Aithal, G.P.; Day, C.P.; DILIGEN Study & International SAE Consortium. (2009) HLA-B*5701 genotype is a major determinant of drug-induced liver injury due to flucloxacillin. *Nature Gent.*, vol. 41, pp. 816-819

Evans, W.E. & Johnson, J.A. (2001) Pharmacogenomics: the inherited basis for interindividual differences in drug response. *Annu. Rev. Genomics Hum. Genet.* vol. 2, pp. 9-39

Evans, W.E. (2004) Pharmacogenetics of thiopurine S-methyltransferase and thiopurine therapy. *Ther. Drug Monit.* Vol. 26, pp. 185-191

Frueh, F.W.; Amur, S.; Mummaneni, P.;, Epstein, R.S.; Aubert, R.E.;, DeLuca, T.M.; Verbrugge, R.R.; Burckart, G.J. & Lesko, L.J. (2008) Pharmacogenomic biomarker information in drug labels approved by the United States food and drug administration: prevalence of related drug use. *Pharmacotherapy*, vol. 28, pp. 992-998

Ge, D.; Fellay, J.; Thompson, A.J.; Simon, J.S.; Shianna, K.V.; Urban, T.J.; Heinzen, E.L.; Qiu, P.; Bertelsen, A.H.; Muir, A.J.; Sulkowski, M.; McHutchison, J.G. & Goldstein, D.B. (2009) Genetic variation in IL28B predicts hepatitis C treatment-induced viral clearance. *Nature*, vol. 461, pp. 399-401

Hibi, T.; Naganuma, M.; Kitahora, T.; Kinjyo, F. & Shimoyama, T. (2003) Low-dose azathioprine is effective and safe for naintenance of remission in patients with ulcerative coltits. *J. Gastroenterol.* Vol. 38, pp. 740-746

Imaoka, T.; Kusuhara, H.; Adachi, M.; Schuetz, J.D.; Takeuchi, K. & Sugiyama, Y. (2007) Functional involvement of multidrug resistance-associated protein 4 (MRP4/ABCC4) in the renal elimination of the antiviral drugs adefovir and tenofovir. *Mol. Pharmacol.*, vol. 71, pp. 619-627

Ishikawa, T.; Sakurai, A.; Hirano, H.; Lezhava, A.; Sakurai, M. & Hayashizaki, Y. (2010) Emerging new technologies in pharmacogenomics: Rapid SNP detection, molecular dynamic simulation, and QSAR analysis methods to validate clinically important genetic variants of human ABC Transporter ABCB1 (P-gp/MDR1). *Pharmacol. Ther.*, vol. 126, pp. 69-81

Kamatani, Y.; Matsuda, K; Okada Y.; Kubo,M.; Hosono, N.; Daigo, Y.; Nakamura, Y. & Kamatani, N. (2010) Genome-wide association study of hematological and biochemical traits in a Japanese population. *Nat. Genet.*, vol. 42, pp. 210-215

Krishnamurthy, P.; Schwab, M.; Takenaka, K.; Nachagari, D.; Morgan, J.; Leslie, M.; Du, W.; Boyd, K.; Cheok, M.; Nakauchi, H.; Marzolini, C.; Kim, R.B.; Poonkuzhali, B.; Schuetz, E.; Evans, W.; Relling, M. & Schuetz, J.D. (2008) Transporter-mediated protection against thiopurine-induced hematopoietic toxicity. *Cancer Res.*, vol. 68, pp. 4983-4989

Krynetski, E.Y.; Schuetz, J.D.; Galpin, A.J.; Pui, C.; Relling, M.V. & Evans, W.E. (1995) A single point mutation leading to loss of catalytic activity in human thioprine S-methyltransferase. *Proc. Natl. Acad. Sci. USA* vol. 92, pp. 694-702

Lee, K.; Klein-Szanto, A.J. & Kruh, G.D. (2000) Analysis of the MRP4 drug resistance profile in transfected NIH3T3 cells. *J. Natl. Cancer Inst.*, vol. 92, pp. 1934-1940

Lee, S.S.; Kim, W.Y.; Jang, Y.J. & Schin, L.G. (2008) Duplex pyrosequencing of the TPMT*3C and TPMT*6 alleles in Korean and Vietnamese populations. *Clin Chem.* Vol. 398, pp. 82-85

Lesko, L.J. (2008) The critical path of warfarin dosing: finding an optimal dosing strategy using pharmacogenetics. *Clin. Pharmacol. Ther.*, vol. 84, pp. 301-303

Lezhava, A.; Ishidao, T.; Ishizu, Y.; Naito, K.; Hanami, T.; Katayama, A.; Kogo, Y.; Soma, T.; Ikeda, S.; Murakami, K.; Nogawa, C.; Itoh, M.; Mitani, Y.; Harbers, M.; Okamoto, A. & Hayashizaki, Y. (2010) Exciton Primer-mediated SNP detection in SmartAmp2 reactions. *Hum. Mutat.*, vol. 31, pp. 208-217

Lichtenstein, G.R.; Sbreu, M.T.; Cohen, R. & Tremaine W. (2006) American Gastroenterological Association Institute technical review on corticosteroids, immunomodulators, and infiximab in inflammatory bowel disease. *Rev. Gastroenterol. Mex.*, vol. 71, pp. 351-401

Mitani, Y.; Lezhava, A.; Kawai, Y.; Kikuchi, T.; Oguchi-Katayama, A.; Kogo, Y.; Itoh, M.; Miyagi, T.; Takakura, H.; Hoshi, K.; Kato, C.; Arakawa, T.; Shibata, K.; Fukui, K.; Masui, R.; Kuramitsu, S.; Kiyotani, K.; Chalk, A.; Tsunekawa, K.; Murakami, M.; Kamataki, T.; Oka, T.; Shimada, H.; Cizdziel, P.E. & Hayashizaki, Y. (2007) Rapid SNP diagnostics using asmmetric isothermal amplification and a new mismatch-suppression technology. *Nature Methods*, vol. 4, pp. 257-262

Mitani, Y.; Lezhava, A.; Sakurai, A.; Horikawa, A.; Nagakura, M.; Hayashizaki, Y. & Ishikawa, T. (2009) A rapid and cost-effective SNP detection method: Application of SmartAmp2 to pharmacogenomics research. *Pharmacogenomics*, vol. 10, pp. 1187-1197

Okada, R.; Ishizu, Y.; Endo, R.; Lezhava, A.; Ieiri, I.; Kusuhara, H.; Sugiyama, Y. & Hayashizaki, Y. (2010) Direct rapid genotyping of glutathione-S-transferase M1 and T1 from human blood specimens using the SmartAmp2 method. *Drug Metab. Dispos.*, vol. 38, pp. 1636-1639

Ota, I.; Sakurai, A.; Toyoda, Y.; Morita, S.; Sasaki, T.; Chishima, T.; Yamakado, M.; Kawai, Y.; Ishidao, T.; Lezhava, A.; Yoshiura, K.; Togo, S.; Hayashizaki, Y.; Ishikawa, T.; Ishikawa, T.; Endo, I. & Shimada, H. (2010) Association between breast cancer risk and the wild-type allele of human ABC transporter ABCC11. *Anticancer Res.*, vol. 30, pp. 5189-5194

Salerno, R. & Lesko, L.J. (2004) Pharmacogenomics in drug development and regulatory decision-making: the genomic data submission. *Pharmacogenomics*, vol. 5, pp. 25-30

Salerno, R. & Lesko, L.J. (2004) Pharmacogenomic data: FDA volutanry and required submission guidance. *Pharmacogenomics*, vol. 5, pp. 503-505

Schaeffeler, E.; Zanger, U.M.; Eichelbaum, M.; Asante-Poku, S.; Shin, J.-G. & Schwab, M. (2008) Highly multiplexed genotyping of thiopurine S-methyltransferase variants using MALDI-TOF mass spectrometry: reliable genotyping in different ethic groups. *Clin. Chem.* Vol. 54, pp. 1637-1647

Schuetz, J.D.; Connelly, M.C.; Sun, D.; Paibir, S.G.; Flynn, P.M.; Srinivas, R.V.; Kumar, A. & Fridland, A. (1999) MRP4: a previously unidentified factor in resistance to nucleoside-based antiviral drugs. *Nature Med.*, vol. 5, pp. 1048-1051

Schuldiner, A.R.; O'Connell, J.R.; Bliden, K.P.; Gandhi, A.; Ryan, K.; Horenstein, R.B.; Damcott, C.M.; Pakyz, R.; Tantry, U.S,; Gibson, Q.; Pollin, T.I.; Post, W.; Parsa, A.; Mitchell, B.D.; Faraday, N.; Herzog, W. & Gurbel, P.A. (2009) Association of cytochrome P450 2C19 genotype with the antiplatelet effect and clinical efficacy of clopidogrel therapy. *JAMA*, vol. 302, pp. 849-857

Scchütz, E.; von Ahsen, N. & Oellerich, M. (2000) Genotyping of eight thiopurine methyltransferase mutations: three-color multiplexing, "two-color/shered" anchor, and fluorescence-quenching hybridization probe assays based on thermiodynamic nearest-neighbor probe design. *Clin. Chem.*, vol. 46, pp. 1728-1737

Stolk, J.N.; Boerbooms, A.M.; de Abreu, R.A.; de Koning, D.G.; van Beusekom, H.J.; Muller, W.H. & van de Putte, L.B. (1998) Reduced thiopurine methyltransferase activity and development of side effects of azathioprine treatment in patients with rheumatoid arthritis. *Arthritis Rheum.*, vol. 41, pp. 1858-1866

Tai, H.L.; Krynetski, E.Y.; Schuetz, E.G.; Yanishevski, Y. & Evans, W.E. (1997) Enhanced proteolysis of thiopurine S-methyltransferase (TPMT) encoded by mutant alleles inn humans (TPMT*3A,TPMT*2): mechanism for genetic polymorphisms of TPMT activity. *Proc. Natl. Acad. Sci. USA*, vol. 94, pp. 6444-6449

Takatsu, N.; Matsui, T.; Murakami, Y.; Ishihara, H.; Hisabe, T.; Nagahama, T.; Maki, S.; Beppu, T.; Takaki, Y.; Hirai, F. & Yao, K. (2009) Adverse reactions to azathioprine cannot be predicted by thiopurine S-methyltransferase genotype in Japanese patients with inflammatory bowel disease. *J. Gastroenterol. Hepatol.*, vol. 24, pp. 1258-1264

The SEARCH Collaborative Group. (2008) SLCO1B1 variants and statin-induced myopathy – a genomewide study. New Eng. J. Med., vol. 359, pp. 789-799

Tian, Q.; Zhang, J.; Tan, T.M.; Chan, E.; Duan, W.; Chan, S.Y.; Boelsterli, U.A.; Ho, P.C.; Yang, H.; Bian, J.S.; Huang, M.; Zhu, Y.Z.; Xiong, W.; Li, X. & Zhou, S. (2005) Human multidrug resistance associated protein 4 confers resistance to camptothecins. *Pharm. Res.* Vol. 22, pp. 1837-1853

Toyoda, Y.; Sakurai, A.; Mitani, Y.; Nakashima, M.; Yoshiura, K.; Nakagawa, H.; Sakai, Y.; Ota, I.; Lezhava, A.; Hayashizaki, Y.; Niikawa, N. & Ishikawa, T. (2009) Earwax, osmidrosis, and breast cancer: why does one SNP (538G>A) in the human ABC transporter ABCC11 gene determine earwax type? *FASEB J.*, vol. 23, pp. 2001-2013

Wang, L.; Sullivan, W.; Toft, D. & Weinshilboum, R. (2003) Thiopurine S-methyltransferase pharmacogentics: chaperone protein association and allozyme degradation. *Pharmacogenetics*, vol. 13, pp. 555-564

Wang, L.; Nguyen, T.V.; McLaughlin, R.W.; Sikkink, L.A.; Ramirwez-Alvarado, M. & Weinshilboum, R. (2005) Human thiopurine S-methylytansferase pharamcogenetics: variant allozyme misfolding and aggresome formation. *Proc. Natl. Acad. Sci. USA*, vol. 102, pp. 9394-9399

Wang, L. & Weinshilboum, R. (2006) Thiopurine S-methyltransferase pharmacogenetics: insights, challenges and future directions. *Oncogene*, vol. 25, pp. 1629-15638

Watanabe, J.; Mitani, Y.; Kawai, Y.; Kikuchi, T.; Kogo, Y.; Oguchi-Katayama, A.; Kanamori, H.; Usui, K.; Itoh, M.; Cizdziel, P.E.; Lezhava, A.; Tatsumi, K.; Ichikawa, Y.; Togo, S.; Shimada, H. & Hayashizaki, Y. (2007) Use of a competitive probe in assay design for genotyping of the UGT1A1*28 microsatellite polymorphism by the smart amplification process. *Biotechniques*, vol. 43, pp. 479-484

Weinshilboum, R.M. & Sladek, S.L. (1980) Mercaptopurine pharamcogenetics: monogenic inheritance of erythrocyte thioprine methyltransferase activity. *Am. J. Hum. Genet.*, vol. 32, pp. 651-662

Wielinga, P.R.; Reid, G.; Challa, E.E.; van der Heijden, I.; van Deemter, L.; de Haas, M.; Mol, C.; Kuil, A.J.; Groeneveld, E.; Schuetz, J.D.; Brouwer C, De Abreu, R.A.; Wijnholds, J.; Beijnen, J.H. & Borst, P. (2002) Thiopurine metabolism and identification of the thiopurine metabolites transported by MRP4 and MRP5 overexpressed in human embryonic kidney cells. *Mol. Pharmacol.*, vol. 62, pp. 1321-1331

Yates, C.R.; Krynetski, E.Y.; Loennechen, T.; Fessing, M.Y.; Tai, H.L.; Pui, C.H.; Relling, M.V. & Evans, W.E. (1997) Molecular diagnosis of thiopurine S-methyltransferase deficiency: genetic basis for azathioprine and mercaptopurine intolerance. *Ann. Internal Med.*, vol. 126, pp. 608-614

Permissions

The contributors of this book come from diverse backgrounds, making this book a truly international effort. This book will bring forth new frontiers with its revolutionizing research information and detailed analysis of the nascent developments around the world.

We would like to thank Dr. James Paxton, for lending his expertise to make the book truly unique. He has played a crucial role in the development of this book. Without his invaluable contribution this book wouldn't have been possible. He has made vital efforts to compile up to date information on the varied aspects of this subject to make this book a valuable addition to the collection of many professionals and students.

This book was conceptualized with the vision of imparting up-to-date information and advanced data in this field. To ensure the same, a matchless editorial board was set up. Every individual on the board went through rigorous rounds of assessment to prove their worth. After which they invested a large part of their time researching and compiling the most relevant data for our readers. Conferences and sessions were held from time to time between the editorial board and the contributing authors to present the data in the most comprehensible form. The editorial team has worked tirelessly to provide valuable and valid information to help people across the globe.

Every chapter published in this book has been scrutinized by our experts. Their significance has been extensively debated. The topics covered herein carry significant findings which will fuel the growth of the discipline. They may even be implemented as practical applications or may be referred to as a beginning point for another development. Chapters in this book were first published by InTech; hereby published with permission under the Creative Commons Attribution License or equivalent.

The editorial board has been involved in producing this book since its inception. They have spent rigorous hours researching and exploring the diverse topics which have resulted in the successful publishing of this book. They have passed on their knowledge of decades through this book. To expedite this challenging task, the publisher supported the team at every step. A small team of assistant editors was also appointed to further simplify the editing procedure and attain best results for the readers.

Our editorial team has been hand-picked from every corner of the world. Their multi-ethnicity adds dynamic inputs to the discussions which result in innovative outcomes. These outcomes are then further discussed with the researchers and contributors who give their valuable feedback and opinion regarding the same. The feedback is then collaborated with the researches and they are edited in a comprehensive manner to aid the understanding of the subject.

Apart from the editorial board, the designing team has also invested a significant amount of their time in understanding the subject and creating the most relevant covers. They scrutinized every image to scout for the most suitable representation of the subject and create an appropriate cover for the book.

The publishing team has been involved in this book since its early stages. They were actively engaged in every process, be it collecting the data, connecting with the contributors or procuring relevant information. The team has been an ardent support to the editorial, designing and production team. Their endless efforts to recruit the best for this project, has resulted in the accomplishment of this book. They are a veteran in the field of academics and their pool of knowledge is as vast as their experience in printing. Their expertise and guidance has proved useful at every step. Their uncompromising quality standards have made this book an exceptional effort. Their encouragement from time to time has been an inspiration for everyone.

The publisher and the editorial board hope that this book will prove to be a valuable piece of knowledge for researchers, students, practitioners and scholars across the globe.

List of Contributors

Fabricio Rios-Santos and Luiz Alexandre V. Magno
Federal University of Mato Grosso & Federal University of Minas Gerais, Brazil

Ayman El-Kattan and Manthena Varma
Pharmacokinetics, Dynamics and Metabolism Department, Pfizer Inc., USA

Petra Jančová
Department of Environmental Protection Engineering, Faculty of Technology, Tomas Bata University, Zlin, Czech Republic

Michal Šiller
Department of Pharmacology and Institute of Molecular and Translational Medicine, Faculty of Medicine and Dentistry, Palacky University, Olomouc, Czech Republic

Adarsh Gandhi and Romi Ghose
Department of Pharmacological and Pharmaceutical Sciences, University of Houston, United States of America

Hanane Akhdar, Claire Legendre, Caroline Aninat and Fabrice Morel
Inserm, UMR991, Liver Metabolisms and Cancer, Rennes, University of Rennes 1, Rennes, France

Viola Tamási and András Falus
Semmelweis University, Hungary

Piotr Czekaj and Rafał Skowronek
Department of Histology, Medical University of Silesia in Katowice, Poland

Jan Jurica and Alexandra Sulcova
Masaryk University, Brno, CEITEC - Central European Institute of Technology, Faculty of Medicine, Department of Pharmacology, Czech Republic

Jinsong Ni and Josh Rowe
Department of Drug Safety Evaluation, Allergan, Inc., Irvine, CA, USA

Alejandro Álvarez-Lueje, Magdalena Pérez and Claudio Zapata
University of Chile, Chile

Atsumu Hirabayashi
Hitachi, Ltd., Japan

Toshihisa Ishikawa and Yoshihide Hayashizaki
Omics Science Canter, RIKEN Yokohama Institute, Japan

www.ingramcontent.com/pod-product-compliance
Lightning Source LLC
Chambersburg PA
CBHW070737190326
41458CB00004B/1200